DATE DUE			
MAY − 5 2001			
JUN 2 5 2005			
MAY 2 0 2006	1914938		
GAYLORD			PRINTED IN U.S.A.

Practical Laboratory Andrology

PRACTICAL LABORATORY ANDROLOGY

David Mortimer, Ph.D.

Scientific Director
Sydney IVF
Australia

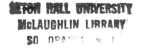
New York   Oxford
OXFORD UNIVERSITY PRESS
1994

Oxford University Press

Oxford   New York   Toronto
Delhi   Bombay   Calcutta   Madras   Karachi
Kuala Lumpur   Singapore   Hong Kong   Tokyo
Nairobi   Dar es Salaam   Cape Town
Melbourne   Auckland   Madrid

and associated companies in
Berlin   Ibadan

Published by Oxford University Press, Inc.
200 Madison Avenue, New York, New York 10016

Library of Congress Cataloging-in-Publication Data
Mortimer, David.
Practical laboratory andrology / David Mortimer.
p.   cm.   Includes bibliographical references and index.
ISBN 0-19-506595-6
1. Infertility, Male–Diagnosis–Laboratory manuals.
2. Diagnosis, Laboratory.
3. Spermatozoa–Analysis–Laboratory manuals.
I. Title.
[DNLM: 1. Infertility, Male–diagnosis. 2. Insemination.
3. Semen–chemistry. 4. Semen Preservation–methods.
5. Spermatozoa–cytology.   WJ 709 M888p]
RC889.M759   1993   616.6′92075–dc20
DNLM/DLC for Library of Congress   92-48921

9 8 7 6 5 4 3 2 1

Printed in the United States of America
on acid-free paper

My impetus to write this book was the discovery of three fetal hearts during an ultrasound examination of my wife Sharon's pregnancy in February 1989. This book is dedicated to my wife Sharon, to our daughters Caitlin and Sara, and to the memory of their sister Rebecca.

Preface

Practical Labaratory Andrology was conceived as a detailed, comprehensive reference source describing techniques used in today's andrology laboratories. The strategy of the book is not only to describe how to perform a particular procedure, but also to describe the technical basis and factors influencing the recommended method(s). In addition, the book explains how the results of each procedure may be interpreted and used in practical situations. Little prior knowledge of the area has been assumed, and the methods should be amenable to implementation by anyone with basic laboratory skills and experience. Considerations of standardization and quality control are fundamental to the author's approach and intrinsic to all recommended methods.

This book is aimed at all scientists and technicians working in the area of infertility diagnosis performing semen analysis and other assessments on infertile men, as well as graduate students and researchers working in human gamete biology and reproductive physiology. It will also provide clinical Fellows and sub-specialist obstetrician-gynecologists and urologists with a comprehensive overview of the services provided by a modern andrology laboratory. The techniques and procedures described in this book are relevant to all hospital, commercial, government, and university laboratories involved in infertility diagnosis and treatment, especially those associated with IVF and other assisted conception programs and sperm banks, as well as reproductive toxicology.

I would like to take this opportunity to express my deepest gratitude to my mentors during the development of my career: Professor Terry G. Baker, Dr. Alan R. Beatty, Professor Georges David, Professor Patrick J. Taylor, and the late Dr. Tom E. Thompson.

Finally, it goes without saying that this book could never have been written without my wife Sharon's unfailing support and editorial assistance.

Sydney, Australia   D.M.
May, 1993

Contents

Section II   Diagnostic Procedures

Section III   Therapeutic Procedures

Section IV Laboratory Management

Appendices

I

Basic Concepts

1

Introduction

The greatly increased interest in andrology over the past two decades has produced a vast increase in our knowledge of male reproductive physiology and the processes leading to conception in vivo and in vitro. It is now obvious that the etiology of human infertility is as often due to the male partner as the female, although in a few socioreligious groups the existence of male infertility is still ignored or even adamantly denied.

Our ability to treat male factor infertility, however, even after the diagnosis of a specific problem, remains limited. Except in the case of azoospermia, where the individual is clearly sterile, the outlook for many men with poor semen quality who want to sire children is bleak. The immediate therapy often prescribed is artificial insemination of their partners with donor semen. If there is a concurrent problem of blocked fallopian tubes, in vitro fertilization using donor semen (IVF-D), might be indicated, as the current success rates with male factor IVF are low. This state of affairs is hardly satisfactory and reflects continuing gaps in our understanding of the pathophysiological basis of many of the apparent defects we are able to identify by modern diagnostic testing.

Although substantial progress has, and is, being made in the endocrine aspects of the hypophyseal-pituitary-testicular axis and the regulation of spermatogenesis, as well as in the microsurgical treatment of partial or complete obstruction of the excurrent ducts, there is little understanding of the fate of the spermatozoa after ejaculation unless a pregnancy occurs. By extrapolation from studies in other eutherian mammals we are able to construct working hypotheses for the various component processes leading to conception in vivo, including sperm and egg transport through the female tract (gamete approximation), sperm capacitation, and gamete interaction resulting in fertilization. At syngamy, the haploid chromosome sets from the male and female gametes are combined to reinstate the normal diploid state, and the resulting zygote begins cleavage as a genetically new potential human being.

The purpose of this monograph is to provide a comprehensive state-of-the-art laboratory manual for diagnostic and therapeutic procedures now being used in the clinical andrology laboratory and in certain areas of assisted reproductive technology, the ever increasing field of infertility treatment that has stemmed from the pioneering work of a few individuals responsible for the first successful IVF procedures. In each chapter the underlying physiology is explained both as a background to the relevant reproductive process(es) and as justification for the choice of certain procedures, methodological details, or biochemical markers. The monograph is divided into four major sections.

I. An introduction with a discussion of some basic philosophical concepts relevant to an understanding of fertility and infertility plus some general background in the form of overviews of sperm production, gamete approximation and interaction (Chapters 1 and 2).
II. Detailed procedural details for the various diagnostic procedures that may be provided by both basic and specialized andrology laboratories, including some aspects that are usually (and best) provided in collaboration with other specialized laboratories (Chapters 3 to 11).
III. Detailed procedural details for many of the therapeutic procedures in which an andrology laboratory may be involved as part of a multidisciplinary infertility service (Chapters 12 to 14).
IV. A discussion of some aspects of laboratory management that enable the reader to establish an andrology laboratory, develop internal standardization, and institute necessary quality control and quality assurance procedures (Chapters 15 and 16).

A bibliography is provided at the end of each chapter. It comprises the primary and other literature considered essential resources in preparing the chapter, as well as recommended reading for those who want to delve deeper into the young science of andrology.

CONVENTIONS USED IN THE BOOK

For ease of reading and conciseness, certain abbreviations, expressions, and conventions are defined here.

Standard Abbreviations

Certain common scientific and andrological abbreviations are used throughout the text without obligatory redefinition. They are listed in Table 1-1. In addition, the large number of abbreviations and acronyms used in assisted reproductive technology are listed in Table 1-2.

Chemical Names and Suppliers

Generic names of chemicals are usually provided. For multinational companies or products available through local distributors worldwide, no address is provided; but for small companies a location is supplied.

For plasticware such as centrifuge tubes and culture dishes, my laboratories, probably similar to most IVF programs around the world, use Falcon plastics. Although other brands may be perfectly suitable, many workers are loathe to change because of the effort required simply to validate the acceptability of a dif-

Table 1–1 Standard abbreviations used in an andrology laboratory

Abbreviation	Explanation
A23187	A calcium ionophore
AIDS	Acquired immunodeficiency syndrome
AR	Acrosome reaction
ASAB	Antisperm antibody
ATP	Adenosine triphosphate
BBT	Basal body temperature
BSA	Bovine serum albumin (Cohn fraction V)
CI	Color index number (for stains)
CZBT	Competitive (sperm-)zona binding test
DMSO	Dimethylsulfoxide (cryoprotectant and carrier molecule for A23187)
DNA	Deoxyribonucleic acid
DPX	Microscopy mountant
FITC	Fluorescein isothiocyanate
FSH	Follicle-stimulating hormone
GEYC	Glycerol–egg yolk–citrate (a modified Ackerman's cryoprotectant medium for freezing human spermatozoa
hCG	Human chorionic gonadotropin
HEPT	(Zona-free) hamster egg penetration test
HIV	Human immunodeficiency virus
HMT	Hyaluronate migration test
HOS test	Hypoosmotic swelling test
HPF	High-power field
HSA	Human serum albumin (Cohn fraction V)
HTF	Human tubal fluid culture medium
HZA	Hemizona assay
IBT	Immunobead test
Ig	Immunoglobulin
IU	International unit[a]
LH	Luteinizing hormone
MAR	Mixed antiglobulin reaction
MI	(Sperm) motility index
NCD	Nuclear chromatin decondensation
PBS	Phosphate-buffered saline
PCT	Postcoital test
PR	(Sperm motility) progression rating
RBC	Red blood cell (erythrocyte)
SCMC test	Sperm–cervical mucus contact test
SD	Standard deviation
SEM	Standard error of the mean; or scanning electron microscopy
SIT	Sperm immobilization test
SMIT	Sperm–mucus interaction test
SPA	Sperm penetration assay (North American term for the HEPT)
TAT	Tray agglutination test
TEM	Transmission electron microscopy
U	(International) unit[a]
UV	Ultraviolet
WBC	White blood cell (leukocyte)
WHO	World Health Organization
XHT	Crossed hostility test
ZBT	(Sperm-)zona binding test

[a]IU for enzymes refers to the conversion of 1 μmol of substrate/minute at 37°C.

Table 1–2   Assisted reproductive technology nomenclature

Term	Group	Explanation
AI	1	Artificial insemination (unspecified source of spermatozoa)
AID	1	Artificial insemination by donor (no longer used, see DI)
AIH	1	Artificial insemination, homologous or by husband
ART		Assisted reproductive technology
CRYO		Cryopreservation or cryopreserved
-D		Added to acronyms to denote the use of donor gametes
DI	1	Donor insemination
DIPI		Direct intraperitoneal insemination
ET		Embryo transfer
FET		Fallopian embryo transfer
GIFT		Gamete intrafallopian transfer (by laparoscopy or minilaparaotomy)
ICSI		Intracytoplasmic sperm injection
IFI		Intrafollicular insemination
ITI		Intratubal insemination
IUI		Intrauterine insemination
IVF(-ET)	2	In vitro fertilization (and embryo transfer)
LAP		Abbreviation for laparoscopy
MAF	3	Mechanically assisted fertilization (also includes zona drilling/tearing/cracking)
MIST	3,6	Microinsemination by sperm transfer (a form of sperm microinjection)
PN		Pronucleus in a zygote
POREC		Programmed oocyte retrieval and embryo cryopreservation
POST	4,5	Pronuclear oocyte stage transfer (by laparoscopy or minilaparotomy); *also* peritoneal oocyte and sperm transfer (ultrasound-guided)
PROST	4,5	Pronuclear stage tubal transfer (by laparoscopy or minilaparotomy)
PZD	3	Partial zona dissection
SMI	3,6	Sperm microinjection (a general term not specifying the site of sperm placement
SUZI	3,6	Subzonal insemination (a form of sperm microinjection)
SZI	3,6	Subzonal insemination (a form of sperm microinjection)
TDI	1	Therapeutic donor insemination (an alternative to DI)
TEST	4	Tubal embryo stage transfer (by laparoscopy or minilaparotomy)
TET	4	Tubal embryo transfer (by laparoscopy or minilaparotomy)
ZIFT	4,5	Zygote intrafallopian transfer (by laparoscopy or minilaparotomy)

Terms in the same group are either closely related or synonymous.

ferent brand. In this regard the reader is also referred to Sample Collection in Chapter 3.

With regard to quality or purity of chemicals, I use primarily AnalaR grade from BDH Chemicals or Sigma Grade biochemicals from the Sigma Chemical Co. In some cases where specific substances are available only from a particular supplier or a particular supplier's product has been found ideal, the supplier and catalogue number are provided.

Water

Water is the major chemical used in all andrology laboratories. Three grades of water are used.

Tap water is the local municipal supply.

Reagent water is either double-distilled, deionized, or now more commonly purified by reverse osmosis. It should be > 10 MΩ/cm resistivity, but no particular attention is paid to the removal of pyrogens or other organics or to its sterility.

Tissue culture grade water is highly purified, "polished" water suitable for tissue culture and, more pertinently, assisted reproductive technology procedures. Many purification systems are available, and their configurations depend on local conditions. However, such water is free of all inorganic and organic substances, including pyrogens, and is produced sterile.

N.B. Multiple-distilled water is *not* considered tissue culture grade, even though in some situations it may be used as such. Distillation is incapable of producing what is generally known as grade 1 water.

CONCEPTS OF FERTILITY, INFERTILITY, AND STERILITY

Although careful and thorough semen analyses are an essential part of the initial investigations of all couples presenting with infertility, the fertility of a population of human spermatozoa cannot be established with certainty. Consequently, probability analysis must be used to assess a man's fertility potential. Such considerations are based on statistical correlations between observed values and normal ranges reported for fertile men, which unfortunately immediately creates three problems.

1. Defining when an individual is fertile
2. Defining the normal ranges
3. Issues of standardization and quality control of semen analysis procedures and for reporting results

Fertility status is subject to many extrinsic factors so the only true definition of a fertile man is one who has recently sired a child, although this criterion assumes, but does not provide for, biological proof of paternity. Ideally, control subjects should be recruited through antenatal clinics or, at worst, postnatal wards. Obviously, it is insufficient to recruit fathers and thereby assume paternity, this being an increasingly dangerous assumption in many modern societies. For example, it is possible that a man may have had a vasectomy since the birth of his last child. Even though this example may be an extreme case, it serves to emphasize the magnitude of the assumption that a group of fathers represent a reliable subgroup of the fertile population.

So who can we define as "normal"? What do terms such as *fertile, infertile,* or *sterile* mean? A logical approach to the use of such terms would at least reduce much of the confusion, and Table 1-3 is provided as a guide for this purpose.

A man with any motile spermatozoa in his semen cannot be described as sterile; he must be credited with some potential for fertility. However, if a man succeeds in siring a child after infertility investigations or treatment, although he was clearly fertile at that time he is by no means necessarily "normal." If the cause of a cou-

Table 1–3   Terminology used for describing human infertility

Observation	Terminology	Do Not Use
One child or more	Father	Fertile
No children, never tried	Fertility unknown/unproven Unsuspected fertility	
No child, trying > 1 year	Suspected or possibly infertile, subfertile	Sterile
Normal semen analyses	Define observations and standards	Fertile
Abnormal semen analyses	Specify and define observations	Subfertile, infertile, sterile
Proven sterile	Sterile	Infertile
Tried > 1 year, unsuccessful, normal investigation, then a non-treatment-related pregnancy	Subfertile	Infertile, sterile

ple's infertility can be identified as a gross female factor, such as anovulation or bilateral tubal occlusion, the male partner may be considered as unsuspect. Or may he? There is no biological or medical rule that prevents both partners from having simultaneous disturbances in their reproductive systems, and the presently accepted figure for combined male and female factor infertility is about 20%, with an additional 33% incidence of "male factors" (World Health Organization, 1990). Consequently, only couples who have never had any reason to consult for infertility and who have achieved a pregnancy within a year of trying should be considered "normally fertile." Even if a pregnancy is achieved after a longer period of trying (without recourse to medical assistance), some men with reduced fertility will have had their "deficiency" compensated for by having partners of above-average fecundity. This concept can be elaborated on in the manner shown in Figure 1-1.

Clearly, any couple that includes at least one sterile partner is not a fertile union. Fertility, or more correctly fecundity, is then a continuum stretching from severely subfertile (functional sterility) through "superfertile." For the present purposes this classification has simply been divided into subfertile and fertile. Couples in which both partners are fertile can achieve a pregnancy, as do many couples in which a subfertile individual is paired with a fertile partner. Some of these couples do not achieve a pregnancy and so consult for infertility, probably with a unifactorial diagnosis. However, in the remaining category, where both partners are subfertile, there are fewer pregnancies; and more of these couples present for infertility investigations, which likely result in multifactorial diagnoses. Hence multifactorial infertility is a relatively common, rather than a rare, diagnosis.

DEFINING NORMAL RANGES

The above discussion is intended as neither exhaustive nor final. Many of our ideas are based on currently accepted definitions, which change (often markedly) with time. Again we return to statistical concepts and probability analysis. Because we are interested in determining a man's fertility potential based on the assessment of

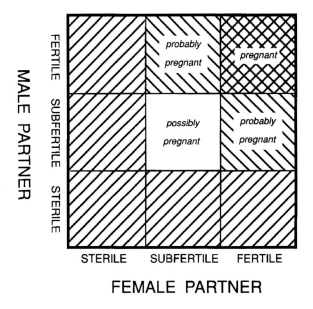

FIGURE (labels):

MALE PARTNER

FERTILE / SUBFERTILE / STERILE

probably pregnant

pregnant

possibly pregnant

probably pregnant

STERILE   SUBFERTILE   FERTILE

FEMALE PARTNER

Figure 1-1   Concept of multifactorial infertility. See text for explanation.

certain indirect criteria, so long as the assumptions are stated (and accepted) this goal may be achieved within the limits of the stated preconditions. However, because statistical analysis requires reliable numbers obtained by objective, standardized techniques, we now face the greatest problem in andrology: Such techniques exist in relatively few laboratories (see Chapter 16).

All diagnostic laboratory procedures demand precision, reproducibility, and sensitivity. Furthermore, if reports produced by one laboratory are to be intelligible to others, standardization is also clearly essential. In addition, clinical interpretation of the results requires normal ranges for the various characteristics reported so deviations from the norm may be evaluated. Although each laboratory should ideally determine its own ranges of normal values, it is clearly not always possible. So long as this basic principle is borne in mind and accepted standard laboratory procedures are employed, results may be interpreted using the WHO normal limits for semen characteristics as shown in Table 1-4 (World Health Organization, 1992).

Although these ranges delimit the lower end of normality, they are not as useful for interpreting semen analysis results as the scheme given in Table 1-5. These values are based on the work of Eliasson (1975, 1977, 1981), with some modification for more modern methods, and are derived from cumulative frequency distribution analyses of populations of fertile men and infertility clinic patients. In simple terms, the point where these two distributions of the values for a semen characteristic start to differ is the transition from "normal" to "doubtful." Where the distributions no longer overlap or are different is the transition from "doubtful" to "pathological." It must be emphasized, however, that when interpreting a semen analysis based on these ranges, conception may still occur even with one (and perhaps even several)

Table 1–4   Semen analysis normal ranges

Semen Characteristic	Units	WHO (1987)	WHO (1992)
Volume	ml	≥ 2.0	≥ 2.0
pH	pH units	7.2–8.0	7.2–8.0
Sperm concentration	10^6/ml	≥ 20	≥ 20
Total sperm count	10^6/ejaculate	≥ 40	≥ 40
Motility (within 60 minutes	% Class a	≥ 25	≥ 25
of ejaculation	% Classes a and b	≥ 50	≥ 50
Morphology	% Normal	≥ 50	≥ 30
Vitality	% Live	≥ 75	≥ 75
Leukocytes (WBCs)	10^6/ml	< 1.0	< 1.0
Immunobead test	% Sperm with beads	≤ 10	< 20
MAR test	% Sperm with RBCs	< 10	< 10
α-Glucosidase (neutral)	mU/ejaculate		≥ 20
Zinc (total)	μmol/ejaculate		≥ 2.4
Citric acid (total)	μmol/ejaculate		≥ 52
Acid phosphatase (total)	U/ejaculate		≥ 200
Fructose (total)	μmol/ejaculate		≥ 13

Source: After World Health Organization.

characteristics in the pathological range. The correct interpretation is that such an event is improbable, but not so improbable as conception if one (or more) semen characteristics are in the doubtful range (see Chapter 11 for further discussion).

So what is a normal semen sample? Perhaps the purest definition is a semen sample that, had it been inseminated into a reproductively normal female at coitus, would have resulted in a successful pregnancy. This definition takes into account not only the classic descriptive characteristics of the semen sample itself but also the intrinsic fertilizing ability of the spermatozoa; it also requires normal fecundity of the female partner.

Table 1–5   Semen analysis: normal ranges

Semen Characteristic	Units	Normal	Borderline	Pathological
Volume	ml	2.0–6.0	1.5–2.0	< 1.5
Sperm concentration	10^6/ml	20–250	10–20	< 10
Total sperm count	10^6/ejaculate	> 80	20–80	< 20
Motility (0.5–2.0 hours after ejaculation)	% Motile	> 50	35–49	< 35
Progression (at 37°C)	Scale 0–4	3 or 4	2	< 2
Morphology	% Normal	≥ 60	35–59	< 35
Head defects	Per 100 sperm	< 35	35–60	> 60
Midpiece defects	Per 100 sperm	≤ 20	21–25	> 25
Tail defects	Per 100 sperm	≤ 20	21–25	> 25
Vitality	% Live	≥ 75	50–74	< 50

Source: Modified from Mortimer (1985).

TERMINOLOGY USED BY ANDROLOGISTS

Numerous jargon words are used by andrologists to describe abnormalities encountered during semen analysis. Because there is no general agreement as to the precise definitions of these terms (notwithstanding methodological questions), and because they are not synonymous with any specific clinical or pathological conditions, their use is discouraged. For example, describing two semen samples with sperm motilities of 39% and 5% as both being asthenozoospermic (defined below) is hiding an important difference. However, because readers frequently encounter the use, and misuse, of these terms, some attempt at clarification is made.

The term *-spermia* refers to the volume of the ejaculate, and *-zoospermia* refers to the spermatozoa in the semen. Therefore *aspermia* means the absence of semen (i.e., zero volume) and *azoospermia* the complete absence of spermatozoa from the ejaculate. Abnormally low and high ejaculate volumes are sometimes described as hypospermia and hyperspermia, with *oligozoospermia* meaning a reduced sperm concentration (usually $< 20 \times 10^6$/ml).

Oligozoospermia is often divided into severe ($< 10 \times 10^6$/ml) and mild (10×10^6 to 20×10^6/ml) forms. The term *cryptozoospermia* is occasionally found describing sperm concentrations of $< 1 \times 10^6$/ml, and *polyzoospermia* simply means a very high sperm concentration ($> 250 \times 10^6$/ml), a situation of uncertain relevance as a defined clinical entity.

Asthenozoospermia means decreased sperm motility (usually $< 40\%$), with the extreme being zero motility. *Teratozoospermia* means an increased number of spermatozoa with abnormal morphology (typically $> 50\%$ abnormal forms), although it must be interpreted in light of the definition of "normal" spermatozoa (see Chapter 3), as well as the fastidiousness of the andrologist responsible for the analysis. *Necrozoospermia* means that many or all of the spermatozoa are dead as defined by vital staining.

Some andrologists use combinations of these terms, such as *oligoasthenoteratozoospermia*. Because all of these aspects of semen quality are interrelated (see Chapter 11) such a finding is not unusual. More importantly, the term neither clearly nor precisely describes the situation, nor does it give any indication of the severity of the problem(s).

For the benefit of everyone concerned, clinical assessments should state the laboratory findings clearly, pointing out any deviations from normal and giving some indication of the severity of any such deviation. Laboratories should report only the results of their measurements and tests; it must remain the responsibility of the physician requesting the tests to interpret the results in relation to the overall clinical picture for the patient.

References and Recommended Reading

Eliasson, R. (1975). Analysis of semen. In Behrman, S. J., and Kistner R. W. (eds): *Progress in Infertility,* 2nd ed. Little, Brown, Boston.

Eliasson, R. (1977). Semen analysis and laboratory workup. In Cockett, A.T.K., and Urry, R. L. (eds): *Male Infertility. Workup, Treatment and Research.* Grune & Stratton, Orlando, FL.

Eliasson, R. (1981). Analysis of semen. In Burger, H., and de Kretser, D. M. (eds): *The Testis.* Raven Press, New York.

World Health Organization (1990). Prevention and management of infertility. *Progress,* **15,** 1.

World Health Organization (1992). *WHO Laboratory Manual for the Examination of Human Semen and Sperm–Cervical Mucus Interaction,* 3rd ed. Cambridge University Press, Cambridge.

2

Sperm Physiology

A comprehensive discussion of male reproductive physiology is outside the scope of this text, and the interested reader is referred to standard texts on reproductive physiology. However, a brief overview is provided, as sperm physiology is fundamental to understanding what follows in Sections II and III of this book.

SPERM PRODUCTION

Testis

The testis, like the ovary, has both endocrine and gametogenic functions. In simple terms, the bulk of the testis comprises the seminiferous tubules, which are looped tubules opening at both ends into the rete testis and hence into the epididymis (Fig. 2-1). The convoluted seminiferous tubules lie within the lobes of the testis separated by fibrous septa and are enclosed by loose connective tissue containing, in addition to the usual blood vessels, lymphatics, and nerves, interstitial or Leydig cells. The wall of each seminiferous tubule is primarily fibrous tissue (including collagen fibers) with some myoid cells giving it limited contractility.

Leydig Cells
The Leydig cell contains a large amount of smooth endoplasmic reticulum and is responsible for the testicular production, under pituitary stimulation by LH, of the male sex steroid testosterone. This androgen is released into the circulation and regulates its own production by negative feedback on the pituitary to modulate or suppress LH secretion (Fig. 2-2).

Seminiferous Epithelium and Sertoli Cells
The adult seminiferous tubule contains a stratified epithelium of five to eight layers of cells of widely different morphology and an irregular lumen. The seminiferous epithelium is organized by the Sertoli cells (tall, irregular-shaped cells with large basal nuclei) that extend from the basement membrane of the tubule wall to the tubule lumen (Fig. 2-3). The various germinal cells are embedded in, and their development is regulated by, the Sertoli cells. In addition, each Sertoli cell has tight junctions with its neighbors to create the blood-testis barrier, which prevents the passage of molecules between the basal and luminal compartments of the seminiferous tubules. This barrier serves to isolate meiotic and postmeiotic germinal cells, which express specific antigens on their surfaces that are not found before puberty

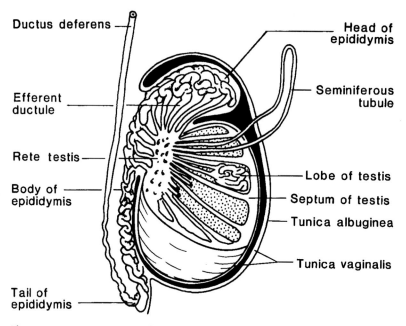

Ductus deferens

Head of epididymis

Efferent ductule

Seminiferous tubule

Rete testis

Body of epididymis

Lobe of testis

Septum of testis

Tunica albuginea

Tunica vaginalis

Tail of epididymis

Figure 2-1   Human testis and epididymis.

(and hence would be considered "foreign" by the adult immune system) in the luminal compartment.

The Sertoli cell is sensitive to FSH from the pituitary (Fig. 2-2). In response to this stimulation, the Sertoli cell produces an androgen-binding protein (ABP), which has a high affinity for testosterone and ensures that a high concentration of this androgen is maintained within the tubule and hence the excurrent ducts of the testis. The Sertoli cell also produces a polypeptide known as inhibin, which provides a negative feedback mechanism on the pituitary to regulate FSH secretion.

The germ cells go through a complicated series of divisions and maturational changes that together constitute the process of spermatogenesis, which produces haploid spermatids. The final transformation of spermatid into spermatozoon is known as spermiogenesis.

Spermatogenesis
The most immature male germinal cell is the spermatogonium. It is the basic, self-renewing stem cell of the male germ cell line. Spermatogonia first undergo mitotic division to increase their number with daughter cells either proceeding into spermatogenesis, forming replacement stem cells, or degenerating. In the human testis, three types of spermatogonium are usually considered: (1) dark type A (or Ad) spermatogonia, which develop into (2) pale type A (Ap) spermatogonia, and then mature into (3) type B or differentiating spermatogonia (Figs. 2-4 and 2-5). Some authors also consider a fourth, "long" type A (or Al) spermatogonium, which may be a reserve stem cell that gives rise to the Ad type.

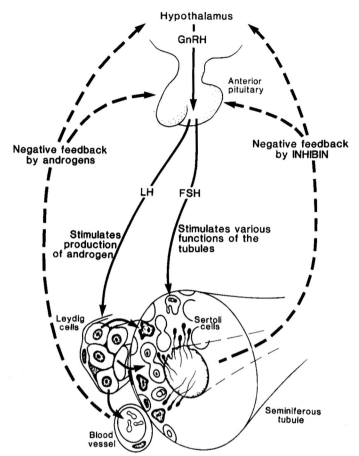

Figure 2-2 Hypothalamic-pituitary-testicular axis. (Adapted from Fawcett, D. W. Gametogenesis in the male: Prospects for its control. In Markert, D. L., and Papaconstantinou, J. (eds): *The Developmental Biology of Reproduction.* Academic Press, Orlando, FL, 1975, p. 25.)

Type B spermatogonia are the immediate precursors of primary spermatocytes, into which they transform before entering the first meiotic division to produce secondary spermatocytes. In turn, secondary spermatocytes go through the second meiotic division to produce haploid spermatids.

Spermiogenesis

Spermiogenesis is the complex maturational process by which a haploid spermatid differentiates into a mature spermatid, i.e., testicular spermatozoon (de Kretser, 1969); (Fig. 2-6).

Basically, the nuclear histones are replaced by protamines, the chromatin condenses, and the smaller nucleus assumes an eccentric position close to the cell membrane. Disulfide bond cross-linking of the protamines makes the inert, con-

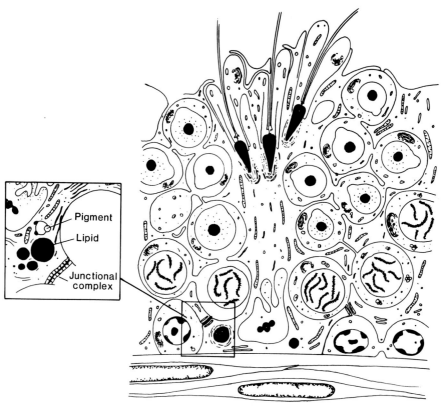

Figure 2-3   Sertoli cell and the blood-testis barrier. (Adapted from Fawcett, D. W. The ultra-structure and functions of the Sertoli cell. In Greep, R.O., and Koblinsky, M.A. (eds): *Frontiers in Reproduction and Fertility Control*. MIT Press, Cambridge, 1977, p. 302.)

densed chromatin resistant to DNAse. The Golgi complex elaborates the acrosome, which is closely applied to that part of the nucleus in contact with the cell membrane. One of the centrioles attaches to the pole of the nucleus opposite the developing acrosome and produces the axial filament. Structures in addition to the simple 9 + 2 structure of the axoneme (typical of cilia and flagella) develop to form the axial filament complex. Cytoplasmic reduction of the spermatid occurs; and the mitochondria, which transform into more tubular, less ovoid structures, become arranged around the proximal part of the axial filament complex of the developing tail.

Residual cytoplasm is shed from the neck region of the mature spermatid as it is released from the seminiferous epithelium into the tubule lumen, a process termed *spermiation* (Fig. 2-7). A small residual cytoplasmic droplet also remains attached to testicular spermatozoa at the point of separation. As the cell undergoes further maturation during epididymal transit, this cytoplasmic droplet migrates along the tail and is finally lost.

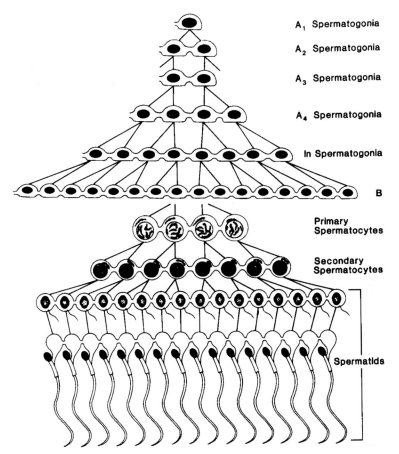

A₁ Spermatogonia

A₂ Spermatogonia

A₃ Spermatogonia

A₄ Spermatogonia

In Spermatogonia

B

Primary Spermatocytes

Secondary Spermatocytes

Spermatids

Figure 2-4 Cascade of cell divisions comprising spermatogenesis. (Adapted from Dym, M., and Fawcett, D. W. Further observation on the numbers of spermatogonia, spermatocytes and spermatids connected by intercellular bridges in the mammalian testis. *Biol. Reprod.* **4,** 195, 1971.)

Human sperm production takes a fixed period of 70 ± 4 days from the commitment of a type A spermatogonium to undergo spermatogenesis to the appearance of the mature spermatid in the seminiferous epithelium (Heller and Clermont, 1964). This rate cannot be altered by exogenous hormonal treatment, extrinsic factors such as temperature, or noxious agents such as radiation. Release of the testicular spermatozoon (spermiation) and its passage through the excurrent ducts of the testis and the epididymis is generally believed to take another 12–21 days (depending on the method of experimental measurement). However, very recent studies have indicated that it may take as little as 3 days. Consequently, a period of 10–12 weeks is required for the production of human spermatozoa from germinal stem cells to a stage where they are ready to be ejaculated.

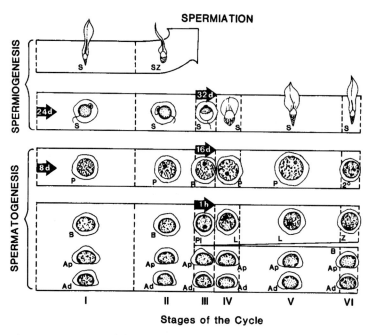

Figure 2-5 Stages of the seminiferous epithelium cycle during human spermiogenesis. (Adapted from Heller, C. G., and Clermont, Y. Spermatogenesis in man: An estimate of its duration. *Science* **140**, 184, 1963.)

Epididymis

The epididymis lies along the dorsolateral border of each testis. It comprises the vasa efferentia, which emanate from the rete testis, and the epididymal ducts (Fig. 2-1). The epididymis opens into the vas deferens, which then passes through the inguinal canal into the peritoneal cavity and opens into the urethra adjacent to the prostate.

The primary functions of the epididymis are the posttesticular maturation and storage of spermatozoa during their passage from the testis to the vas deferens. The epididymal epithelium, which is androgen-dependent, has both absorptive and secretory functions, and the epididymis is generally divided into three functionally distinct (although anatomically less so) regions: head, body, and tail, or caput epididymidis, corpus epididymidis, and cauda epididymidis. Their functions can be described simplistically as the concentration, maturation, and storage of the spermatozoa, respectively.

Much of the testicular fluid that transports spermatozoa from the seminiferous tubules is resorbed in the caput so the concentration of the spermatozoa is increased some 10- to 100-fold. The epididymal plasma, in which the spermatozoa are suspended within the epididymis, is also secreted by the epididymal epithelium. It is a complex fluid whose composition changes along the length of the epididymis; hence the spermatozoa experience a series of sophisticated microenvironments that regulate their maturation.

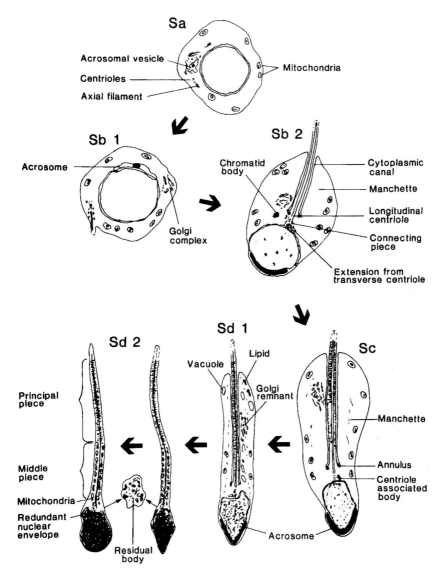

Figure 2-6 Differentiation of the round spermatid into a spermatozoon during spermio-genesis. (Adapted from de Kretser, D. M. Ultrastructural features of human spermiogenesis. *Z. Zellforsch. Mikrosk. Anat.* **98,** 477, 1969.)

Posttesticular Sperm Maturation

Posttesticular sperm maturation involves an intricate combination of morphological, biochemical, biophysical, and metabolic changes. Physiologically, the spermatozoa develop motility and become capable of fertilizing, contingent on the final maturational process of capacitation (see below).

The most striking morphological change involves loss of the cytoplasmic droplet.

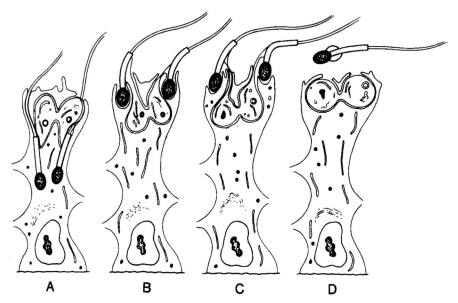

Figure 2-7 Process of spermiation, the release of spermatozoa from the seminiferous epithelium at the end of spermiogenesis. (Adapted from Fawcett, D. W. Ultrastructure and function of the Sertoli cell. In Hamilton, D. W., and Greep, R. O. (eds): *Handbook of Physiology. Sect. 7. Endocrinology. Vol. V. Male Reproductive System.* American Physiological Society, Washington, DC, 1975, p. 21.)

Additional changes in the sperm surface alter the spermatozoa's electrophoretic properties and their agglutination by lectins, indicating glycosylation modifications to cell surface glycoproteins. The acrosome acquires its final shape; final chromatin condensation and stabilization occurs; and the axonemal complex "matures" or is modified.

Metabolically, the spermatozoa become more active and show increased fructolysis. This is associated with a weak, uncoordinated, vibratory pattern of nonprogressive motility that may be stimulated by their suspension in seminal plasma or a physiological saline or culture medium. The capacity for motility increases as the spermatozoa are transported through the epididymis, so spermatozoa stored in the cauda are capable of normal progressive motility upon entry into seminal plasma or resuspension in appropriate artificial media.

Spermatozoa taken from the caput or proximal corpus are generally incapable of fertilization, whereas those from the distal corpus and the cauda are able to undergo capacitation and achieve normal gamete interaction (Moore et al., 1983). Reports that human spermatozoa aspirated from the proximal epididymides of men with congenital agenesis of the vasa deferentia can fertilize human oocytes in vitro (Temple-Smith et al., 1985; Silber et al., 1990) cannot be taken as evidence for epididymal maturation being nonessential. These patients had substantial pathology; and such observations, albeit of clinical importance, cannot be considered physiologically relevant (Cooper, 1990).

Epididymal Sperm Storage

As many as half of the spermatozoa released from the testis die and disintegrate within the epididymis and are resorbed by the epididymal epithelium. The remaining mature spermatozoa are stored in the caudae epididymides, which contain about 70% of all the spermatozoa present in the male tract. The vasa deferentia are not a physiological site of sperm storage and contain only about 2% of the total spermatozoa in the male tract.

Although the environment of the cauda is adapted for sperm storage, it is not a perfect storage organ, and the spermatozoa do not remain in a viable state indefinitely. After prolonged sexual inactivity, caudal spermatozoa first lose their fertilizing ability, followed by their motility and then their vitality; they finally disintegrate. Unless these older, senescent spermatozoa are eliminated from the male tract at more or less regular intervals, their relative contribution to the next ejaculate(s) increases, thereby reducing semen quality, even though such ejaculates do have a high sperm concentration. This process is one of the reasons for the proscribed 3-day period of sexual abstinence prior to collection of ejaculates for semen analysis (see Chapter 3). Caudal spermatozoa are also sensitive to increased external temperature, as in cryptorchidism or artificial scrotal heating (e.g., prolonged periods spent seated or immersed in hot water), which causes deterioration in sperm quality.

Accessory Sexual Glands

The accessory glands of the human male reproductive system are highly specialized structures under both endocrine (androgen) and neural control. Their physiological roles in male fertility remain unclear, but it has long been considered unreasonable to assume that a compound secretion as complex as seminal plasma should serve only as a vehicle for the spermatozoa between the caudae epididymides and the vagina. Furthermore, dysfunction of the accessory glands, often associated with clinical or subclinical infections, does cause impaired fertility.

Seminal Vesicles

The paired seminal vesicles lie on the dorsal face of the bladder. Each is a convoluted glandular sac or tube about 5–6 cm in length (about 15 cm if unraveled), arising from the vas deferens just below the ampulla of the vas (Fig. 2-8 and 2-9). The yellowish, viscous, alkaline secretion of the seminal vesicles is called the vesicular fluid. It is the last fraction of the semen ejaculated and contributes about 70% of the ejaculate volume. A single ejaculate essentially depletes these glands, as an immediate repeat ejaculate contains little fructose, a marker specific for the vesicular fluid where it is present in unusually high concentrations. Other major constituents of vesicular fluid include ascorbic acid, inorganic phosphorus, and potassium, which is the principal cation present, sodium being virtually absent.

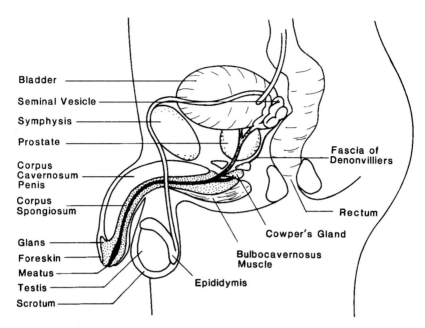

Figure 2-8 Sagittal view of the human male urogenital system. (Adapted from Spring-Mills, E., and Hafez, E.S.E. Male accessory sexual organs. In Hafez, E.S.E. (ed): *Human Reproduction. Conception and Contraception,* 2nd ed. Harper & Row, Hagerstown, MO, 1979, p. 60.)

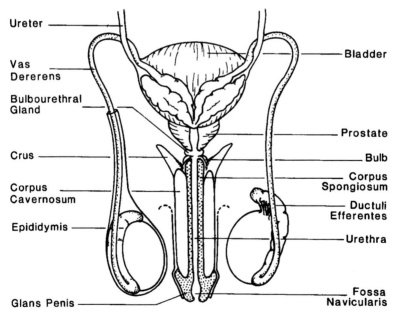

Figure 2-9 Ventral view of the human male urogenital system. (Adapted from Dym, M. The male reproductive system. In Weiss, L., and Greep, R. O. (eds): *Histology.* McGraw-Hill, New York, 1977.)

Prostaglandins in human semen also come almost exclusively from the seminal vesicles, but their concentrations are more or less independent of seminal fructose. This point indicates that the seminal vesicles are functionally multiglandular and that more than a single marker substance, such as the commonly measured fructose, should be assayed to assess their secretory function reliably.

Because the seminal vesicles and vas deferens have the same embryonic origin, congenital absence of the vas is associated with agenesis of the seminal vesicles. This fact can be used in the differential diagnosis of azoospermia, as only in cases of excretory azoospermia due to congenital absence of the vas is there an absence of seminal fructose. In cases of secretory azoospermia (i.e., due to defective spermatogenesis) or excretory azoospermia due to blockage at the epididymal level, seminal fructose is in the normal range.

The seminal vesicles are not a site of functional sperm storage.

Prostate

The prostate is the largest human male accessory gland (3.5–4.0 cm in diameter; 20 g in weight) and completely surrounds the urethra below the neck of the bladder. In adults the prostate is continuously active, producing 0.5–2.0 ml of prostatic fluid per day. Expressed prostatic fluid is a homogeneous, serous, slightly milky fluid that is often slightly acidic (pH 6.8) or just on the alkaline side of neutral (pH 7.2). In men with prostatitis it is often more alkaline (pH 7.5–8.0).

Prostatic secretion is produced primarily by the merocrine mechanism of exocytosis. However, there is some evidence for an apocrine mechanism (blebbing of apical cytoplasm from columnar epithelial cells), as is highly pronounced in the rabbit. The latter process may be increased with prostatitis and contribute to increased anucleate cytoplasmic debris in the semen.

Most of the balance of the ejaculate volume (almost 30%) is contributed by the prostate and constitutes the first fraction of the ejaculate proper. It contains most of the spermatozoa and does not coagulate spontaneously upon emission, e.g., as when collected as part of a split ejaculate. The prostatic fluid contains the fibrinolytic enzymes responsible for liquefaction of coagulated vesicular secretion.

Essentially all the citric acid and zinc found in human seminal plasma come from the prostatic fluid. Acid phosphatase, which may be involved in sperm metabolism by converting glycerylphosphorylcholine (also primarily from the prostate) into choline, is another major constituent; and sodium is the major cation. Prostatic fluid also enhances sperm motility by contributing certain factors, perhaps albumin, to seminal plasma that stimulate the motility of epididymal and washed ejaculate spermatozoa.

Again, the prostate is functionally multiglandular, and adequate assessment of its secretory function requires measurement of several marker substances.

Bulbourethral Glands

The bulbourethral (Cowper's) glands are two small lobulated glands located dorsal to the bulb (base) of the penis whose excretory ducts open into the penile urethra.

The secretion of these glands is clear and mucoid, rich in sialoprotein, and discharged during erection and perhaps at ejaculation (prior to ejaculation of spermatozoa). The primary function of this secretion is traditionally described as the lubrication of the urethra, which is probably better expressed as the neutralization of any acidic urinary residue in the urethra before ejaculation of the sperm-rich first fraction of the ejaculate proper. Acidic pH is detrimental to human spermatozoa, whereas high pH (e.g., pH 8.4) is well tolerated.

Other Accessory Glands

Additional small, barely studied—and hence poorly understood—glands are scattered throughout the male reproductive tract. They include the ampullary, urethral (Littre's), and preputial (Tyson's) glands.

EJACULATION AND INSEMINATION

At ejaculation, spermatozoa are transferred from storage in the caudae epididymides (contributing 5–10% of the ejaculate volume), mixed with the secretions of the accessory glands in a precise sequence (first prostatic and then vesicular fluids), and emitted to the exterior along the penile urethra that has been prepared by the bulbourethral glands' secretion. The first part of the ejaculate proper contains most of the spermatozoa suspended in more or less pure prostatic fluid (obviously including a small volume of epididymal fluid). The subsequent fraction is transitional between prostatic fluid and vesicular fluid, so the last fraction contains only the residual spermatozoa mobilized from the epididymal reserves suspended in pure vesicular fluid. The proportion of the ejaculate volume occupied by the spermatozoa themselves (the "spermatocrit") is only of the order of 1–5%.

Spontaneous coagulation of the human ejaculate occurs rapidly after ejaculation due to components of the vesicular secretion. Subsequent liquefaction is effected by factors contributed by the prostatic secretion.

Although the whole ejaculate is involved in coagulum formation when semen is collected by masturbation into a specimen container in vitro (or a Silastic condom in vivo), the precise nature of events in vivo (i.e., when semen is ejaculated per vaginam around the external cervical os during intercourse) is not amenable to investigation. One highly pertinent observation, however, comes from studies using the immediate postcoital test, when spermatozoa have been reported within the cervical mucus as soon as 1.5 minutes after ejaculation, at a time when coagulated semen was seen elsewhere in the vagina (Sobrero and MacLeod, 1962). From the evolutionary aspect, the phenomenon of coagulation of the vesicular secretion is well known in rodents, pigs, and some primates where a "copulatory plug" is formed to prevent leakage of the sperm-rich fraction of the ejaculate from the female tract.

Consequently, the human situation may represent an evolutionary vestige so that under in vivo conditions the spermatozoa migrate into the cervical mucus from that part of the noncoagulated sperm-rich fraction deposited around the external os of the cervical canal. It is certainly inappropriate to assume that the collection of an ejaculate as a single, mixed specimen reflects physiology, even though it is the only practicable standard test procedure.

SPERMATOZOON

The male human is unusual, perhaps unique, among mammals in the degree of morphological heterogeneity or pleomorphism of his gametes. Normal fertile men produce ejaculates containing as many as 50% grossly abnormal spermatozoa, displaying defects in one or several regions of the cell including head size and shape, chromatin condensation and the presence of nuclear vacuoles, persistent cytoplasmic droplets, tail defects, and even duplicate or conjoined ("siamese twin") spermatozoa. Although it was once suggested that human sperm head shape was obviously bimodally distributed, reflecting X- and Y-chromosome-bearing cells, it is not the case.

In the absence of adequate direct observations on human spermatozoa performing their ultimate function of fertilization under in vivo conditions, spermatologists and andrologists have had to resort to describing the modal (i.e., most frequently occurring) morphological form of spermatozoa seen in human semen samples (Figs. 2-10 and 2-11). Confirmation of the validity of this approach has been provided by examining postcoital cervical mucus samples where the spermatozoa generally have this "typical" morphological appearance.

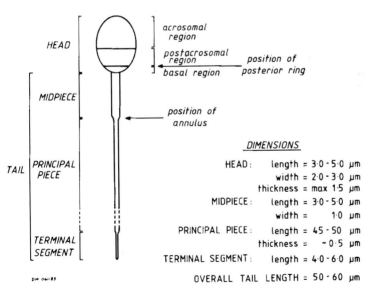

Figure 2-10 Morphometry of the human spermatozoon. (From Mortimer, D. The male factor in infertility Part I. Semen analysis. *Curr. Probl. Obstet. Gynecol. Fertil.* Vol. VIII (7), 87 pp. Year Book Medical Publishers, Chicago, 1985. With permission.)

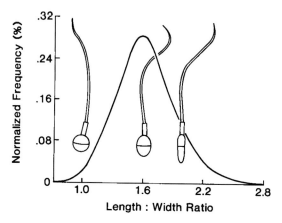

Figure 2-11 Frequency distribution of human sperm head shape, illustrating the concept of the modal "oval form." (Adapted from Van Duijn, C. Cytological details and size-frequency distribution in human spermatozoa. *Int. J. Fertil.* 9, 533, 1964.)

Sperm Morphology and Morphometry

A normal, mature human spermatozoon (Fig. 2-10) is typically described as possessing an oval head of regular outline (3–5 μm long, 2–3 μm wide) with clearly defined pale anterior (acrosomal) and darker posterior regions in stained preparations. Slightly tapering or pear-shaped heads are not necessarily abnormal, as they may represent the extremes of the normal distribution (Fig. 2-11) for that individual (or be typical of a man who is an extreme case of the population distribution); nor is the presence of a few small vacuoles (weakly stained areas) within the head abnormal. However, obviously tapered, pyriform, or otherwise misshapen heads, large or small heads, highly vacuolated heads, or heads lacking the two defined regions (i.e., more or less uniformly dark-staining) are abnormal. The single sperm tail, about 50 μm overall length, is inserted into a symmetrically located shallow depression at the base of the head. The head should not come to a point here; otherwise it is considered pyriform, indicating a weakness of the neck region. Immediately behind the head the tail is slightly thickened to form the midpiece region (7–8 μm long, maximum width 1 μm). Immature spermatozoa often show a cytoplasmic droplet in the neck region, at other locations along the tail, or even at the tip of the tail.

  Determination of the precise quantitative morphology of the spermatozoon, its morphometry, is not usually considered a routine procedure. Of significance, however, is the observation that fixed and stained spermatozoa are slightly smaller than those in wet preparations (Katz et al., 1986), which means that morphometric descriptions must also include the state of the cells measured (Table 2-1). An all-encompassing description must cover the range of both stained and unstained spermatozoa (e.g., World Health Organization, 1992). The use of reliable descriptions is important for the "strict criteria" morphological classification from Tygerberg,

Table 2–1   Head morphometry of fixed and unfixed human spermatozoa

Measurement	Katz et al. (1986)		Schrader et al. (1990)
	Wet Preparations	**Stained Preparations**	**Stained Preparations**
Head length (μm)	5.26 ± 0.61	4.54 ± 0.50	4.57 ± 0.76
Head width (μm)	3.37 ± 0.41	2.82 ± 0.25	2.85 ± 0.42
Head area (μm²)	13.91 ± 2.69	9.79 ± 1.43	8.72 ± 2.09
Aspect ratio[a]	1.59 ± 0.24	1.63 ± 0.26	0.64 ± 0.12

Values are means ± SD.

[a]Aspect ratio = L/W for Katz et al. (1986) but W/L for Schrader et al. (1990).

which requires that sperm head morphometry be used for determining whether a cell is morphologically normal (see Chapter 3).

Sperm ultrastructure is discussed in Chapter 8.

Sperm Motility

Testicular spermatozoa of humans, as for all other eutheria, are either motionless or feebly motile. This immotility, which is true even if testicular spermatozoa are sampled by micropuncture and suspended in culture medium, is apparently due to the "immaturity" of the plasmalemma, as demembranated spermatozoa can be induced, under appropriate conditions, to move almost as actively as mature spermatozoa from the the cauda (Mohri and Yanagimachi, 1980). During passage through the epididymis, spermatozoa undergo substantial maturational changes that result in their acquisition of motility. Although motile spermatozoa from the cauda are capable of progressive motility when suspended in culture medium in vitro, they remain essentially immotile in vivo. Only at ejaculation, when they are mixed with the secretions of the accessory glands, do spermatozoa undergo motility activation.

The motility of ejaculated spermatozoa has long been recognized as an important functional characteristic that must be evaluated as an integral part of semen analysis. More recently, major influences of sperm motility on the cervical mucus penetrating ability and the fertilizing potential of human spermatozoa have been demonstrated. It is not just the proportion of spermatozoa that are motile or even their concentration that is of greatest importance. The objective and quantitative measurement of sperm movement characteristics derived from observations on individual cells has been found to be more predictive of functional ability and hence a man's potential fertility (see Chapters 7 and 11). Consequently, in recent years increasing attention has been paid to the evaluation of sperm motility at more than the crude level of determining the proportion of motile spermatozoa, and it is apparent that we need to concentrate on those approaches that provide objective and accurate measurements of specific aspects of sperm movement, not just simple motility.

SPERM TRANSPORT IN THE FEMALE TRACT

Spermatozoa in the Vagina

At the moment of insemination, 2–6 ml of semen containing some 200 million to 300 million spermatozoa are deposited around the external cervical os and in the posterior fornix of the vagina (Fig. 2-12). Around midcycle the pH of the vagina is strongly acidic, a situation highly detrimental to spermatozoa. Fortunately, seminal plasma has a strong buffering capacity and is able, within seconds of ejaculation, to raise the vaginal pH to at least neutral and to maintain this state for up to 2 hours. Perhaps this is the function of the vesicular fraction?

The vaginal pool of liquefied semen probably plays little or no significant part in sperm transport for several reasons: (1) most of the spermatozoa that are to penetrate the cervical mucus have done so within 15–20 minutes of ejaculation; (2) most of the ejaculate is often lost from the vagina soon after coitus; (3) vaginal spermatozoa are quickly inactivated (spermatozoa exposed to the vaginal environment for 35 minutes are incapable of penetrating cervical mucus); (4) any prolonged exposure of spermatozoa to seminal plasma results in marked declines in both their motility and vitality, as well as in their subsequent functional potential; and (5) recolonization of the cervix from the vagina is apparently minimal. Some motile spermatozoa may remain in the vagina for up to 24 hours, although as the postcoital interval increases the incidence of sperm-positive cases (irrespective of motility) decreases. See Mortimer (1983) for a more detailed review.

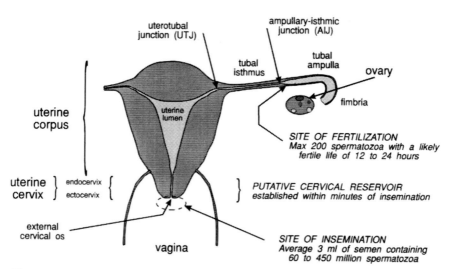

Figure 2-12   Sperm transport through the female tract. (Redrawn from Mortimer, 1985.)

Spermatozoa in the Cervix

When cervical mucus and liquefied semen come into contact in vitro, the phenomenon of phalanges formation occurs (Fig. 2-13), and it has been assumed to occur in vivo. This rheological property is not exclusive to these two biological fluids, but in this particular case it may well serve to entrap some of the first sperm-rich fraction of the ejaculate within the periphery of the cervical mucus at the external os. There is then gradual penetration of progressively motile spermatozoa into the mucus column from these repositories protected from the vaginal milieu.

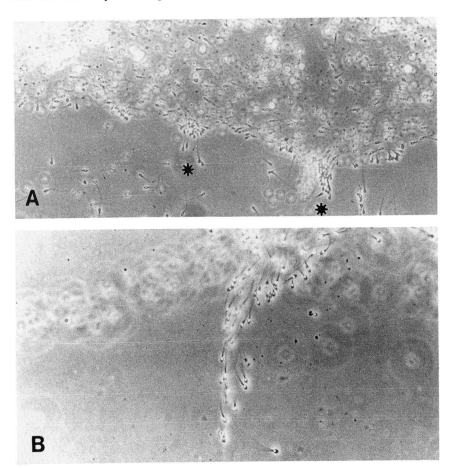

Figure 2-13 Photomicrographic series to illustrate the formation of phalanges at the interface between human semen (upper part of each figure) and cervical mucus (lower part of each figure). (**A**) Two phalanges of spermatozoa can be seen beginning to penetrate the mucus phase. (**B**) Two major phalanges of spermatozoa are progressing away from the semen phase, one in focus and a second (to the left at right angles) out of focus.

Some component of seminal plasma is important for efficient entry of human spermatozoa across the mucus interface (Overstreet et al., 1980), and successful penetration into cervical mucus has been related to specific patterns of sperm movement (see Chapters 7 and 11). Furthermore, penetration of the mucus column by spermatozoa causes some change(s) in the mucus so the motility of "following" spermatozoa is altered compared to that of the "vanguard" spermatozoa (Katz et al., 1982).

The nature of the mucous secretion of the cervix varies with the phase of the menstrual cycle, the secretion produced under the influence of high circulating estrogen levels being the most ideal for sperm penetration (Fig. 2-14). Consequently, the receptivity of cervical mucus to penetration by spermatozoa is cyclic, increasing over a period of about 4 days before ovulation and decreasing rapidly (within 2 days) after, with receptivity being maximal on the day before and the day of the LH peak.

The concept of a cervical sperm reservoir originates mainly from work in sheep. Although it is an attractive hypothesis, and has been widely promulgated for all species with vaginal insemination, there is little evidence for any such process in the human female tract. Certainly spermatozoa populate the crypts of the cervical epithelium, but a successive shift from the lower to upper levels of the cervix has not been demonstrated (Insler et al., 1980). Because continuous migration from the vaginal pool into the lower crypts, which might mask such an upward transfer of spermatozoa, is known not to happen (see above), we are forced to accept that spermatozoa stored in any particular crypt remain there until being either transferred directly to the uterus or disposed of, probably by phagocytosis because there is pronounced leukocytosis from the cervical epithelium after insemination (Pandya and Cohen, 1985; Barratt et al., 1990). In the continued absence of definite evidence that any spermatozoa leave a crypt after entering it, there is no sound basis for considering the crypts of the cervical mucosa as organs of sperm storage in the human.

A more plausible hypothesis is that because spermatozoa swimming in cervical mucus are constrained to follow the lines of the mucin structure, it may be that those spermatozoa that follow this orientation back its secretory origin in the crypts are those that are later found there, and they have reached the (dead-)end of their journey. Only those spermatozoa that continue to swim within the mucus column to the internal os eventually reach the uterine cavity. This population of spermatozoa, each swimming at their own speed, may well be the real "cervical reservoir," a concept supported by various observations on the dynamics of sperm distributions within the cervical mucus (review: Mortimer, 1983).

"Rapid" Sperm Transport

The occurrence of a phase of "rapid" sperm transport, whereby spermatozoa are transported by the actions of the female tract from the site of insemination to the fallopian tubes within a few minutes of insemination, has been based on studies in other species that are probably of minimal relevance to the human situation and on

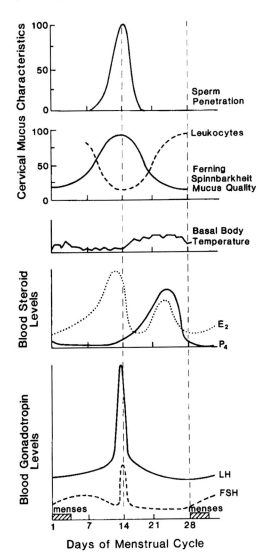

Figure 2-14 Cyclical changes in cervical mucus during the ovarian cycle. (Adapted from Hafez, E.S.E. Sperm transport. In Behrman, S. J., and Kistner, R. W. (eds): *Progress in Infertility*, 2nd ed. Little, Brown, Boston, 1975, p. 143.)

poorly controlled studies in women. This literature has been extensively and critically reviewed elsewhere (Mortimer, 1983; Hunter, 1987), and the existence of such a physiological process cannot be substantiated for human spermatozoa. Indeed, even in the rabbit, where rapid sperm transport has been unequivocally demonstrated, the rapidly transported spermatozoa are nonfunctional and do not participate in fertilization.

Spermatozoa in the Uterus

Spermatozoa probably enter the uterine cavity from the internal cervical os by virtue of their own motility. This theory is in accordance with the 1.5-hour delay reported between insemination and the appearance of spermatozoa in the uterine cavity.

In the adult nulliparous state, the uterine cavity is merely a slit, more of a potential than an actual lumen, although it remains somewhat larger in parous women. Spermatozoa entering the uterine cavity are probably suspended in the small volume of uterine fluid. Their intrinsic motility may help maintain them in suspension while the fluid is mixed throughout the uterus by segmental pattern myometrial contractions. A more or less uniform distribution of spermatozoa throughout the uterine cavity would therefore be established. There is no evidence to support or disprove this hypothesis.

Likewise, only theories exist as to how spermatozoa traverse the uterotubal junction (UTJ) to reach the tubal isthmus. The UTJ is clearly a barrier of some sort, as pressure must be exerted to force fluid through it. Sperm motility is probably also important, and there is some evidence that the UTJ constitutes a barrier to spermatozoa with impaired motility (review: Mortimer, 1978).

Isthmic Sperm Reservoir

Critical review of all careful studies to date on the dynamics of sperm transport in the eutherian female tract has supported the common existence of a sperm reservoir in the lower isthmus, a phenomenon most clearly demonstrated in the rabbit (review: Hunter, 1987). These isthmic reservoir spermatozoa apparently show reduced motility, which switches to the hyperactivated pattern (see Capacitation, below) upon transfer into ampullary fluid or culture medium. This quiescence may be regulated by a high extracellular potassium ion concentration.

Spermatozoa from this isthmic reservoir are redistributed during the immediate periovulatory phase, so they appear in the ampulla of the fallopian tube (the site of fertilization) synchronously with the egg. This system is regulated in some way by local messengers produced by the ovary (Hunter, 1989).

GAMETE INTERACTION AND FERTILIZATION

Capacitation

Eutherian spermatozoa (including man), unlike those of lower species, cannot penetrate the zona pellucida immediately after ejaculation. A final stage of maturation, which has been termed capacitation and is defined as the process by which spermatozoa acquire the capacity to undergo the acrosome reaction and fertilize eggs, is required (review: Yanagimachi, 1988). It is essential for fertilization both in vivo and in vitro, in the homologous in vitro test of sperm–zona binding, and even in the heterologous test of sperm fertilizing ability using zona-free hamster oocytes (see Chapter 10). Although capacitation starts with the separation of spermatozoa from the seminal plasma, it is more than just liberation from inhibition because a period of time, usually in the female tract, is required. This complex environment changes with the female's endocrine state relative to ovulation and with the anatomical region of the tract.

Capacitation serves to regulate the occurrence of the acrosome reaction within the female tract, probably having evolved as a result of changes in the oocyte-cumulus complex (Bedford, 1983). A high fertilization rate soon after ovulation may demand further temporal coordination of capacitation with the arrival of the egg(s) at the site of fertilization than the intrinsic character of the spermatozoon can provide. Regulation of achievement of the capacitated state must therefore be closely integrated with sperm transport and storage in the female tract. The time needed for capacitation varies among species and between the in vivo and in vitro situations. The time required for human sperm capacitation in vitro appears to be widely variable (Perreault and Rogers, 1982) and is unknown for the in vivo situation.

Capacitation probably involves the removal of cholesterol from the sperm plasma membrane by sterol acceptors present in the female tract secretions. Sterol sulfatase, which is also associated with cumulus cells, may be involved (Langlais and Roberts, 1985). Morphological concomitants of capacitation are difficult to define, although changes in chlortetracycline fluorescence and modifications of sperm surface glycoproteins (monitored using lectins) associated with the time sequence of capacitation and the acrosome reaction have been described (see Chapter 10).

In all eutheria, including humans, a marked change in sperm motility is associated with capacitation. An extremely vigorous but nonprogressive pattern, termed *hyperactivated motility,* develops as a result of a Ca^{2+} influx, causing increased flagellar curvature (Lindemann and Kanous, 1989) and hence extreme lateral movements of the sperm head. Hyperactivated motility is essential for the fertilization of intact oocyte-cumulus complexes in vitro and in vivo (reviews: Yanagimachi, 1988; Katz et al., 1989).

Acrosome Reaction

The acrosome is a membrane-bound organelle that covers the anterior one-half to two-thirds of the sperm head. Upon completion of capacitation, spermatozoa are ready to undergo the acrosome reaction (review: Yanagimachi, 1988), an exocytotic event involving localized fusions between the outer acrosomal and sperm plasma membranes that results in formation of vesicles; the acrosome contents, mainly the enzymes hyaluronidase and acrosin, are then released through the holes between them (Fig. 2-15). Intraacrosomal changes, perhaps related to the activation of proacrosin to acrosin (Harrison, 1983), may precede membrane vesiculation (Nagae et al., 1986).

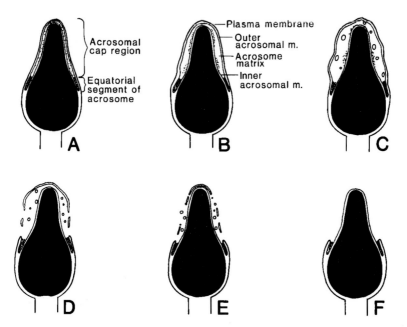

Figure 2-15 Probable sequence of morphological events in the human sperm acrosome reaction.

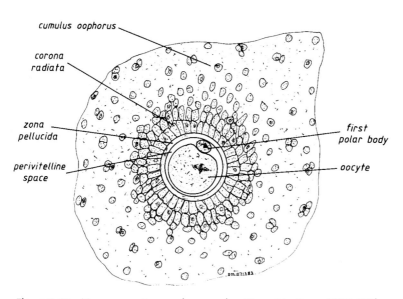

Figure 2-16 Human oocyte-cumulus complex. (From Mortimer, 1985. With permission.)

Although hyaluronidase has traditionally been considered to facilitate sperm penetration through the cumulus mass surrounding the freshly ovulated oocyte (Fig. 2-16), studies have now suggested not only that this enzyme may be nonessential for cumulus penetration but that an acrosome reaction prior to cumulus penetration may even be detrimental (Talbot, 1985). Although hyaluronidase may have some indirect involvement, it is believed that acrosin, a trypsin-like enzyme, is primarily responsible for softening the zona pellucida glycoprotein. Although an essential role for acrosin as a "zona lysin" has been questioned (Talbot, 1985), the fact remains that the acrosome reaction is essential for eutherian fertilization.

The roles of ion transport and hydrolytic enzymes in the eutherian acrosome reaction are complex and outside the scope of this monograph (reviews: Meizel, 1978, 1984; Yanagimachi, 1988). In brief, there is a massive influx of Ca^{2+} ions due to either activation of plasma membrane Ca^{2+} carrier proteins or inactivation of the Ca^{2+} "pump" (Ca^{2+}-ATPase). Elevated intracellular Ca^{2+} inactivates plasma membrane Na^+,K^+-ATPase, resulting in a rapid increase in intracellular Na^+. This action causes an H^+ efflux (through an Na^+/H^+ antiporter), producing a rise in intracellular pH that precedes the morphological events of the acrosome reaction. The roles of calcium channels and calmodulin are uncertain. These ion transport events are mediated by cyclic nucleotides, and indeed both they and phosphodiesterase inhibitors stimulate capacitation and the acrosome reaction. High intraacrosomal pH may allow activation or maximal activity of acrosomal enzymes such as phospholipase A_2, which has been implicated in the final destabilization of the apposed outer acrosomal and plasma membranes, ultimately causing membrane fusion, by producing a lysophospholipid fusogen from phospholipid (review: Langlais and Roberts, 1985).

Physiological Regulation of Sperm Fertilizing Ability

The classic concept of the eutherian acrosome reaction is in question. Some workers are of the opinion that some component of the products of ovulation induces the natural acrosome reaction, whereas others believe that neither the oviduct, the egg or its vestments, nor follicular fluid is essential for a normal acrosome reaction. Yet others consider that the fertilizing spermatozoon undergoes its acrosome reaction on the zona pellucida, not prior to or during cumulus penetration (reviews: Bavister 1982; Bedford, 1983; Wassarman, 1987).

Clearly this discussion is well outside the scope of the present text except to say that although evidence for the stimulation of human sperm fertilizing ability by cumulus cells, follicular fluid, or oviduct fluid does exist in vitro specific roles in in vivo fertilization remain unproven.

Most recently, attention has focused on the ability of progesterone to cause an increase in intracellular calcium levels and so induce the acrosome reaction in vitro. Again, there is no evidence for a significant role for this phenomenon in vivo (review: Mortimer, 1991).

Sperm–Egg Interaction

Although it was classically accepted that the acrosome reaction occurred prior to the spermatozoon's penetration of the cumulus (review: Yanagimachi, 1988), there is increasing support for a "modern" hypothesis that the acrosome reaction is induced by some component(s) of the zona pellucida (review: Wassarman, 1987).

Acrosome-intact and acrosome-reacted human spermatozoa can be seen within the cumulus as well as bound to, or partially embedded in, the zona pellucida of oocytes fertilized in vitro. However, only acrosome-reacted spermatozoa are found deep in the zona pellucida, and all those in the perivitelline space show completed acrosome reactions (Sathananthan et al., 1982). Completion of the acrosome reaction is also necessary for fertilization after sperm microinjection into the perivitelline space (review: Mortimer, 1993). These findings, in conjunction with the ability of acid-solubilized human zonae pellucidae to induce an acrosome reaction in capacitated spermatozoa (Cross et al., 1988), support the concept that the fertilizing human spermatozoon also undergoes its acrosome reaction in contact with the zona pellucida.

There is more or less species-specific binding between sperm surface glycoproteins and receptor components of the zona pellucida perhaps involving glycosyltransferases (reviews: Wassarman, 1987; Macek and Shur, 1988; Yanagimachi, 1988). Sperm penetration through the zona matrix into the perivitelline space is primarily a mechanical process, aided by the extra power output generated by the hyperactivated motility pattern with probably some role for acrosin in softening the zona matrix (review: Katz et al., 1989).

Sperm–Oocyte Fusion and Syngamy

Emerging from the inner face of the zona pellucida, the fertilizing spermatozoon is in the perivitelline space surrounding the oocyte. At this stage the spermatozoon has completed the acrosome reaction, so the inner acrosomal membrane is revealed over the anterior cap region of the sperm head, but the equatorial segment remains intact. After attachment to the oolemma, perhaps involving a carbohydrate lectin-hapten-type recognition process and the postacrosomal region of the sperm head, sperm motility ceases. Fusion is then initiated between the oolemma and the equatorial segment, leading ultimately to complete engulfment of the spermatozoon, including the sperm tail, by the oocyte (Fig. 2-17).

As the sperm head is incorporated into the ooplasm, the carefully packaged chromatin within its nucleus is decondensed, and the protamines are replaced by histones derived from the oocyte. A new nuclear envelope is formed, also from components derived from the oocyte, and the male pronucleus is created. The fertilized oocyte is now termed a *zygote*.

At the moment of sperm-oocyte contact, the oocyte initiates the cortical reaction, a process whereby the contents of numerous secretory granules located in the

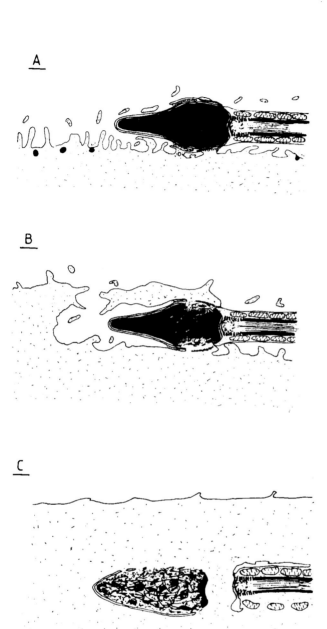

Figure 2-17 Probable sequence of morphological events during incorporation of the fertilizing spermatozoon into the human oocyte. (From Mortimer, 1985. With permission.)

peripheral, cortical region of the ooplasm (the cortical granules) are released into the perivitelline space. This reaction, which spreads out over the surface of the oocyte from the point of sperm-oocyte fusion, is the basis of the block to polyspermy, i.e., the process whereby further spermatozoa are prevented from penetrating the oocyte.

The male and female pronuclei move toward each other, and their nuclear envelopes break down. The chromosomes from the male and female gametes are released into the ooplasm, and the first cleavage division is initiated. This intermingling of parental genetic material is the completion of syngamy, the creation of a genetically new individual.

References and Recommended Reading

Barratt, C. L. R., Bolton, E. A., and Cooke, I. D. (1990). Functional significance of white blood cells in the male and female reproductive tract. *Hum. Reprod.* **5,** 639.

Bavister, B. D. (1982). Evidence for a role of post-ovulatory cumulus components in supporting fertilizing ability of hamster spermatozoa. *J. Androl.* **3,** 365.

Bedford, J. M. (1983). Significance of the need for sperm capacitation before fertilization in eutherian mammals. *Biol. Reprod.* **28,** 108.

Cooper, T. G. (1986). *The Epididymis, Sperm Maturation and Fertilization.* Springer-Verlag, Heidelberg.

Cooper, T. G. (1990). In defense of a function for the human epididymis. *Fertil. Steril.* **54,** 965.

Cross, N. L., Morales, P., Overstreet, J. W., and Hanson, F. W. (1988). Induction of acrosome reactions by the human zona pellucida. *Biol. Reprod.* **38,** 235.

De Kretser, D. M. (1969). Ultrastructural features of human spermiogenesis. *Z. Zellforsch. Mikrosk. Anat.* **98,** 477.

Hafez, E. S. E. (ed.) (1976). *Human Semen and Fertility Regulation in Men.* Mosby, St. Louis.

Hafez, E. S. E. (ed.). (1980). *Human Reproduction. Conception and Contraception,* 2nd ed. Harper & Row, Hagerstown, MD.

Harrison, R. A. P. (1983). The acrosome, its hydrolases, and egg penetration. In André, J. (ed): *The Sperm Cell.* Martinus Nijhoff, The Hague.

Heller, C. G., and Clermont, Y. (1964). Kinetics of the germinal epithelium in man. *Recent Prog. Horm. Res.* **20,** 545.

Hunter, R. H. F. (1987). Human fertilization *in vivo*, with special reference to progression, storage and release of competent spermatozoa. *Hum. Reprod.* **2,** 329.

Hunter, R. H. F. (1989). Ovarian programming of gamete progression and maturation in the female genital tract. *Zool. J. Linn. Soc.* **95,** 117.

Insler, V., Glezerman, M., Zeidel, L., Bernstein, D., and Misgav, N. (1980). Sperm storage in the human cervix: a quantitative study. *Fertil. Steril.* **33,** 288.

Katz, D. F., Brofeldt, B. T., Overstreet, J., and Hanson, F. W. (1982). Alteration of cervical mucus by vanguard human spermatozoa. *J. Reprod. Fertil.* **65,** 171.

Katz, D. F., Drobnis, E. Z., and Overstreet, J. W. (1989). Factors regulating mammalian sperm migration through the female reproductive tract and oocyte vestments. *Gamete Res.* **22,** 443.

Katz, D. F., Overstreet, J. W., Samuels, S. J., Niswander, P. W., Bloom, T. D., and Lewis, E.

L. (1986). Morphometric analysis of spermatozoa in the assessment of human male fertility. *J. Androl.* **7,** 203.

Langlais, J., and Roberts, K. (1985). A molecular membrane model of sperm capacitation and the acrosome reaction of mammalian spermatozoa. *Gamete Res.* **12,** 183.

Lindemann, C. B., and Kanous, K. S. (1989). Regulation of mammalian sperm motility. *Arch. Androl.* **23,** 1.

Macek, M. B., and Shur, B. D. (1988). Protein-carbohydrate complementarity in mammalian gamete recognition. *Gamete Res.* **20,** 93.

Meizel, S. (1978). The mammalian sperm acrosome reaction: a biochemical approach. In Johnson, M. H. (ed): *Development in Mammals,* Vol. 3. Elsevier/North Holland, Amsterdam.

Meizel, S. (1984). The importance of hydrolytic enzymes to an exocytotic event; the mammalian sperm acrosome reaction. *Biol. Rev.* **59,** 125.

Mohri, H., and Yanagimachi, R. (1980). Characteristics of motor apparatus in testicular, epididymal and ejaculated spermatozoa: A study using demembranated models. *Exp. Cell Res.* **127,** 191.

Moore, H. D. M., Hartman, T. D., and Pryor, J. P. (1983). Development of the oocyte-penetrating capacity of spermatozoa in the human epididymis. *Int. J. Androl.* **6,** 310.

Mortimer, D. (1978). Selectivity of sperm transport in the female genital tract. In Cohen, J., and Hendry, W. F. (eds): *Spermatozoa, Antibodies and Infertility.* Blackwell, London.

Mortimer, D. (1983). Sperm transport in the human female reproductive tract. In Finn, C. A. (ed): *Oxford Reviews of Reproductive Biology,* Vol. 5. Oxford University Press, Oxford.

Mortimer, D. (1985). The male factor in infertility Part II. Sperm function testing. *Curr. Probl. Obstet. Gynecol. Fertil.* Vol. VIII (8), 75 pp. Year Book Medical Publishers, Chicago.

Mortimer, D. (1991). Behaviour of spermatozoa in the human oviduct. *Arch. Biol. Med. Exp.* **24,** 339.

Mortimer, D. (1993). Techniques for the preparation of spermatozoa and the need for capacitation and the acrosome reaction. In Fishel, S. B., and Symonds, E. M. (eds): *Gamete and Embryo Micromanipulation in Human Reproduction.* Edward Arnold, Sevenoaks, Kent, UK (in press).

Nagae, T., Yanagimachi, R., Srivastava, P. N., and Yanagimachi, H. (1986). Acrosome reaction in human spermatozoa. *Fertil. Steril.* **45,** 701.

Overstreet, J. W., Coats, C., Katz, D. F., and Hanson, F. W. (1980). The importance of seminal plasma for sperm penetration of human cervical mucus. *Fertil. Steril.* **34,** 569.

Pandya, I. J., and Cohen, J. (1985). The leukocytic reaction of the human cervix to spermatozoa. *Fertil. Steril.* **43,** 417.

Perreault, S. D., and Rogers, B. J. (1982). Capacitation pattern of human spermatozoa. *Fertil. Steril.* **38,** 258.

Sathananthan, A. H., Trounson, A. O., Wood, C., and Leeton, J. F. (1982). Ultrastructural observations on the penetration of human sperm into the zona pellucida of the human egg *in vitro. J. Androl.* **3,** 356.

Schrader, S. M., Turner, T. W., and Simon, S. D. (1990). Longitudinal study of semen quality of unexposed workers: sperm head morphometry. *J. Androl.* **11,** 32.

Silber, S. J., Ord, T., Balmaceda, J., Patrizio, P., and Asch, R. H. (1990). Congenital absence of the vas deferens: the fertilizing capacity of human epididymal sperm. *N. Engl. J. Med.* **323,** 1788.

Sobrero, A. J., and MacLeod, J. (1962). The immediate postcoital test. *Fertil. Steril.* **13,** 184.

Talbot, P. (1985). Sperm penetration through oocyte investments in mammals. *Am. J. Anat.* **174,** 331.

Temple-Smith, P. D., Southwick, G. J., Yates, C. A., Trounson, A. O., and de Kretser, D. M. (1985). Human pregnancy by in vitro fertilization (IVF) using sperm aspirated from the epididymis. *J. In Vitro Fert. Embryo Transf.* **2,** 119.

Wassarman, P. M. (1987). Early events in mammalian fertilization. *Annu. Rev. Cell Biol.* **3,** 109.

World Health Organization (1992).*WHO Laboratory Manual for the Examination of Human Semen and Sperm-Cervical Mucus Interaction,* 3rd ed. Cambridge University Press, Cambridge.

Yanagimachi, R. (1988). Mammalian fertilization. In Knobil, E., Neill, J. D., Ewing, L. L., Markert, C. L., Greenwald, G. S., and Pfaff, D. W. (eds): *The Physiology of Reproduction,* Vol. 1. Raven Press, New York.

II

Diagnostic Procedures

3

Semen Analysis

The intention of this chapter is to provide detailed descriptions of the basic technical procedures for performing a routine semen analysis. A general schedule and sample Laboratory Report Form for this whole procedure are provided in Appendix I. This evaluation of the classic "descriptive" semen characteristics is fundamental to the operation of an andrology laboratory that provides diagnostic or therapeutic services. It provides the criteria on which most initial clinical decisions are based, thereby necessitating accuracy and precision. Reliable methods must be used for semen analysis as for any other laboratory test, and there is no substitute for thorough training and experience. It has become apparent that reliable semen analysis requires staff with good observational powers and critical ability. Matters of training, standardization, quality control, and quality assurance are dealt with in Chapter 16.

GENERAL PRINCIPLES

Standardization of semen analysis begins with the method of collecting the semen specimen and its delivery to the laboratory.

Patient Instructions

Patients should be provided with a simple but comprehensive instruction sheet explaining not only what should (and should not) be done but also giving some indication why. Patients comply with instructions more readily if given an explanation for what might otherwise appear to be unimportant requests. The following specific points should be made.

1. The need for a proscribed period of abstinence (usually 3 days), including an honest statement of the actual period of abstinence (see Chapter 11)
2. The need to produce the specimen by masturbation directly into the sterile plastic container provided
3. That contraceptive condoms cannot be used because their lubricant is spermicidal, and that withdrawal (coitus interruptus) is unacceptable because the first, sperm-rich part of the ejaculate is easily lost
4. That contamination of the specimen container should be minimized by removing its lid only at the moment of collection of the ejaculate, replacing it immediately after completing the collection

5. The need to have the patient's name written on the specimen container, along with the date and time of collection of the specimen

N.B. If the specimen cannot be produced adjacent to the laboratory, it must be delivered to the laboratory as quickly as possible, certainly within 1 hour of collection. During this journey the sample must be kept warm, usually by carrying it next to the body, avoiding excessive heating or chilling (i.e., outside the range 25°–40°C).

Sample Collection

Semen specimens for diagnostic or therapeutic use should be produced by masturbation directly into the container, ideally in a room specially provided for the purpose, adjacent to the laboratory. Other methods of sample production (e.g., withdrawal or in contraceptive condoms) are unacceptable (see above).

When samples are produced at the laboratory, the patient's name (or donor reference number) should be written on the container before handing it to him. This first step is important for eliminating any chance of confusing samples.

Obviously, wide-mouthed containers should be used for collecting ejaculates. The easiest way of ensuring that only suitable containers are used is to provide them. Most laboratories nowadays use plastic containers because they are disposable and available sterile, but the containers must be tested for suitability because many plasticizers and mold release agents are spermicidal. Notwithstanding this limitation, plastic containers are preferable to glass because, for reasons of economy, glass containers are normally reused. Ensuring thorough rinsing to remove all traces of detergent (which is spermicidal) and subsequent sterilization are significant negative factors when considering the use of glass containers. Containers whose lids have rubber or waxed cardboard liners should not be used.

Specialized graduated tubes with detachable funnels are also available commercially (Recosperme: BICEF, L'Aigle, France) (Fig. 3-1). For individuals with religious or moral objections to masturbation, Silastic condoms (e.g., Seminal Collection Device: HDC Corporation, Mountainview, CA, USA: Fig. 3-2) may be used. In cases of paraplegia or erectile impotence, mechanical stimulation using a vibrator has been found to be of benefit (review: Brindley, 1983). Also see Chapter 13 for a discussion of retrograde ejaculation.

Split Ejaculates

On occasions it is necessary to collect an ejaculate in two or more fractions so the first fraction, which contains most of the spermatozoa, may be analyzed or used for therapeutic purposes without dilution by, or exposure to, the later fractions of the ejaculate (which consists primarily of seminal vesicle secretions). Such a collection is usually achieved by taping the required number of containers together (Fig. 3-3); a dual Recosperme holder is available if this specimen collection system is being

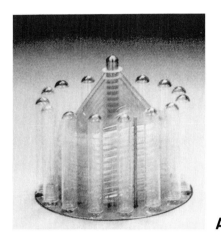

A

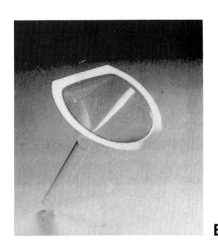

B

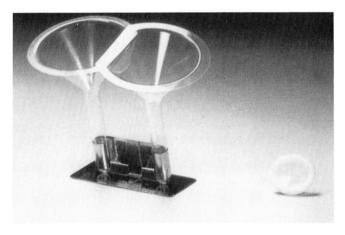

C

Figure 3-1 (A) Recosperme semen collection system: ready-use "cloche." (B) Graduated collection tube with funnel attached. (C) Split ejaculate collection device. (Photographs courtesy of BICEF, L'Aigle, France.)

45

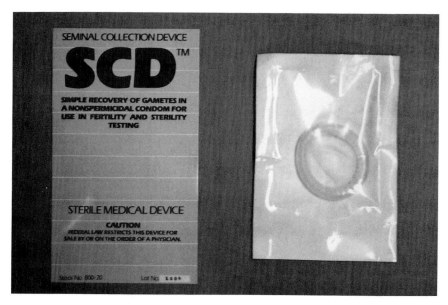

Figure 3-2 Seminal Collection Device. (HDC Corporation, Mountainview, CA, USA.)

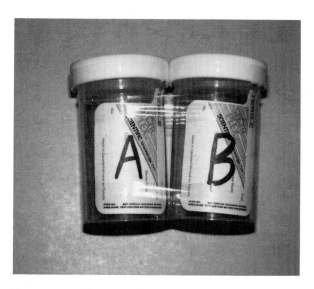

Figure 3-3 Collection of a two-fraction split ejaculate using two specimen jars taped together.

used (Fig. 3-1). Reliable collection of a split ejaculate sample often takes some practice on the part of the patient.

Liquefaction

Authorities recommend incubation of the sample at either ambient temperature or 37°C for completion of liquefaction. Although normal samples should liquefy within 20 minutes even at ambient temperature, reliable assessment of sperm progressivity and measurement of movement characteristics using the new automated analyzers (see Chapter 7) require that the sample be at 37°C at the time of analysis. Consequently, it is probably best to use 37°C throughout.

At the end of the proscribed incubation period (usually 20 or 30 minutes) the sample should be checked for the completion of liquefaction. If a specimen is not fully liquefied, it should be returned to the incubator for an additional few minutes. However, prolonged exposure of spermatozoa to seminal plasma can permanently diminish their functional capacity, a factor of great importance if the spermatozoa are to be used for sperm function testing or therapeutic purposes (see Chapter 10). A semen analysis should be commenced by 1 hour after ejaculation.

The technique of *needling* (passing the sample once or twice through a 19-gauge syringe needle) has been used to reduce the viscosity of incompletely liquefied samples. It causes deterioration in motility (Knuth et al., 1989), however, and therefore must not be applied to samples to be used for sperm function testing or therapeutic purposes. Because needling can induce deterioration in sperm motility, and thereby influence semen analysis results, it should probably be avoided altogether (see also Chapter 12).

Mixing

Obviously, a semen sample must be thoroughly mixed after liquefaction has been completed before any analysis commences. The use of cradles or roller systems is ideal, although it can be difficult if the sample also has to be maintained at 37°C. Thorough mixing can be achieved by swirling the sample around the inside of the container for 20–30 seconds. Vortex mixing should be avoided with live spermatozoa.

PHYSICAL CHARACTERISTICS

Appearance

The specimen's appearance is assessed in terms of its color, opacity/translucence, and the presence of mucus streaks or visible clumps of cells. Human semen is normally an off-white to grayish-yellow opalescent fluid.

Urine Contamination

Contamination of the semen with urine (e.g., in men with bladder neck dysfunction) may produce a more pronounced yellow discoloration. This problem is readily identified by the reduced viscosity of the sample along with the toxic effects of disturbed osmolarity and urea upon the spermatozoa (Crich and Jequier, 1978). Significant urine contamination also causes samples to have a marked uriniferous odor.

Blood Contamination

Discoloration of semen due to contamination with blood (sometimes called hematospermia) is dependent on both the amount of blood relative to the ejaculate volume and the age of the blood. Traces of fresh blood color the semen pink or even reddish, and old blood (when bleeding into the genital tract has occurred hours or even days previously) colors the semen more brown.

Other Contaminants

Bilirubin contamination of semen associated with jaundice may result in bright yellow ejaculates.

Liquefaction and Viscosity

It is important that abnormalities of liquefaction not be confused with abnormalities of viscosity. *Incomplete liquefaction* results in a heterogeneous sample consisting of gelatinous material in a fluid base. Viscosity relates to the fluid nature of the whole sample, which can be essentially normal even though liquefaction may be incomplete.

Precise quantitation of viscosity is possible using either a microviscosimeter or by measuring the time it takes for a known volume of semen to run out of a pipette that has been calibrated using oils of standard viscosities. Such measurements are clearly excessive, and, consequently, objective measurements and definitions of semen viscosity are uncommon. Generally, viscosity is rated subjectively according to the length of the thread produced by the semen as it runs out of the pipette used to measure the ejaculate volume.

Although the clinical significance of altered semen viscosity remains uncertain, increased viscosity may be associated with infertility by virtue of its impairment of sperm movement and hence sperm penetration of cervical mucus. Highly viscous semen samples may be treated with trypsin (Cohen and Aafjes, 1982) or diluted with culture medium before attempting swim-up preparations for use in sperm function tests or for therapeutic purposes.

Odor

The ability to smell semen is variable. Whereas some people find that normal semen has no smell at all, others find it to have a strong, even highly unpleasant, odor. Clearly with such variability, little may be done for its routine assessment. However, if there is a strong smell of urine or putrefaction, it should be noted. Also, a semen sample produced after a long period of abstinence (i.e., several weeks) probably has a stronger smell than one produced after a few days' abstinence.

Ejaculate Volume

The volume of semen sample can be determined either by its collection into a graduated container such as the Recosperme or using a warmed disposable pipette of the "graduated to contain" or "blow out" types. Usually 5-ml pipettes are sufficient, although some 10-ml pipettes are needed for samples of larger than average volume. Some plastic syringes contain a lubricant, which is detrimental to sperm motility and should therefore be checked before acceptance into routine use (de Ziegler et al., 1987).

Semen pH

The pH of liquefied semen is normally determined using test strips; the Merck ColorpHast type, pH 6.5–10.0, has been found most suitable for this purpose. Normal semen pH is in the range 7.2–8.2, although pH does tend to increase with time after ejaculation, at least in the short term. Inflammatory disorders of the prostate or seminal vesicles may result in pH values outside this range (see Chapter 2).

ASSESSMENT OF THE WET PREPARATION

A drop of about 10 μl of thoroughly mixed, liquefied semen placed on a clean, warmed microscope slide and covered with a 22 × 22 mm No. 1½ warmed coverslip. Examination of this "wet preparation," which has a depth of approximately 20 μm (Table 3-1), should commence as soon as any flow within it has stopped. If examination is not begun within a minute, the preparation is discarded and another

Table 3–1 Depths of wet preparations obtained using fixed volume slide and coverslip preparations

| Volume of drop (μl) | Depth of Preparation (μm), by Coverslip Size | | | | | |
	18 × 18 mm	22 × 22 mm	22 × 32 mm	16 mm ∅	19 mm ∅	22 mm ∅
5.0	15.4	10.3	7.1	24.9	17.6	13.2
6.0	18.5	12.4	8.5	29.8	21.2	15.8
7.0	21.6	14.5	9.9	34.8	24.7	18.4
7.5	23.2	15.5	10.7	37.3	26.5	19.7
8.0	24.7	16.5	11.4	39.8	28.2	21.0
9.0	27.8	18.6	12.8	44.8	31.7	23.7
10.0	30.9	20.7	14.2	49.7	35.3	26.3
12.5	38.6	25.8	17.8	62.2	44.1	32.9
15.0	46.3	31.0	21.3	74.6	52.9	39.6

one made. Phase-contrast optics are essential for this procedure, and a heated microscope stage is a definite advantage. If phase-contrast optics are not available, brightfield (Köhler) illumination may be used if the microscope is first set up correctly and then the condenser defocused downward until sufficient contrast is obtained.

If there is no more than the occasional spermatozoon per 40× objective field, as large a part of the sample as possible is centrifuged at 1000 g for 15 minutes in a disposable, conical plastic centrifuge tube (e.g., Falcon 2095, 2096, or 2097) and most of the supernatant removed. The exact volumes of semen initially transferred to the tube and supernatant removed (and therefore the volume of the resuspended pellet by subtraction) are used to calculate the correct sperm concentration in the original sample. The resuspended pellet is then used for the remainder of the analysis, including the stained preparations for vitality and morphology assessments.

N.B. *It must be emphasized that this procedure is for diagnostic purposes only. Centrifugal pelleting of unselected sperm populations must be avoided under all circumstances where the spermatozoa are to be used for sperm function testing or therapeutic purposes* (review: Mortimer, 1991; also see Chapter 11).

Careful standardization of this wet preparation, so the volume contained within a microscope field of view, between slide and coverslip, is 1 nl, allows estimation of the approximate sperm concentration, as the number of spermatozoa per field approximates their concentration in millions per milliliter. Microscope field areas can be easily calculated using the formula πr^2, where r is the radius of the field of view, measured using a stage micrometer (see Appendix II).

Sperm Motility

The first aspect assessed on the wet preparation is sperm motility, and this assessment must be completed before the preparation either cools or dries out too much, as these changes affect sperm progression. Several scoring systems exist for sperm motility assessments; some consider qualitative progression as a modal characteristic of the motile spermatozoa (e.g., Belsey et al., 1980), whereas others rank the progression of individual spermatozoa and count them separately (e.g., MacLeod, 1965; World Health Organization, 1987, 1992). Various motility indices can be calculated from these scores, which although mathematically impure often facilitate clinical interpretation.

If more than 10–15% of the spermatozoa are involved in clumping (see Sperm Aggregation and Agglutination, below), the motility assessed is based on *free spermatozoa only,* which is noted on the report form. It is always advisable to repeat the motility count on a second wet preparation, especially if the sperm concentration or motility is high.

Modal Progression Rating
In the modal progression rating system the forward progression exhibited by the largest proportion of the *motile,* not just progressive, spermatozoa is rated on a

semisubjective scale. Traditionally, a 0–4 scale of progression ratings (PR values) (Table 3-2A), has proved most satisfactory for routine use in terms of minimizing intra- and interobserver variability (Mortimer et al., 1986). Use of a 0–10 scale, or one with plus and minus subcategories is not standardizable in practice. Assignment of the PR value is the first step upon examination of the wet preparation and is based on the visual appraisal of at least 10 fields away from the coverslip edge.

Practically, sperm motility is determined by counting the numbers of motile and immotile spermatozoa in several randomly selected fields under a 40× objective until *at least 200* spermatozoa have been counted. Within each field the number of *progressively motile* spermatozoa is counted first, counting only those spermatozoa that were in the field at one moment in time. If the number of progressively motile spermatozoa in the whole field is too great for rapid visual counting, a small area of the field should be defined using an eyepiece graticule. After the progressive spermatozoa have been counted, the numbers of *nonprogressively motile and immotile spermatozoa present within the same area* are counted. The three figures are expressed as the percentages of progressive, nonprogressive, and immotile spermatozoa. Report the values as integers only, adding up to 100%, with any correction for rounding-off errors being made in the largest class(es).

A normal semen sample contains at least 50% motile spermatozoa, with most of

Table 3–2   Sperm progression rating systems

Rank	Explanation
A. Modal progression rating of motile spermatozoa	
0	None = absence of forward progression
1	Poor = weak or sluggish forward progression
2	Moderate = definite forward progression
3	Good = good forward progression
4	Excellent = vigorous, rapid forward progression
B. Traditional individual spermatozoon progression rating	
0	None = absence of forward progression
1	Poor = weak forward progression
2	Good = moderate forward progression
3	Excellent = very active forward progression
C. WHO 1987 progression classification system	
Class a	Rapid, linear progressive motility
Class b	Slow or sluggish linear, or nonlinear motility
Class c	Nonprogressive motility
Class d	Immotile
D. WHO 1992 progression classification system	
Class a	Rapid progressive motility
Class b	Slow or sluggish progressive motility
Class c	Nonprogressive motility
Class d	Immotile

them exhibiting at least good forward progression. Any abnormal movement pattern, e.g., highly irregular or circular trajectories or movement similar to the "shaking" pattern indicative of attachment phenomena (see Chapter 9), should be noted, along with the approximate percentage of motile spermatozoa affected.

For the modal progression rating system of scoring sperm motility the following *motility index* (MI) has been used.

$$MI = (\% \text{ progressive} \times PR \times 2.5) + \% \text{ nonprogressive}$$

The weighting factor of 2.5 is used to emphasize the importance of the quality of progression and gives a range of MI values between 0 and 1000 (Pandya et al., 1986).

Individual Sperm Progression Scoring

In the individual sperm progression scoring system each motile spermatozoon is attributed a motility/progression rating as it is counted. Traditionally, the system described in Table 3-2B has been used, although the WHO for a while recommended the system described in Table 3-2C. Such systems are more difficult to standardize among observers, and the WHO version lacked definitions for "linear" and "nonlinear," thereby making its implementation inconsistent (e.g., Dunphy et al., 1989). Consequently, in the latest edition of its *Laboratory Manual,* the WHO has deleted this system and recommended the system described in Table 3-2D (World Health Organization, 1992).

Practically, sperm motility is determined by examining several randomly selected fields away from the coverslip edge under a $40\times$ objective and counting only those spermatozoa that were in the field at one moment in time. *At least 200* spermatozoa must be counted, and each is tallied in its appropriate category. If the number of spermatozoa in a field is too great for rapid visual counting, a small area of the field should be defined using an eyepiece graticule. The four figures are expressed as integer percentages, adding up to 100%, with any correction for rounding-off errors being made in the largest class(es).

A normal semen sample contains at least 50% progressively motile spermatozoa (progression classes 3 and 4, or WHO classes *a* and *b*). Any abnormal movement pattern, e.g., highly irregular or circular trajectories or movement similar to the shaking pattern indicative of attachment phenomena (see Chapter 9), should be noted, along with the approximate percentage of motile spermatozoa affected.

For the individual sperm progression scoring system of assessing sperm motility, the motility index (MI) may be calculated by multiplying the incidence of each category by its ranking (Table 3-2B) and finding the total score.

Sperm Aggregation and Agglutination

Several randomly selected fields away from the coverslip edge are examined, and the proportion of spermatozoa involved in clumps is expressed as an approximate percentage to the nearest 5%. It must be emphasized that *agglutination* is strictly reserved to describe spermatozoa that are stuck to each other by antibodies. Such spermatozoa are mostly motile, and there is usually only minimal involvement of other cells or debris. If the latter elements are substantially involved in the clumps, the situation is probably *aggregation,* where, in addition, the spermatozoa are usually dead. Small aggregates of spermatozoa and other material often occur in normal semen, although the presence of large clumps, often involving many hundreds of spermatozoa each, is abnormal (Fig. 3-4).

Spermagglutination usually occurs in a specific manner such as head-to-head (H-H), midpiece-to-midpiece (MP-MP), tail-to-tail (T-T), or tail-tip-to-tail-tip (tt-tt). Occasionally mixed forms of agglutination occur, such as head-to-tail (H-T); or the agglutination may be so massive it is impossible to identify any specific pattern. Tests for the detection and titration of antisperm antibodies are discussed in Chapter 5.

Other Cellular Components and Debris

Even normal semen samples from fertile donors often contain substantial numbers of other cells and debris contamination.

Round Cells
It is important to differentiate round cells into leukocytes, immature germinal line cells, and large, usually anucleate, bodies of residual cytoplasm coming from the seminiferous epithelium. If more than one round cell is seen per 40× objective microscope field (because this number is equivalent to a concentration of about 1×10^6/ml), a specific test for the presence of leukocytes is indicated (see Identification of Leukocytes in Semen, below). However, the concentration of round cells in general can be determined by comparison of their relative frequency to the spermatozoa (in either the wet preparation or the stained smear used for morphology assessment), whose concentration is determined by hemocytometry (see below). For practical purposes, anucleate cytoplasmic masses larger than a sperm head are considered round cells, whereas those smaller than a sperm head are considered debris (see below).

Epithelial Cells
Epithelial cells are usually present in most semen samples in small numbers (Fig. 3-5), and even the presence of numerous such cells cannot be associated with any specific dysfunction or infection. Semen specimens collected by withdrawal invariably contain many (vaginal) epithelial cells. In addition, samples collected using Silastic condoms may show increased numbers of epithelial cells, perhaps due to exfoliation from the urethra or glans. The presence of epithelial cells may, for routine purposes, be coded as shown in Table 3-3.

Erythrocytes
Red blood cells (erythrocytes) should not be present in semen, although a few are occasionally found without indicating any pathology. The presence of many erythrocytes is often associated with a pink discolouration of the ejaculate, a definitely

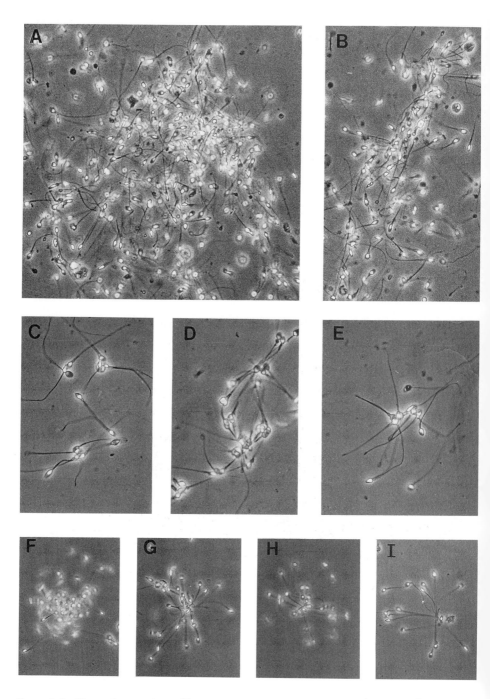

Figure 3-4 Photomicrographs to illustrate sperm aggregation (**A, B**) and spermagglutination of the head-to-head (**C–E**), tail-to-tail (**F–H**) and tail tip-to-tail tip (**I**) types. (From Mortimer, 1985. With permission.)

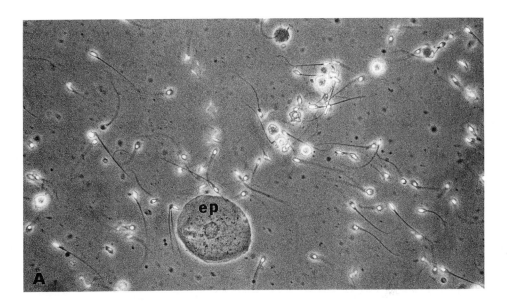

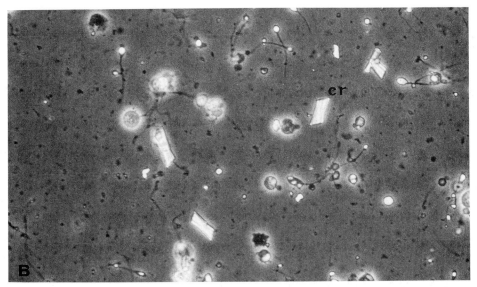

Figure 3-5 Appearance of grade 1 debris contamination (**A**), grade 2 debris contamination (**B**), and grade 3 debris contamination (**C**). Note the presence of crystals (*cr*), unspecific round cells (*rc*), and epithelial cells (*ep*) in these samples. (From Mortimer, 1985. With permission.)

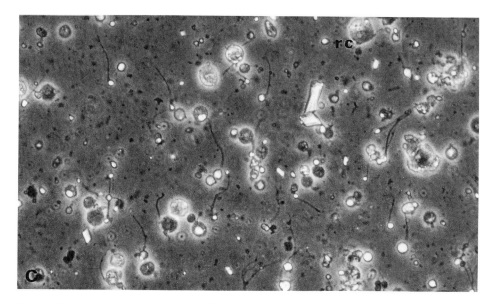

Figure 3–5(C) Appearance of grade 3 debris contamination. Note the presence of crystals (*cr*), unspecific round cells (*rc*), and epithelial cells (*ep*) in these samples. (From Mortimer, 1985. With permission.)

Table 3–3 Semiobjective ranking system for scoring the prevalence of epithelial cells, erythrocytes, round cells, and leukocytes in human semen samples[a]

Score	Meaning	Per HPF[b]	Per mm^{2c}	Per mm^{3d}	Comment
Epithelial cells					
0	None	0	0	0	Usual situation
1	Few	< 1	1–4	< 250	Not unusual
2	Many	> 1	≥ 5	≥ 250	Unusual
Erythrocytes					
0	None	0	0	0	Usual situation
1	Few	< 1	1–4	< 250	Abnormal
2	Many	> 1	≥ 5	≥ 250	Highly abnormal
Round cells/leukocytes[e]					
0	None	0	0	0	Quite rare
1	Few	≤ 4	1–20	< 1000	Typical situation
2	Many	≥ 5	> 20	≥ 1000	Abnormal

[a]Assuming 20 μm deep wet preparations.

[b]HPF = 40 × objective with field area of approximately 0.2 mm^2.

[c]See Appendix II.

[d]See Appendix II; per mm^3 = per microliter; multiply by 10^3 for per milliliter.

[e]Nucleated cells seen under phase contrast with no specific identification of leukocytes.

abnormal condition. For routine purposes, the incidence of erythrocytes may be coded using the simple scheme shown in Table 3-3.

Particulate Debris

Particulate debris, which for practical purposes includes anucleate cytoplasmic masses smaller than a sperm head, may be plentiful even in normal semen samples. There is no objective means to assess debris contamination, which is usually evaluated in routine practice over a number of fields and expressed according to the scheme described in Table 3-4. Care should be taken to distinguish between particulate debris showing brownian motion and bacterial infection of the semen.

Bacteria and Protozoa

Bacteria and protozoa are not usually seen in human semen, but their presence in large numbers is probably associated with an infection of the male genital tract. After noting their presence, samples containing bacteria should be sent for microbiological assessment (see Chapter 6). Further advice may be sought from other medical laboratories, particularly those involved with sexually transmitted diseases, and reference microbiology laboratories.

IDENTIFICATION OF LEUKOCYTES IN SEMEN

The simplest method to identify leukocytes in serum is use of a cytochemical stain for peroxidase activity. Two simple staining methods are available, one using benzidine-cyanosine, the other *o*-toluidine blue. In addition, fluorescence-labeled monoclonal antibody reagents are now available not only for identifying all leukocytes (using a panleukocyte antigen) but also for their subclassification.

Peroxidase Staining Using Benzidine-Cyanosine

Principle

Peroxidase staining using benzidine-cyanosine results in only those cells that contain peroxidase activity staining brown; all other cells counterstain pink (Belsey et al., 1980).

Table 3–4 Semiobjective ranking system for scoring the presence of debris[a] in human semen samples

Score	Explanation	Comment
0	No debris at all	Rare situation
1	Slight debris contamination	Typical condition
2	Moderate debris contamination	Not necessarily abnormal
3	Heavy debris contamination	Abnormal
4	Very heavy debris contamination	Abnormal

[a]Particulate matter and small anucleate cytoplasmic masses (see Fig. 3–5).

Reagents

A stock stain solution is prepared by mixing a solution of 125 mg benzidine in 50 ml 96% (v/v) methanol with a solution of 150 mg cyanosine (phloxine) in 50 ml reagent water; it is stored in a dark bottle at 4°C. The working solution, which is stable for up to 1 day at ambient temperature, is prepared by adding 50 µl hydrogen peroxide (6%, or 20 volumes) to 1.0 ml of the stock solution.

Method

1. Mix 10 µl liquefied semen and 10 µl working solution on a clean slide and cover with a 22 × 22 mm coverslip.
2. Examine under a 40× objective using brightfield optics. If more than one brown (peroxidase-positive) cell is seen per five fields, proceed according to instructions 3–5, below; if not, enter a value of zero on the report form.
3. Mix another 10 µl liquefied semen and 10 µl working solution on a porcelain spotting place.
4. Transfer 4.5 µl of the mixture onto a Makler chamber (see Specialized Counting Chambers, below); apply the cover glass and press down firmly until inference fringes can be seen between the apposed glass surfaces at the four support pillars.
5. Examine the preparation under a 40× objective using brightfield optics. Count the number of peroxidase-positive (brown) cells in the ruled area.

Peroxidase Staining Using *o*-Toluidine Blue

Principle

Using *o*-toluidine blue, only those cells that contain peroxidase activity will be stained; all other cells remain unstained (World Health Organization, 1987).

Reagents

The working solution, which is stable for up to 1 day at ambient temperature, is prepared by mixing:

1.0 ml saturated (25 g/100 ml) NH_4Cl solution
1.0 ml 5.0% (w/v) Na_2EDTA solution in pH 6.0 phosphate buffer
9.0 ml aqueous 0.025% (w/v) solution of *o*-toluidine
50 µl 3% (or 10 volumes) hydrogen peroxide in reagent water

Method

1. Mix 0.1 ml liquefied semen and 0.9 ml working solution and shake for 2 minutes.

2. Leave for 20–30 minutes at ambient temperature.
3. Shake again and transfer about 10 µl onto a clean slide, cover with a 22 × 22 mm coverslip, and examine under a 40× objective using brightfield optics. If more than one stained (peroxidase-positive) cell is seen per five fields, proceed according to instructions 6 and 7, below; if not, enter a value of zero on the report form.
4. Transfer 4.5 µl of the mixture onto a Makler chamber; apply the cover glass and press down firmly until inference fringes can be seen between the apposed glass surfaces at the four support pillars.
5. Examine the preparation under a 40× objective using brightfield optics. Count the number of peroxidase-positive cells in the ruled area.

Peroxidase Staining Results

For either method described above, divide the number of peroxidase-positive cells per ruled area by 5.0 to obtain their concentration in the original semen sample in millions per milliliter. Concentrations of $\geq 10^6$ leukocytes/ml (often described as pyospermia) are considered abnormal. Microcells may be used in place of a Makler chamber (see Appendix II).

Immunocytochemical Identification

Principle

All classes of human leukocytes express a specific antigen (HLe-1, now called CD45) that can be detected using an appropriate monoclonal antibody. Specific recognition of the different types of leukocyte (e.g., macrophages, neutrophils, B or T cells, or even T cell subsets) can be achieved using specific monoclonal antibodies. By choosing a suitable second antibody the labeled cells can be visualized cytochemically (e.g., by alkaline phosphatase) or by fluorescence microscopy. The method described here (World Health Organization, 1992) uses a cytochemical approach.

Reagents

Phosphate-buffered saline (PBS) is prepared as described for the direct Immunobead test (see Chapter 5).

AMF fixative is a mixture of 10 ml acetone, 95 ml methanol, and 95 ml formaldehyde (40% v/v solution).

Tris-buffered saline (TBS) is prepared by dissolving 60.55 g Tris base and 85.20 g NaCl in about 800 ml reagent water. Adjust the pH to 8.6 using 1 N HCl, then make up to 1000 ml with additional reagent water.

Alkaline phosphatase substrate is prepared by dissolving 2.0 mg naphthol AS-MX phosphate, 0.2 ml dimethylformamide, 0.1 ml 1 M levamisole in 9.7 ml 0.1 M Tris buffer, pH 8.2 (dissolve 1.21 g Tris base in reagent water, adjust to pH 8.2

with 1 N HCl, and make up to 100 ml with additional reagent water). Filter through a 0.22-μm membrane filter, and store in clean glass bottles (labeled *AP substrate* with the date and your initials) at 4°C until use. Discard if there are any signs of contamination or sedimentation. Add fast red TR salt 1 mg/ml just before use.

Primary antibody is a monoclonal antibody against the common leukocyte antigen (sometimes *panleukocyte antigen*) known as CD45 (previously HLe-1). It is widely available commercially.

Second antibody is an antimouse immunoglobulin antibody raised in rabbit. The dilution used depends on the titer of the specific commercial preparation, e.g., 1:25 for the Z259 antibody manufactured by DAKO (DAKO Corporation, Carpinteria, CA, USA).

APAAP complex is an alkaline phosphatase–antialkaline phosphatase complex, also purchased commercially. Again its dilution for use depends on the specific commercial preparation, e.g., 1:50 for DAKO's D651 complex.

Hemotoxylin is purchased commercially. If Papanicolaou staining is used for sperm morphology assessments, the same hemotoxylin can be used.

Mounting medium is Apathy's aqueous mounting medium.

Procedure

1. Dilute 500 μl liquefied semen with 2.5 ml PBS and centrifuge at 500 *g* for 5 minutes at ambient temperature.
2. Discard the supernatant and gently resuspend the pellet in 2.5 ml fresh PBS.
3. Centrifuge at 500 *g* for 5 minutes at ambient temperature.
4. Discard the supernatant and gently resuspend the pellet in 2.5 ml fresh PBS.
5. Centrifuge at 500 *g* for 5 minutes at ambient temperature.
6. Discard the supernatant and gently resuspend the pellet in 500 μl fresh PBS.
7. Depending on the original sperm concentration, dilute the washed sperm suspension two- to fivefold with additional PBS to achieve a sperm concentration of the order 50×10^6/ml.
8. Duplicate 5-μl aliquots of the suspension are then air-dried onto a clean glass microscope slide. These preparations may be either stained and examined immediately or wrapped in aluminum foil and stored at −70°C for subsequent analysis.
9. Fix the air-dried cells with the AMF fixative for 90 seconds.
10. Rinse the slides twice with TBS and allow to drain.
11. Each spot of fixed cells is covered with 10 μl primary antibody and incubated in a humid chamber for 30 minutes at ambient temperature.
12. Rinse the slides twice with TBS and allow to drain.
13. Cover each spot of fixed cells with 10 μl second antibody and incubate in a humid chamber for 30 minutes at ambient temperature.
14. Rinse the slides twice with TBS and allow to drain.
15. Add 10 μl APAAP complex to each spot of fixed cells and incubate in a humid chamber for 30 minutes at ambient temperature.

16. Rinse the slides twice with TBS and allow to drain.

N.B. To intensify the reaction product, a repeat round of staining with the second antibody and APAAP can be performed using a shorter (15-minute) incubation period with each reagent.

17. Add 10 μl alkaline phosphatase substrate to each spot of fixed cells and incubate at ambient temperature in a humid chamber for 18 minutes.
18. Rinse the slides twice with TBS and allow to drain.
19. After the alkaline phosphatase color reaction has developed, the slides are washed with TBS and finally counterstained for a few seconds with hemotoxylin before being washed in tap water and mounted using Apathy's aqueous mounting medium.
20. From several fields, count the number of leukocytes (identified by the brown alkaline phosphatase reaction product) and spermatozoa.

Immunocytochemical Staining Results

The concentration of leukocytes, or [WBCs], in the original sample is calculated using the known sperm concentration (as 10^6/ml) according to the following equation:

$$[\text{WBCs}] = \frac{\text{No. of WBCs counted}}{\text{No. of sperm counted}} \times \text{semen sperm concentration}$$

Present the results as the concentration of leukocytes (as 10^6/ml), in the original semen specimen. Any value of 1×10^6/ml or greater is considered clinically significant.

SPERM CONCENTRATION

Accurate determination of the sperm concentration (millions of spermatozoa per milliliter of semen) and the total sperm count (millions of spermatozoa per ejaculate) are important parameters for evaluating the quantitative aspects of spermatogenesis. The most accurate method for determining sperm concentration applicable in the routine laboratory situation is volumetric dilution and hemocytometry. Because of the highly viscous nature of human semen the only type of sampling device that provides a precise volume aliquot of semen for dilution is the positive displacement-type pipette (Fig. 3-6). Although commonly used, WBC pipettes and automatic pipettes that rely on air displacement are *not* accurate enough for making careful volumetric dilutions of such viscous material as semen (Mortimer et al., 1989). However, the aqueous diluent, as well as the diluted preparation, may be measured using the more typical automatic pipettes with the disposable plastic tips. Alternative methods using various specialized counting chambers intended for rapid semen analysis are discussed under Specialized Counting Chambers, below.

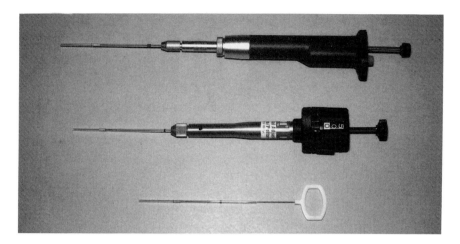

Figure 3-6   Various types of positive displacement pipettes.

Hemocytometry

Principle

Hemocytometry involves diluting a fixed-volume aliquot of liquefied semen and counting the preserved sperm suspension in a hemocytometer chamber. Although a 1 + 19 (i.e., 1:19, 1/20, or 1 in 20) dilution is usually employed, if the preliminary examination of the semen indicates that the concentration of spermatozoa present is either excessively high or low, the extent to which the sample is diluted should be adjusted accordingly. For samples containing fewer than 20×10^6 spermatozoa per milliliter, a 1 + 9 (1/10) dilution may be used, and for samples containing more than 100×10^6 spermatozoa per milliliter, a 1 + 49 (1/50) dilution may be appropriate.

Dilutions should be made in small, clean, glass or plastic vials (e.g., autoanalyzer cups) with tight-fitting caps if the diluted sample is to be left for more than a few minutes before loading into a hemocytometer. Extreme care must be taken when making the volumetric dilutions and preparing the hemocytometer.

Reagents

The diluent consists of 50 g $NaHCO_3$, 10 ml 36–40% formaldehyde solution, and 0.25 g trypan blue (CI 23850) dissolved in reagent water and made up to 1000 ml. This solution is filtered through Whatman No. 1 papers into a clean bottle and stored at $+4°C$.

Method

N.B.   If the estimated sperm concentration seen in the wet preparation was less than 10×10^6/ml, an aliquot of semen should be concentrated by centrifugation and reduction of the supernatant volume (see above) prior to making the dilution.

1. Add 50 μl liquefied semen (after ensuring thorough mixing of the specimen) to the 950 μl diluent in a capped 2-ml polystyrene autoanalyzer cup. A positive displacement pipettor *must* be used to ensure accurate handling of the viscous semen.
2. These dilutions may be stored at 4°C for up to 4 weeks but normally are counted within 2 days.
3. Fix the hemocytometer coverslip over the chambers. Interference fringes should be visible between the apposed glass surfaces.
4. Before loading into the hemocytometer, vortex the diluted sample for 10 seconds, then transfer about 10 μl to each of the hemocytometer chambers. Each dilution is counted in duplicate.
5. Leave the hemocytometer in a humid chamber (to prevent drying out) for 10–15 minutes. During this time the spermatozoa settle down onto the counting grid.
6. Count the spermatozoa using a 20× objective and preferably phase-contrast optics. The central square of the grid in an Improved Neubauer hemocytometer contains 25 large squares, each with 16 smaller squares (Fig. 3-7). The number of squares counted on each grid depends on the number of spermatozoa seen in the first *large* square counted. For samples containing fewer than 10 spermatozoa per square, the whole grid (i.e., 25 squares) is counted; for samples containing 10–40 spermatozoa per square, 10 squares (two horizontal or vertical rows)

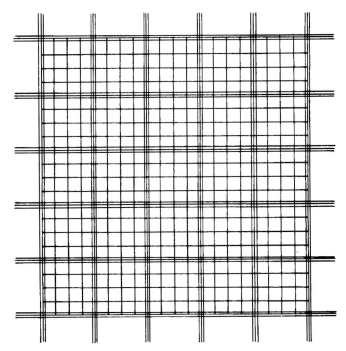

Figure 3-7 Central ruled area of the Improved Neubauer hemocytometer showing the 25 large squares, each comprising 16 small squares.

are assessed; and for samples containing more than 40 spermatozoa per square, five squares (the four corners plus the center) are counted

If a spermatozoon lies on the line dividing two adjacent squares, it is counted only if it is on the upper or the left side of the square being assessed. Only recognizable spermatozoa are counted. Free or "loose" heads, other germinal line cells, and free tails must *not* be counted (World Health Organization, 1992). Pinhead spermatozoa (see Sperm Morphology, below) are considered free tails and are not counted.

Results

If the counts of the two hemocytometer chambers are not within 5% of their average (i.e., the difference between them exceeds 1/20 of their sum), they should be discarded, the sample remixed, and another hemocytometer prepared. In other words, for a count to be acceptable, the following equation must be true:

$$\text{(Higher value} - \text{lower value)} \leq \text{(sum of values} \div 20)$$

Otherwise, the *total* number of spermatozoa (i.e., the sum of the two chambers) is divided by the appropriate correction factor (Table 3-5) to give the sperm concentration in the original semen sample in millions per milliliter. The total sperm count (millions per ejaculate) is calculated as the product of the sperm concentration and the ejaculate volume (in milliliters). Although it is accepted that the expression of sperm concentrations in millions per milliliter does not follow the International System of Units (SI) guidelines, which require results to be expressed per liter, it is the system used by andrology laboratories around the world.

The older term "sperm density" should be avoided, as it may lead to confusion with the density (specific gravity) of spermatozoa. Sperm counting is a general term that describes the procedure for determining sperm concentration and hence the total sperm count of a semen specimen.

Specialized Counting Chambers

Of the several specialized counting chambers for rapid semen analysis that have become available in recent years (Fig. 3-8), the Makler chamber (Sefi Medical

Table 3–5 Correction factors for hemocytometry counts using the Improved Neubauer chamber

Dilution (semen + diluent)	Correction Factors		
	2×25^a	2×10^a	2×5^a
1 + 9	20	8.0	4.0
1 + 19	10	4.0	2.0
1 + 49	4	1.6	0.8

[a]Number of counts × number of large squares counted.

Instruments, Haifa, Israel) has certainly gained the widest acceptance and usage. Others include the less expensive Horwell Fertility counting chamber (A. R. Horwell, London, UK), which has the same basic design as the Makler chamber but seems to be manufactured to a lower precision and uses a standard hemocytometer coverglass.

Both of these chambers have a depth of 10 μm and a ruled area of 1 mm^2 divided into 100 squares. Hence the number of spermatozoa seen in 10 squares corresponds to the concentration in millions per milliliter (e.g., 345 spermatozoa seen across the whole grid = 34.5 × 10^6/ml). Great care must be taken not to overfill these chambers, and a maximum sample volume of 5 μl must be used. Although such chambers are convenient in that they can be used on undiluted semen, it appears that in routine use they are prone to substantial errors. Hence although they may simplify the work for less specialized laboratories, they lack the accuracy of hemocytometry and cannot be recommended for laboratories wishing to perform semen analyses to presently accepted standards (Mortimer, 1990).

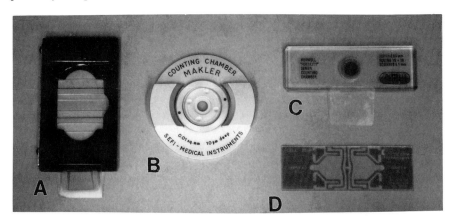

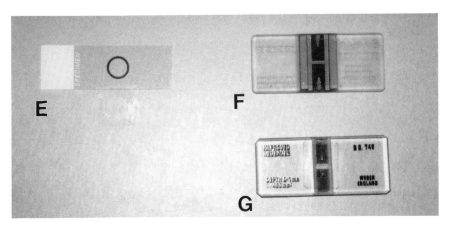

Figure 3-8 Specialized counting chambers. (**A**) Petroff-Hausser chamber. (**B**) Makler chamber. (**C**) Horwell chamber. (**D**) Microcell. (**E**) Chartpak slide. (**F, G**) Hemocytometers.

Most recently there has appeared the disposable μ-Cell or Microcell chamber (Fertility Technologies, Natick, MA, USA) (Fig. 3-8). Microcells are available in 12, 20, and 50 μm depths, are disposable, and seem to show adequate precision (Ginsburg and Armant, 1990). For sperm concentration determinations they must be used in conjunction with an eyepiece graticule or reticle to define a square of known area (and hence volume) for counting. Reticles with a 10 × 10 box pattern similar to a Makler chamber grid are available from Fertility Technologies to fit most major makes of microscope. The manufacturer provides complete calibration instructions to derive the appropriate correction factor for any combination of microscope optics.

The Petroff-Hausser bacterial counting chamber (20 μm depth) (Fig. 3-8) has also been used for sperm motility studies. Its relative expense and difficult cleaning are significant disadvantages in its routine use.

Finally, disposable chambers of approximate 32–33 μm depth can be made by pressing dry transfer circles (13 mm ∅; No. RDC49: Chartpak, Leeds, MA, USA) (Fig. 3-8) onto thoroughly cleaned ordinary microscope slides. Five microliters of sample are placed in the center of this circle and an ordinary coverslip (No. 1.^{1}/$_2$) applied firmly, forcing the sample to spill over the side of the O-ring. Although the depth of these preparations is too imprecise for volumetric use, they have the advantage of being effectively sealed, thereby minimizing drying out, and have proved useful in sperm motility studies (see Chapter 7).

SPERM VITALITY, INTEGRITY, AND LONGEVITY

The term *sperm vitality* is preferred to *sperm viability,* as it not only reflects the characteristic of the spermatozoa being tested, it minimizes possible confusion with aspects of sperm longevity. Sperm vitality is normally measured by testing cellular integrity, assessing the ability of the sperm plasma membrane to exclude extracellular substances such as dyes or fluorochromes (see below), or measuring the leakage of intracellular markers, particularly enzymes (see Chapter 4).

"Longevity" is commonly used to describe the duration of sperm motility. However, it is important to remember that the fertile life of a spermatozoon, the persistence of its motility, and the duration of its vitality are different aspects of the cell.

Although sperm vitality is not assessed routinely in all andrology laboratories, it does allow the rare situation of necrozoospermia to be distinguished from total sperm immotility (e.g., Kartagener syndrome) (see Transmission Electron Microscopy in Chapter 8). Vitality assessment also provides a check on the accuracy of motility assessments, as the percentage of live spermatozoa should slightly exceed the total percentage of motile spermatozoa. The proportion of cytologically intact "live" cells can be determined using any of several vital staining techniques, including eosin Y, trypan blue, or the Hoechst fluorochrome H33258 (see below).

The hypoosmotic swelling (HOS) test, although originally described as a test of sperm function, is now more appropriately considered an additional test of sperm integrity. It is included below as another procedure for evaluating sperm vitality.

Sperm Vitality Assessment Using Eosin-Nigrosin

The eosin-nigrosin test is probably the simplest and least expensive technique for assessing sperm vitality. Although eosin Y can be used without a counterstain, it makes the unstained live cells difficult to see unless phase-contrast optics (preferably negative phase contrast) are used.

Principle
Intact cells exclude eosin, whereas dead cells (i.e., those with damaged plasma membranes) take up the red color of eosin. Nigrosin is used as a counterstain to facilitate visualization of the unstained (white) live cells.

Reagents
The eosin-nigrosin (E-N) stain is prepared by dissolving 0.67 g eosin Y (CI 45380) in 100 ml tap water. This solution is heated gently, and 10.0 g nigrosin (CI 50420) is added and dissolved before being brought to the boil. The stain is allowed to cool, filtered using Reeve grade 802 papers, and stored in a stoppered glass bottle at 4°C. The stain is warmed to ambient temperature before use.

New batches of stain are checked against the old batch before being accepted for use. On at least 10 semen samples two parallel sets of vitality smears are prepared, coded, and scored blind. The percentages of live cells should not be significantly different (by paired t-test). If the difference is significant, discard the new batch of stain and prepare another.

Method

1. Mix equal volumes of liquefied semen and E-N stain (1 or 2 drops, or about 50 μl of each is sufficient) on a spotting plate and leave for 30 seconds.
2. Transfer about 50 μl of the mixture onto a clean microscope slide and smear. Do not make the smears too thick or the counterstain will be too dark for visualizing the spermatozoa.
3. Allow to air-dry and mount with DPX or equivalent mountant as soon as is convenient. These slides may be stored indefinitely at ambient temperature.
4. At least 100 (preferably 200) spermatozoa are examined at a magnification of 1000× (or 1250×) under oil immersion using a high-quality *non-phase-contrast* objective and correctly adjusted brightfield (Köhler illumination) optics. Spermatozoa that are white (unstained) are counted as live and those showing any degree of pink or red coloration as dead.

Sperm Vitality Assessment Using the H33258 Fluorochrome

The fluorochrome H33258, which binds strongly to DNA, is excluded from intact cells but taken up by dead cells. Although the H33258 method can be used on washed seminal spermatozoa, it is better suited to vitality assessments on prepared populations of already washed or migrated spermatozoa in culture medium. The method described below provides easy to read preparations with minimal residual background fluorescence. Reducing or eliminating the washing steps results in increased background fluorescence that may hinder or even prevent reliable scoring. For quick counting, the special antifade mountant may be omitted and 1:1 glycerol/PBS used instead.

Principle
Whereas live cells show only faintly under the fluorescence microscope, dead cells fluoresce a bright blue or even blue-white.

Reagents

H33258 (bis-benzimide) is prepared as a 1000× concentrated aqueous stock solution at a concentration of 1 mg/ml in reagent water. This solution may be stored frozen in small Eppendorf tubes covered with aluminum foil to protect the H33258 from light, which would cause loss of fluorescence. For use, a working solution is prepared by diluting the stock H33258 solution at 1 µl/ml in the same medium as used for the sperm suspension to be stained.

PVP-40 washing column is prepared as a 2.0% (w/v) solution of 40,000 MW polyvinylpyrrolidone in PBS (see Chapter 5, Direct Immunobead Test, for PBS recipe).

Mountant refers to a special mountant for fluorescence microscopy that greatly reduces fluorochrome fading (see Appendix III).

Method

1. The suspension to be stained should be of washed spermatozoa to eliminate seminal plasma proteins, at a concentration of 5×10^6 to 20×10^6 spermatozoa/ml.
2. Add 1.0 ml of the H33258 working solution to 0.5 ml of sperm suspension and leave at ambient temperature for 7 minutes. This step and all following steps should be carried out under subdued lighting with aluminum foil wrapped around the tubes.
3. Layer the 1.5 ml of sperm suspension with H33258 onto a 4-ml column of PVP-40 and centrifuge at 900 *g* for 5 minutes.
4. Aspirate and discard the supernatant.
5. Resuspend the spermatozoa to about 20×10^6/ml in culture medium.
6. Spread 20-µl aliquots of the stained sperm suspension over the end 2 cm of cleaned microscope slides and allow to air-dry.
7. Fix in 95% (v/v) ethanol for 5 minutes and allow to air-dry again.
8. Mount with a drop of fluorescence mountant and 22 × 22 mm coverslip and observe under an epifluorescence microscope using an appropriate filter set (see Appendix III).
9. Count at least 100 (preferably 200) spermatozoa and classify according to the

intensity of their fluorescence. Live cells appear a faint to moderate blue, and dead cells appear bright blue or even blue-white.

Sperm Vitality Results
The result from either method is the "percent live" or "percent vital" spermatozoa, expressed as an integer. The proportion of vital cells is usually slightly greater than that of the motile spermatozoa seen in the wet preparation.

Sperm Osmotic Fragility: The Hypoosmotic Swelling Test

Although the hypoosmotic swelling (HOS) test was originally described as a test of sperm function with a good correlation with the zona-free hamster egg penetration test (Jeyendran et al., 1984), this correlation has not been confirmed by several other studies. Others, however, have found the HOS test capable of discriminating fertile from infertile semen samples. Nonetheless, some workers believe the HOS test has clinical value, although it is probably most appropriately considered as an additional aspect of sperm vitality (because it assesses the osmoregulatory ability of the spermatozoa, an aspect of membrane functional integrity). Consequently, a standard technique is provided below.

Principle
The HOS test is based on the ability of live spermatozoa to withstand moderate hypoosmotic stress. Dead spermatozoa whose plasma membranes are no longer intact do not show swelling. In addition, dead spermatozoa retaining their plasma membranes, as well as senescent spermatozoa with poor osmoregulatory capacity, show uncontrolled swelling that rapidly results in rupture of their overdistended plasma membranes. Consequently, the proportion of spermatozoa that show controlled swelling under test conditions is considered the good fraction with low osmotic fragility.

Reagents
The HOS test diluent consists of 7.35 g sodium citrate ($Na_3Cit \cdot 2H_2O$) and 13.51 g fructose dissolved in 1000 ml reagent water, giving an osmolarity of 150 mOsm/kg.

Method
1. Mix 0.1 ml of liquefied semen (or washed sperm preparation) with 1.0 ml of HOS diluent in a small stoppered tube.
2. Incubate at 37°C for at least 30 (preferably 60) minutes.
3. Remix the tube and transfer one drop (about 30 μl) to a clean microscope slide and mount using a 22 × 22 mm coverslip.
4. Examine using phase-contrast microscopy at a magnification of 400× to 500× and count at least 100 (preferably 200) spermatozoa. Each spermatozoon is scored as either normal or showing swelling of the tail region (Fig. 3-9).

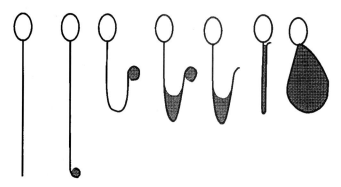

Figure 3-9 Swelling patterns seen in the HOS test. Shaded areas denote regions of tail swelling. (Adapted from Jeyendran et al., 1984.)

N.B. a. If the sperm concentration is very low, the concentrated sample (see Assessment of the Wet Preparation, above) should be used. However, such results may be biased owing to the effects of peroxidative damage to the sperm plasma membrane induced by reactive oxygen species within the pellet (see Chapter 12). This condition could make the plasma membrane less fluid and the cell therefore less able to swell without bursting.

b. For seminal spermatozoa, a wet preparation of the fresh semen should also be examined at the start of the HOS incubation to determine whether substantial numbers of the spermatozoa already have swollen tails. If so, the wet preparation should be scored as for the post-HOS test preparation and the proportion of swollen spermatozoa subtracted from the HOS test score.

Results

The result of the test is expressed as the percent swollen cells, equivalent to the proportion of osmotically competent spermatozoa. Osmotically incompetent and dead spermatozoa swell so much that the plasma membrane bursts, allowing the tail to straighten out again.

Sperm Longevity Assessments

The persistence of motility and the duration of cellular integrity reflect important aspects of sperm quality. Therefore their evaluation as part of a semen analysis may provide valuable insight into the potential etiology of a couple's infertility. Although those spermatozoa that migrate successfully into the cervical mucus after insemination in vivo spend less than 30 minutes in seminal plasma (see Chapter 2), it can be helpful to reevaluate the motility and vitality of spermatozoa in a semen specimen 2–3 hours after the initial examination (see Appendix I).

Because it is known that sperm functional ability and, to a lesser extent, motility and vitality decrease with prolonged exposure to seminal plasma, it may be considered more of a stress test. However, a normal fertile man's semen rarely shows significant changes in either motility or vitality over such a short time frame. Consequently, a rapid decline in either or both the quantitative or qualitative motility or the vitality may be diagnostically helpful.

True sperm longevity would probably be better assessed using a prepared motile sperm population in culture medium and some aspect of sperm function (see Chapter 10) as the endpoint. Unfortunately, no defined assay has yet been established that might be amenable to routine use in a diagnostic andrology laboratory. Although several laboratories have reported associations between the maintenance of sperm motility in IVF preparations and the likelihood of fertilization, there is no consensus as to what the association should be.

SPERM MORPHOLOGY

An assessment of the morphological characteristics of the spermatozoa is as important for complete evaluation of the semen sample as are the count and motility. Although, ideally, sperm morphology should be assessed on unfixed, unstained preparations using phase-contrast microscopy, the small size of the human sperm head makes it impractical. It is therefore mandatory to prepare an air-dried smear from the fresh semen at the same time as the smears for vitality staining are made. A wise precaution is to make at least two smears in case of accidents or problems when one is being stained. These smears are made on thoroughly cleaned microscope slides and then are fixed, stained, and mounted. The method of fixation depends on the staining technique to be used.

Frequently used staining procedures for human spermatozoa include the Papanicolaou, Giemsa, Shorr, and modified Bryan-Leishman methods. Giemsa staining provides smears that are less easy to assess than the Papanicolaou method. The Bryan-Leishman method, although it permits better differentiation of the other cell types present in semen, is also less ideal than the Papanicolaou method for differential sperm morphology assessments. A simplified Papanicolaou method (World Health Organization, 1987) has not been found to be a successful staining method for human spermatozoa and should not be used.

Should it prove impossible to use such a technique, special prestained slides (e.g., Testsimplets: Boehringer, Mannheim, Germany), prestained coverslips (e.g., Sangodiff: Merck, Darmstadt, Germany), or a rapid staining technique such as Diff-Quik (Dade Diagnostics, Miami, FL, USA) may be used, although the slides are not as clean and easy to read as, for example, with the Papanicolaou method.

A basic morphological assessment of the spermatozoa can also be performed on the eosin-nigrosin vitality smears. Although the latter method has the extra advantage that the percentage of morphologically normal live spermatozoa can be determined, it is difficult to classify germinal cells and leukocytes.

Papanicolaou Staining

The most widely used staining technique is that of Papanicolaou. It provides probably the best differential staining of the spermatozoa.

Principle

The Papanicolaou stain clearly distinguishes between basophilic and acidophilic cell components and allows detailed examination of the chromatin pattern. It has proved useful for evaluation of human sperm morphology and of immature germinal cells.

Reagents

Fixative

For Papanicolaou staining the best fixation is achieved using a *freshly prepared* solution of equal parts of analytical grade absolute ethanol and diethyl ether. The solvents are mixed in a stoppered measuring cylinder. If fixing is performed in Coplin jars, prepare enough fixative for all jars at the same time (each Coplin jar takes 50 ml).

Ethanol Dehydration Series

Various strengths of analytical grade ethanol in aqueous solution are required: 50%, 70%, 80%, 95%, and 99.5% (v/v). They are prepared by volumetric dilution of absolute ethanol with reagent water and are stored in well-stoppered glass bottles at ambient temperature.

Staining Solutions

Harris hematoxylin, EA50, and *OG6* stains, which may be purchased ready prepared (e.g., Ortho Diagnostics), are stored at ambient temperature. The hemotoxylin should be filtered (Reeve grade 802 papers) immediately before use. Alternatively, one can prepare the stains in the laboratory at considerable savings (Belsey et al., 1980).

Acid ethanol is prepared by mixing 300 ml 95% (v/v) ethanol and 2.0 ml concentrated hydrochloric acid (36% HCl v/v) in 100 ml reagent water.

Scott's solution is prepared by dissolving 3.5 g $NaHCO_3$ and 20.0 g $MgSO_4 \cdot 7H_2O$ in reagent water to a total volume of 1000 ml.

Method

1. Allow the smears to air-dry.
2. Fix for 30 minutes and then allow to air-dry.
3. One smear from each pair is kept in reserve; the other is stained and scored.
4. Half-fill staining dishes with the various solutions (see sequence below).

5. Arrange the slides face-out in staining racks.
6. Proceed with the staining according to the sequence below (a "dip" corresponds to an immersion of about 1 second duration):

Ethanol 80%	10 dips
Ethanol 70%	10 dips
Ethanol 50%	10 dips
Distilled water	10 dips
Harris hematoxylin	3 minutes exactly
Running tap water	2 dips
Acid ethanol	2 dips
Running tap water	3–5 minutes
Scott's solution	4 minutes
Distilled water	1 dip
Ethanol 50%	10 dips
Ethanol 70%	10 dips
Ethanol 80%	10 dips
Ethanol 95%	10 dips
Orange G 6	2 minutes
Ethanol 95%	10 dips
Ethanol 95%	10 dips
EA-50	5 minutes
Ethanol 95%	5 dips
Ethanol 95%	5 dips
Ethanol 95%	5 dips
Ethanol 99.5%	2 minutes
Xylene (3 dishes)	approximately 1 minute per dish; change xylene if it turns milky

7. Mount at once with DPX or other equivalent mountant. Leave at least overnight for the mountant to set. Slides may be stored indefinitely at ambient temperature.
8. At least 100 (preferably at least 200) spermatozoa are counted from each smear at a magnification of 1000–1250× under oil immersion using a high quality 100× *non-phase-contrast* objective and correctly adjusted brightfield (Köhler illumination) optics. Each spermatozoon is tallied according to the scoring system being used (see Sperm Morphology Classification Systems, below).
9. At the same time the spermatozoa are being counted, the numbers of other germinal line cells and white blood cells are tallied in each field scored. In this way their incidences can be expressed in terms of per 100 spermatozoa, or their concentrations in the original semen are calculated using the sperm concentration obtained by hemocytometry.

N.B. a. If, for any reason, the stained smear is difficult to read or looks strange, the reserve smear should be stained using fresh batches of stains.

b. If the smear seems to have disappeared during the staining process, and no seminal material can be seen under the microscope, the smear was probably too thick—a not uncommon problem, so beware!

c. The appearance of tiny bluish-black crystals on the stained smear probably indicates that the hematoxylin stain was not filtered before use.

Results

Numerous schemes exist for classifying human sperm morphology. They are discussed under Sperm Morphology Classification Systems, below.

Bryan-Leishman Staining

Principle

The Bryan-Leishman staining method has been widely used in hematology for differential white blood cell counts. It has also proved useful for differentiating the other cellular elements found in human semen, in addition to providing adequate staining of the spermatozoa for differential morphology scoring (Belsey et al., 1980).

Regents

Fixative

No fixative is used for this method; the air-dried smears are processed directly. The alcoholic formalin step constitutes the initial fixation of the smears.

Alcoholic formalin is prepared by mixing 10 ml 36–40% formaldehyde solution with 90 ml 95% (v/v) ethanol. Optionally, 0.05 g calcium acetate may be added to ensure neutral pH.

Ethanol Dehydration Series

Various strengths of analytical grade ethanol in aqueous solution are required: 50%, 70%, and 80% (v/v). They are prepared by volumetric dilution of absolute ethanol with reagent water and stored in well-stoppered glass bottles at ambient temperature.

Staining Solutions

Modified Bryan's stain is prepared by dissolving 0.5 g eosin Y (CI 45380), 0.5 g fast green FCF (CI 42053), and 0.5 g naphthol yellow (CI 1316) in 1500 ml aqueous 1.0% glacial acetic acid. The solution is mixed thoroughly and stored in a tightly stoppered bottle. It is filtered using Reeve grade 802 papers immediately before use.

Leishman's blood stain is initially prepared as a *stock solution* comprising 0.5 g eosinated methylene blue in 300 ml absolute methanol. This solution is mixed thoroughly and allowed to age in the dark at ambient temperature for 7 days. At the end of this time, the stain is placed in a 35°–37°C incubator for 2 days, after which it is ready to use. It should be stored in a tightly stoppered dark bottle away from heat and light. Alternative, commercially available blood stain solutions are Jenner's or Wright's stains, although the timing involved with these stains must be varied empirically to achieve optimum results. The *working solution* is prepared immediately before use by mixing 50 ml of the filtered stock solution with 150 ml of a pH 6.8 buffer solution (two pH 6.8 phosphate-buffered tablets, e.g., BDH B33193, in 200 ml reagent water immediately before use).

α-Naphthol is prepared as a stock solution comprising 1.0 g α-naphthol in 100 ml 40% (v/v) ethanol. Immediately before use, add 0.2 ml 3.0% hydrogen peroxide.

Pyronin Y solution is made by dissolving 0.1 g pyronin Y (CI 45005) and 4.0 ml aniline in 96.0 ml 40% (v/v) ethanol. Filter immediately before use.

Sodium citrate buffer consists of 7.0 g $Na_3Cit·2H_2O$ and 9.0 g NaCl dissolved in reagent water to 1000 ml. The pH is adjusted to 7.5 using either 1 N sodium hydroxide or 1 N hydrochloric acid.

Method

1. Allow the smears to air-dry completely.
2. Arrange the slides face out in staining racks.
3. Proceed with the staining according to the sequence below (a dip corresponds to immersion of about 1 second duration).

Alcoholic formalin	1 minute	fresh every time
Ethanol 80%	5 minutes	change after 30 slides
Ethanol 70%	5 minutes	change after 30 slides
Ethanol 50%	5 minutes	change after 30 slides
α-Naphthol	4 minutes	change every 3 days
Running tap water	15 minutes	running slowly
Pyronin Y	4 minutes	fresh each week
Running tap water	3 dips	running slowly
Sodium citrate buffer	3 minutes	fresh each time
Distilled water	1 minute	fresh each time
Mod. Bryan's stain	15 minutes	fresh every other time
Acetic acid 1%	2 dips	fresh each time
Running tap water	1 minute	running slowly
Leishman's stain	30 minutes	fresh each time
Running tap water	1–2 dips	running slowly

4. Allow to air-dry, do not blot.
5. Mount with DPX or other equivalent mountant. Leave at least overnight for the mountant to set. Slides may be stored indefinitely at ambient temperature.
6. At least 100 (preferably at least 200) spermatozoa are counted from each smear at a magnification of 1000–1250× under oil immersion using a high quality 100× *non-phase-contrast* objective and correctly adjusted brightfield (Köhler illumination) optics. Each spermatozoon is tallied according to the scoring sys-

tem being used (see Sperm Morphology Classification Systems, below). At the same time the spermatozoa are being counted, the numbers of other germinal line cells and white blood cells are tallied in each field scored. In this way their incidences can be expressed in terms of per 100 spermatozoa or their concentrations in the original semen calculated using the sperm concentration obtained by haemocytometry.

N.B.   a. If, for any reason, the stained smear is difficult to read or looks strange, the reserve smear should be stained using fresh batches of stains.
   b. If the smear seems to have disappeared during the staining process and no seminal material can be seen under the microscope, the smear was probably too thick—a not uncommon problem, so beware!
   c. The final stain intensity can be increased by staining for a longer time in the buffered Leishman's stain; it can be decreased by repeated washing in tap water. Check for the desired intensity under the microscope before mounting the slides.

Results

Numerous schemes exist for classifying human sperm morphology. They are discussed under Sperm Morphology Classification Systems, below.

Shorr Staining

Although widely used in France for many years, the Shorr stain has only recently been employed more widely in other countries. Because of the work of Jeulin et al. (1986) the Shorr staining method is being used by an increasing number of andrology laboratories, particularly those working in conjunction with IVF programs.

Principle
The Shorr stain has proved particularly useful for evaluating abnormalities of the sperm head and acrosome.

Reagents

Fixative: A 75% (v/v) solution of ethanol is used. It is prepared by volumetric dilution of absolute ethanol with reagent water.

Ethanol dehydration series: Various strengths of analytical grade ethanol in aqueous solution are required: 70%, 95%, and 96% (v/v). They are prepared by volumetric dilution of absolute ethanol with reagent water and are stored in well-stoppered glass bottles at ambient temperature.

Staining solutions:

Shorr stain is purchased from Merck.

Hematoxylin is the same stain as that used for the Papanicolaou method.

Ammonium alcohol is made by mixing 5 ml NH_4OH (specific gravity 0.88 or 0.91, i.e., about 24–25% v/v) with 95 ml 75% (v/v) ethanol.

Method

1. Allow the smears to air-dry.
2. Fix for 1 minute in 75% (v/v) ethanol.
3. Proceed with the staining according to the sequence below (a dip corresponds to an immersion of about 1-second duration).

Running water	12–15 dips
Hematoxylin	1.5 minutes
Running water	12–15 dips
Ammonium alcohol	5 passages of 5 minutes each
Running water	12–15 dips
Ethanol 70%	5 minutes
Ethanol 95%	5 minutes
Shorr stain	45–60 seconds
Ethanol 96%	5 minutes
Absolute ethanol	2 passages of 5 minutes each
Toluene	2 passages of 5 minutes each

4. Mount with DPX or other equivalent mountant. Leave at least overnight for the mountant to set. Slides may be stored indefinitely at ambient temperature.
5. Score at a magnification of 1000–1250× under oil immersion using a high-quality 100× *non-phase-contrast* objective and correctly adjusted brightfield (Köhler illumination) optics. Each spermatozoon is tallied according to the scoring system being used (see Sperm Morphology Classification Systems, below).

Results

Numerous schemes exist for classifying human sperm morphology.

Sperm Morphology Classification Systems

The major problem of morphological assessment is the pleomorphism of human spermatozoa (Figs. 3-10 and 3-11). Studies on the selection of spermatozoa in vitro and within the female reproductive tract in vivo have helped define the limits of a normal human spermatozoon (Mortimer et al., 1982; see also Chapter 2).

In general terms, only recognizable spermatozoa should be included in the count; immature germinal cells up to and including the Sd_1 stage (see Fig. 2-5) should not be counted as spermatozoa. Loose sperm heads are counted (as abnormal forms because they lack tails), but free tails are *not*. Pinhead forms are considered free tails and are not counted as spermatozoa, as they rarely contain any head structures anterior to the basal plate, which attaches the connecting piece of the neck region to the nucleus of the sperm head. If a high incidence of pinheads (or any other specific defect category, see below) is seen in a sample, it should be noted.

Some systems consider coiled tails separately from other tail defects because a

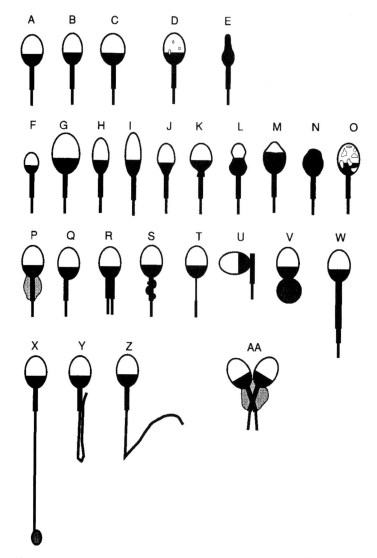

Figure 3-10 Abnormal forms of human spermatozoa. (**A–C**) Variations of normal head shape. (**D**) Normal spermatozoon with a low incidence of vacuoles. (**E**) Normal head seen in side view. (**F–O**) Head defects: **F** = microcephalic or small head; **G** = macrocephalic or large head; **H, I** = tapering forms; **J, K** = pyriform; **L** = constricted; **M** = reduced acrosomal region; **N** = amorphous or dense staining; **O** = vacuolated). **P** Cytoplasmic droplet; (**Q**) Asymmetrical tail insertion. (**R**) Double or duplicate tail. (**S**) Abnormal midpiece. (**T**) Thin midpiece due to the absence of mitochondria. (**U**) Noninserted tail (neck defect). (**V–Z**) Tail defects: **V** = coiled tail; **W** = short-tailed form; **X** = terminal droplet on the tail; **Y** = hairpin tail; **Z** = broken tail. (**AA**) Conjoined form.

large number of coiled tails may indicate that the spermatozoa have been exposed to hypotonic stress, although tail coiling is also associated with sperm senescence. A distended midpiece region could denote either a midpiece defect or the presence of a residual cytoplasmic droplet (residual cytoplasm stains green in a Papanicolaou-stained preparation, whereas abnormal midpieces often stain red) indicative of sperm immaturity. Some immature spermatozoa may show a cytoplasmic droplet at other locations along the tail or even at the tip of the tail.

For current practical purposes, many clinical requirements can be satisfied by a simple statement of the "percent normal forms," although specific defects should be noted if they occur in more than about 20% of the spermatozoa in the sample.

In domesticated species, several "sterilizing defects" have been described. In these cases essentially all the spermatozoa from an individual show a specific structural defect that causes sperm dysfunction. A few similar cases have been described in men, probably the best known of which is the round-head defect, or globozoospermia (Fig. 3-12), where the condensed chromatin, which lacks a nuclear envelope, is surrounded by a "cloud" of cytoplasm out of which protrudes a tail. There are no acrosomal or postacrosomal structures, and these spermatozoa are incapable of fertilization (Aitken et al., 1990).

Because many morphologically abnormal spermatozoa possess multiple defects, differential morphological assessments should ideally be multiparametric rather than the older single-entry scoring methods that assign priorities to the "major" defect on the assumption that the head is more important than the midpiece, and the midpiece is more important than the tail. In multiple-entry scoring schemes, although each defect is tallied independently, the total number of cells evaluated increases by only one for each normal or abnormal spermatozoon. Consequently, the total number of defects scored exceeds the number of abnormal cells.

Indices of the extent of morphological abnormality present in a sperm population have attracted interest. To date, two schemes have been described: the multiple anomalies index (MAI) (Jouannet et al., 1988) and the teratozoospermia index (TZI) (Mortimer, 1990). Each is calculated as the mean number of defects per

$$\longrightarrow$$

Figure 3-11 Photomicrographs of morphologically normal and abnormal human spermatozoa taken from Papanicolaou-stained preparations. **1** = normal form; **2** = normal form in side view; **3** = vacuolated head; **4** = small head (but with "normal" acrosomal region); **5** = small head (but with no acrosomal region); **6, 7** = large heads; **8, 9** = tapering heads; **10** = tapering pyriform head; **11** = pyriform head; **12–14** = dense staining "amorphous" heads; **15** = tapering abnormal head with neck defect and residual cytoplasmic droplet; **16** = "lysed" form; **17** = double conjoined form with tapering heads; **18** = triple coinjoined form with essentially normal heads; **19** = cytoplasmic droplet (immature form); **20** = asymmetrically inserted tail (neck defect); **21, 22** = noninserted tails (neck defects); **23** tailless pyriform head (neck defect); **24** = tailless tapered head (neck defect); **25** = free tail, sometimes referred to as a "pinhead form" (not counted as a spermatozoon in a morphology count); **26** = thickened midpiece; **27** = thin midpiece; **28, 29** = coiled tails; **30** = bent or broken tail; **31** = hairpin tail; **32** = short tail; **33, 34** = double tails; **35, 36** (upper cell) = midpiece defects with short tails. (See pages 80 and 81.)

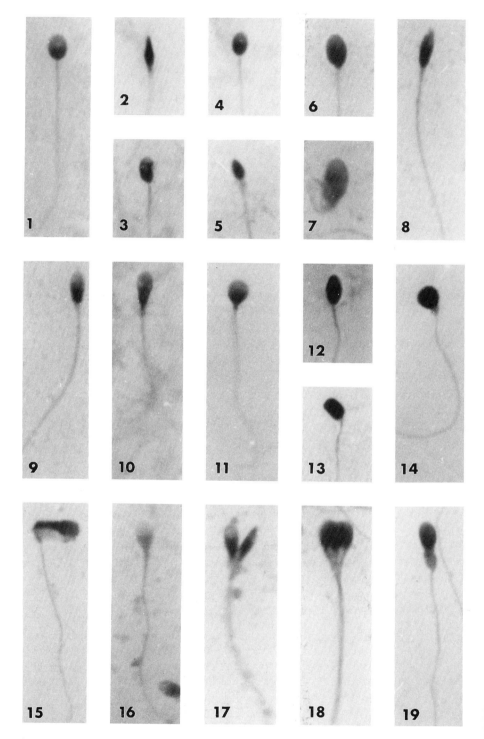

Fig. 3-11

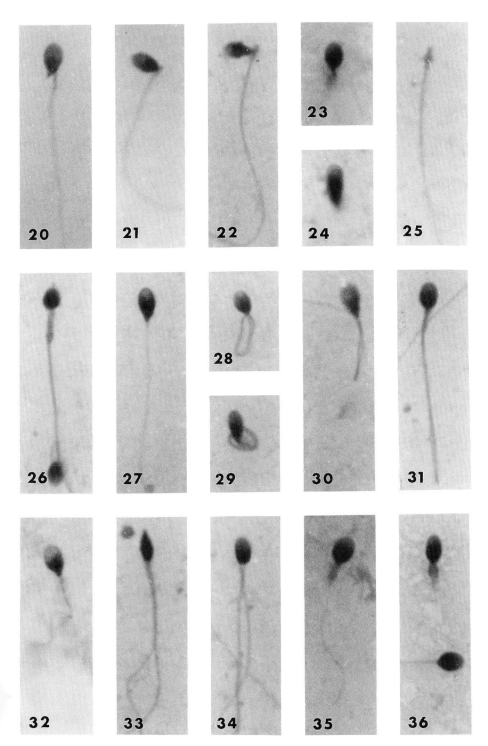

Fig. 3-11 *(cont.)*

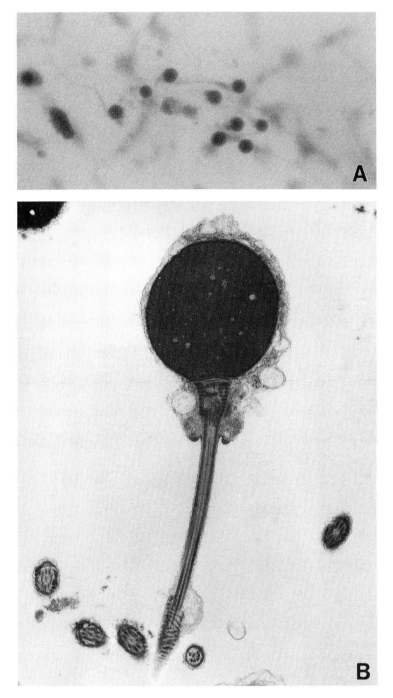

Figure 3-12 **(A)** Photomicrograph and **(B)** electronmicrograph (×18K) of the round-head defect, or globozoospermia. Note the absence of acrosomal and midpiece structures. (Micrographs courtesy of Mr. Ross Boadle, EM Unit, Westmead Hospital, Sydney, Australia.

abnormal spermatozoon from the results of multiple-entry differential sperm morphology scoring. In a prospective study on 394 infertile men, the MAI was the most significant predictor of fertility (Jouannet et al., 1988). This concept has now been adopted by the WHO in the latest edition of its *Laboratory Manual* (see WHO 1992 Classification, below).

WHO 1980 Classification
In the first edition of the WHO *Laboratory Manual* (Belsey et al., 1980) it was unclear whether a single- or multiple-entry scoring system was to be used. The classification scheme, which was apparently based on the early work of MacLeod (1964), and expected frequencies of the various defects in normal, fertile individuals are provided in Table 3-6. From the high expected frequency of morphologically normal spermatozoa and the low incidences of the various defects, it is clear that this classification scheme was based on leniency when assigning a rating of normality.

WHO 1987 Classification
In the second edition of the WHO *Laboratory Manual* (World Health Organization, 1987) the expected frequencies of the various categories were not provided, and the system was modified. Although it was again not specified as to whether single- or multiple-entry scoring was to be used, the latter was implied. Consequently, morphological assessments were separated into the three categories of head, midpiece, and tail, including a subclassification of "normal" available for each. The defects considered were as follows.

Head: normal, large oval, small oval, tapering, pyriform, duplicate/double, amorphous, round, or pin
Midpiece: normal, abnormal, and cytoplasmic droplet
Tail: normal or abnormal

Table 3–6 Prevalence of morphological defects in human spermatozoa

Defect 1980[b]	David et al., 1967[a]	WHO, 1980[b]
Large oval head	1.7	0.3 (0–5.2)
Small oval head	5.2	1.4 (0–13.5)
Tapering head	6.9	0.4 (0–6.2)
Pyriform head	1.5	2.0 (0–21.8)
Duplicate head	1.2	1.5 (0–8.3)
Amorphous head	6.3	6.5 (0–24.9)
Tail defect	15.0	5.2 (0–37.4)
Cytoplasmic droplet	5.0	2.2 (0–14.5)

Values are means; ranges are given where available.

[a]David et al. (1975): data from 50 fertile men.

[b]Belsey et al. (1980): based on 602 ejaculates from 73 men who were fathers.

David's Multiple-Entry Classification

The multiple-entry classification system developed in France in the laboratory of Prof. Georges David (David et al., 1975) is a complex multiple-entry scheme that separates each defect in each region of the spermatozoon so no defect is underestimated in its final incidence per 100 spermatozoa. A single cell may show up to a maximum of four defects. Thirteen specific defects are identified and tallied separately.

Head: tapered (length > 6.0 μm; incorporating simple tapering, pyriform, clapper-shaped, and slender/pointed forms), thin, small, large, amorphous, double, and those in a state of "lysis"
Midpiece: cytoplasmic droplets, bent tail (with an angle of at least 90 degrees between the long axis of the head and that of the tail)
Tail: absent, short, coiled, and double

Simplified Multiple-Entry Classification

This simplified multiple-entry scoring system developed in Calgary, retains the major categories of the earlier WHO schemes but uses a maximum of eight categories to facilitate its implementation using the standard laboratory counter, which has eight tallies plus totalizer (Mortimer, 1985). Papanicolaou staining is used routinely.

Each spermatozoon is scored as either normal or abnormal, with each of the following defects being tallied independently: tapering heads, abnormal heads, immature spermatozoa (i.e., cytoplasmic droplets), midpiece defects, tail defects, coiled tails, and free (tailless) heads. Cytoplasmic droplets are counted only if they are stained green by the Papanicolaou method and are larger than half the area of the sperm head.

Modified David Multiple-Entry Classification

The original system of David et al. (1975) has been modified (Prof. P. Jouannet, personal communication). Spermatozoa in a state of lysis are no longer included in the differential count but are noted as other elements along with germinal line and other cells. The multiple-entry principle of the system remains generally the same, except that now 15 defects are identified and tallied separately.

Head: tapered, thin, small, large, multiple (including double), abnormal base (more or less equivalent to pyriform), and abnormal or absent acrosome
Midpiece: cytoplasmic droplets, thin midpiece, or bent tail
Tail: absent, short, irregular width, coiled, or multiple

Tygerberg Strict Criteria Classification System

Originally described by Kruger et al. (1986), the strict criteria system of classifying human sperm morphology includes routine morphometric analysis (using an eyepiece micrometer) to determine if a sperm head falls within a strictly defined normal size range (see Chapter 2). A spermatozoon is considered normal when the head has a smooth, oval shape with a well-defined acrosome comprising 40–70% of the head area. Morphometrically, the sperm head must be 5.0–6.0 μm long and 2.5–3.5 μm wide. In addition, there must be no neck, midpiece, or tail defects and no cytoplasmic droplets of more than half the size of the sperm head. In contrast to other classification schemes, the Kruger scheme requires that all "borderline" forms be considered abnormal. The general defects recognized are reported according to the WHO 1980 classification (Menkveld et al., 1990).

Head: large, small, tapering, duplicate, or amorphous (with or without neck, midpiece, or tail defects)

Others: neck defects (a bend of > 30 degrees), midpiece defects, tail defects (double or coiled), loose heads, and immature forms (cytoplasmic droplets) noted separately (reported per 100 spermatozoa)

This scheme has been used successfully on preparations stained using either the Papanicolaou of Diff-Quik methods. Typically, normal men show more than 14% normal forms by this strict scoring system.

WHO 1992 Classification

Considering all the above schemes for classifying human sperm morphology, it seemed appropriate to consider a revised system that incorporated the best aspects of each. Clear, objective definitions were needed for each defect in a system using multiple-entry scoring. Given these basic concepts, a combination of the original and modified David and Tygerberg systems was considered potentially ideal. However, the need to divide the results into multiple subcategories serves little purpose when calculating a multiple anomalies or teratozoospermia index, although each functional region of the spermatozoon should be represented. Consequently, based on the description of a normal spermatozoon presented in Chapter 2, the following list of categories is considered.

Head shape/size defects: large, small, tapering, pyriform, amorphous, vacuolated (> 20% of the head area occupied by unstained vacuolar areas), reduced acrosome (< 40% of the head area), absent acrosome, double head, or any combination of these characteristics

Neck and midpiece defects: absent tail ("free" or "loose" head), noninserted or bent tail (tail forms an angle of ≥ 90 degrees to the long axis of the head), distended/irregular midpiece, abnormally thin midpiece (i.e., no mitochondrial sheath), or any combination.

Tail defects: short, multiple, hairpin, broken (angulation of ≥ 90 degrees), irregular width, terminal droplet, coiled, or any combination (**N.B.** For reasons discussed earlier, the proportion of coiled tails should be noted separately if it exceeds 10% of the spermatozoa.)

Immature forms: cytoplasmic droplets more than one-third the area of a normal sperm head

Conjoined forms are distinct from double-headed or multiple-tailed spermatozoa in that they are clearly two (or more) spermatozoa that are conjoined ("siamese twins") due to defective spermiation. Defects in each cell are scored independently, including the region of fusion as being abnormal.

This scheme allows a simplified counting system to be used that requires only five tally counters, although the four defect categories must be tallied independently, and only one cell is contributed to the total counted for an abnormal spermatozoon's combination of defects. All "borderline" or "doubtful" spermatozoa are considered abnormal, and an eyepiece micrometer may be used to ensure accurate application of morphometric criteria. Because spermatozoa lying on their sides should be excluded from the analysis, great care must be taken when preparing the smears not to make them too thick. Highly viscous specimens should be diluted with an isoosmotic medium, i.e., equivalent to seminal plasma, not blood (about 360 mOsm, not 290 mOsm) before smearing.

A (modified) teratozoospermia index can be calculated to represent the average number of defects per abnormal spermatozoon in the sample, although it now has a range of 1.00–4.00.

References and Recommended Reading

Aitken, R. J., and West, K. M. (1990). Analysis of the relationship between reactive oxygen species production and leucocyte infiltration in fractions of human semen as separated on Percoll gradients. *Int. J. Androl.* **13,** 433.

Aitken, R. J., Kerr, L., Bolton, V., and Hargreave, T. (1990). Analysis of sperm function in globozoospermia: implications for the mechanism of sperm-zona interaction. *Fertil. Steril.* **54,** 701.

Barratt, C. L. R., Bolton, A. E., and Cooke, I. D. (1990). Functional significance of white blood cells in the male and female reproductive tract. *Hum. Reprod.* **5,** 639.

Belsey, M. A., Eliasson, R., Gallegos, A. J., Moghissi, K. S., Paulsen, C. A., and Prasad, M.R.N. (1980). *Laboratory Manual for the Examination of Human Semen and Semen-Cervical Mucus Interaction.* Press Concern, Singapore.

Brindley, G. S. (1983). Physiology of erection and management of paraplegic infertility. In Hargreave, T. B. (ed): *Male Infertility.* Springer-Verlag, Berlin.

Cohen, J., and Aafjes, J. H. (1982). Proteolytic enzymes stimulate human spermatozoal motility and in vitro hamster egg penetration. *Life Sci.* **30,** 899.

Crich, J. P., and Jequier, A. M. (1978). Infertility in men with retrograde ejaculation: the action of urine on sperm motility, and a simple method for achieving antegrade ejaculation. *Fertil. Steril.* **30,** 572.

David, G., Bisson, J. P., Czyglik, F., Jouannet, P., and Gernigon, C. (1975). Anomalies morphologiques du spermatozoïde humain. 1. Propositions pour un système de classification. *J. Gynecol. Obstet. Biol. Reprod.* **4(Suppl. I),** 17.

De Ziegler, D., Cedars, M. I., Hamilton, F., Moreno, T., and Meldrum, D. R. (1987). Factors influencing maintenance of sperm motility during in vitro processing. *Fertil. Steril.* **48,** 816.

Dunphy, B. C., Neal, L. M., and Cooke, I. D. (1989). The clinical value of conventional semen analysis. *Fertil. Steril.* **51,** 324.

Ginsburg, K., and Armant, D. R. (1990). The influence of chamber characteristics on the reliability of sperm concentration and movement measurements obtained by manual and videomicrographic analysis. *Fertil. Steril.* **53,** 882.

Jeulin, C., Feneux, D., Serres, C., Jouannet, P., Guillet-Rosso, F., Belaisch-Allart, J., Fryd-man, R., and Testart, J. (1986). Sperm factors related to failure of human in-vitro fertil-ization. *J. Reprod. Fertil.* **76**, 735.

Jeyendran, R. S., Van der Ven, H. H., Perez-Pelaez, M., Crabo, B., and Zaneveld, L.J.D. (1984). Development of an assay to assess the functional integrity of the human sperm membrane and its relationship to other semen characteristics. *J. Reprod. Fertil.* **70**, 219.

Jouannet, P., Ducot, B., Feneux, D., and Spira, A. (1988). Male factors and the likelihood of pregnancy in infertile couples. I. Study of sperm characteristics. *Int. J. Androl.* **11**, 379.

Knuth, U. A., Neuwinger, J., and Nieschlag, E. (1989). Bias to routine semen analysis by uncontrolled changes in laboratory environment—detection by long-term sampling of monthly means for quality control. *Int. J. Androl.,* **12**, 375.

Kruger, T. F., Menkveld, R., Stander, F.S.H., Lombard, C. J., Van der Merwe, J. P., Van Zyl, J. A., and Smith, K. (1986). Sperm morphologic features as a prognostic factor in in vitro fertilization. *Fertil. Steril.* **46**, 1118.

MacLeod, J. (1964). Human seminal cytology as a sensitive indicator of the germinal epithe-lium *Int. J. Fertil.* **9**, 281.

MacLeod, J. (1965). Seminal cytology in the presence of varicocele. *Fertil. Steril.* **16**, 735.

Menkveld, R., Stander, F.S.H., Kotze, T.J.vW., Kruger, T. F., and van Zyl, J. A. (1990). The evaluation of morphological characteristics of human spermatozoa according to stricter criteria. *Hum. Reprod.* **5**, 586.

Mortimer, D. (1985). The male factor in infertility Part I. Semen analysis. *Curr. Probl. Obstet. Gynecol. Fertil.* Vol. VIII (7), 87 pp. Year Book Medical Publishers, Chicago.

Mortimer, D. (1990). Objective analysis of sperm motility and kinematics. In Keel, B. A., and Webster, B. W. (eds): *Handbook of the Laboratory Diagnosis and Treatment of Infertility.* CRC Press, Boca Raton, FL.

Mortimer, D. (1991). Sperm preparation techniques and iatrogenic failures of in-vitro fertil-ization. *Hum. Reprod.* **6**, 173.

Mortimer, D., Leslie, E. E., Kelly, R. W., and Templeton, A. A. (1982). Morphological selec-tion of human spermatozoa *in vivo* and *in vitro. J. Reprod. Fertil.* **64**, 391.

Mortimer, D., Mortimer, S. T., Shu, M. A., and Swart, R. (1989). A simplified approach to sperm-cervical mucus interaction using a hyaluronate migration test. *Hum. Reprod.* **5**, 835.

Mortimer, D., Shu, M. A., and Tan, R. (1986). Standardization and quality control of sperm concentration and sperm motility counts in semen analysis. *Hum. Reprod.* **1**, 299.

Mortimer, D., Shu M. A., Tan, R., and Mortimer, S. T. (1989). A technical note on diluting semen for the haemocytometric determination of sperm concentration. *Hum. Reprod.* **4**, 166.

Pandya, I. J., Mortimer, D., and Sawers, R. S. (1986). A standardized approach for evaluating the penetration of human spermatozoa into cervical mucus *in vitro. Fertil. Steril.* **45**, 357.

Wolff, H., and Anderson, D. J. (1988). Immunohistologic characterization and quantitation of leukocyte subpopulations in human semen. *Fertil. Steril.* **49**, 497.

World Health Organization (1987). *WHO Laboratory Manual for the Examination of Human Semen and Semen-Cervical Mucus Interaction,* 2nd ed. Cambridge University Press, Cambridge.

World Health Organization (1992). *WHO Laboratory Manual for the Examination of Human Semen and Sperm-Cervical Mucus Interaction,* 3rd ed. Cambridge University Press, Cambridge.

4

Biochemistry of Spermatozoa and Seminal Plasma

As discussed in Chapter 2, human seminal plasma is a complex secretion containing numerous substances some of which are specific for the accessory gland, which contributed a fraction of the ejaculate. These substances in particular can be diagnostically useful as markers for the presence or absence, dysfunction, or infection of particular accessory glands. It is now generally accepted that seminal plasma biochemical markers are expressed in quantities per ejaculate rather than per milliliter (e.g., World Health Organization, 1992) as it is considered to better reflect the secretory capacity of the particular accessory gland.

Because the prostate and seminal vesicles are essentially multiglandular (see Chapter 2), more than one biochemical marker should be monitored for each. In addition, for quantitative biochemical investigations of the seminal plasma to be meaningful it is important that several basic conditions be met.

1. The ejaculate must be complete and produced after a standard period of sexual abstinence.
2. The aliquots for biochemical assay must be taken at a standard time after ejaculation from a well-mixed, completely liquefied specimen.
3. A set of biochemical analyses should be performed (at the very minimum fructose and acid phosphatase are assayed).
4. Any abnormal or unusual values must be confirmed before drawing definite conclusions and making clinical management decisions.

In addition, there are a number of substances that are specific to the spermatozoa in an ejaculate; and their levels in seminal plasma, originating in their leakage from the spermatozoa, may be used to assess sperm integrity.

BIOCHEMISTRY OF SPERMATOZOA

Although there is a vast literature on the structural and functional components of spermatozoa, it is not relevant to the present text to discuss the biochemical composition of human spermatozoa. Rather, an overview of some biochemical aspects of human spermatozoa is provided that may be useful diagnostically for determining sperm integrity (see also Sperm Vitality in Chapter 3) and sperm function or functional potential.

Acrosin

Acrosin, a trypsin-like protease, is essential for fertilization in vivo and in vitro; it is specific to the acrosome, where it is present in its zymogen form, proacrosin. Conversion of proacrosin to acrosin may occur within the acrosome as an early feature of the acrosome reaction prior to membrane vesiculation (see Chapter 2). An acrosin inhibitor is also present, and determinations of total acrosin must take this into account, as well as ensuring full conversion of proacrosin to acrosin (optimal at alkaline pH, e.g., 8.0).

Quantitative Enzymatic Determination

Acrosin activity is assayed using its hydrolysis of benzoyl arginine ethyl ester (BAEE) as substrate after extraction from spermatozoa at acidic pH (e.g., 2.5–3.0 to dissociate the acrosin–inhibitor complex). The reaction is followed spectrophotometrically at 253 nm, the point of maximum absorption difference between BAEE and benzoyl arginine. Acrosin activity is usually expressed as micromoles of BAEE hydrolyzed (i.e., international enzyme units) per 10^6 or 10^9 spermatozoa (Polakoski and Zaneveld, 1977).

A simplified assay that incorporates benzamidine inhibition to ensure that the enzymatic activity measured in entirely due to acrosin (the only benzamidine-sensitive protease found in spermatozoa) has been described (Kennedy et al., 1989), and a kit is commercially available (Accu-Sperm: OEM Concepts, Toms River, NJ, USA). "Fertile" men had acrosin levels of 14–60 µIU/10^6 spermatozoa (Kennedy et al., 1989), and total acrosin levels correlate with IVF success (Tummon et al., 1991).

Gelatin Film Lysis Test

The gelatin film lysis test allows investigation of the relative acrosin content of individual spermatozoa. It is based on the leakage of active acrosin from spermatozoa dried onto a gelatin film substrate. The enzyme lyses an area of the film around each sperm head, and the diameter (or area) of the lysed circle is more or less proportional to the amount of enzyme that was contained in the spermatozoon's acrosome (Ficsor et al., 1983). Although this test is relatively simple to perform and has a great advantage in that it assesses acrosin content at the individual cell level, its clinical relevance remains unproven.

ATP Content

The adenosine triphosphate (ATP) content of human semen has been proposed as a quantitative estimate of sperm fertilizing potential (Comhaire et al., 1983). Although much effort has been expended in measuring ATP and attempting to correlate it with other measures of sperm function and with fertility, the final conclusion is that it is only another facet of the number of live spermatozoa and probably has little clinical relevance (Irvine and Aitken, 1985).

Chromatin Condensation Assessments

Although mammalian sperm chromatin is highly condensed and inactive, the degree of condensation varies widely among cells. Two approaches have been used to evaluate this parameter as a possible test of sperm structural and functional status.

Aniline Blue Staining

Simple staining of the sperm nucleus by aniline blue reveals disturbed chromatin condensation by increased intensity staining of the sperm head. The method briefly described below is modified from Dadoune et al. (1988) and Auger et al. (1990).

Either seminal spermatozoa or a prepared sperm population (e.g., swim-up from semen or Percoll gradient methods) is adjusted to 5×10^6 to 10×10^6 spermatozoa/ml. Aliquots of 25 µl volume are spread over the end 1–2 cm of at least two clean microscope slides and allowed to air-dry. The slides are then fixed in 3% (v/v) glutaraldehyde (12.5 ml of 25% v/v glutaraldehyde in 87.5 ml PBS) for 30 minutes at ambient temperature. Aniline blue stain is a 5.0% (w/v) solution of aniline blue (CI 42775) in PBS; this solution is about pH 3.5 and should be filtered using a Whatman No. 2 paper before use). Slides are stained for 5 minutes at ambient temperature, rinsed in PBS, and allowed to air-dry before being mounted using DPX.

Slides are examined under brightfield optics (Köhler illumination) at 1000× magnification. Cells are considered normal if the aniline blue stain has not been taken up by the sperm head (i.e., nucleus). Results are expressed as the percentage of spermatozoa with unstained heads (i.e., mature nuclei). Differentiation of degrees of aniline blue staining is of unknown value, although distinction between morphologically normal and abnormal spermatozoa may clearly have some relevance.

Acridine Orange Fluorescence

Acridine orange can be used to distinguish between spermatozoa with native DNA (green fluorescence) and single-stranded DNA (orange-red fluorescence) as a marker for abnormal chromatin condensation. The method briefly described below is modified from Royere et al. (1988).

Seminal spermatozoa or a prepared sperm population (e.g., swim-up from semen or Percoll gradient methods) is adjusted to 5×10^6 to 10×10^6 spermatozoa/ml. Aliquots of 25 µl volume are spread over the end 1–2 cm of at least two clean microscope slides and allowed to air-dry. A further aliquot of at least 200 µl is boiled (100°C) for 30 minutes, mixed thoroughly, and used to prepare slides as before. The slides are fixed in Carnoy's solution (1:3 glacial acetic acid/absolute methanol) for 2 hours.

Pairs of slides are then stained in acridine orange at pH 2.5 for 5 minutes at ambient temperature in the dark (e.g., in a foil-covered Coplin jar). The staining solution comprises 10.0 ml 0.1% (w/v) acridine orange (CI 46005) in reagent water, 40 ml 0.1 M citric acid, and 2.5 ml 0.3 M disodium orthophosphate (the stock acridine orange solution may be stored frozen at $-20°C$ until needed).

Acridine orange-stained slides must be kept in the dark. They are mounted using a special mountant and examined under epifluorescence using an appropriate filter set (see Appendix III). Count at least 200 spermatozoa, assessing each cell for the abnormal presence of orange-red fluorescence indicative of single-stranded DNA. Express the results as the percentage incidence of cells with "normal" and "abnormal" DNA, perhaps incorporating a distinction between morphologically normal and abnormal spermatozoa.

Of particular interest for the routine application of acridine orange staining is that it can also be assessed using flow cytometry. Application of this sperm chromatin structure assay has shown it to be an objective, biologically stable, sensitive measure of semen quality in toxicological studies (Evenson et al., 1991).

Creatine Kinase Content

The levels of creatine kinase (CK) in human sperm populations has been shown to be a good predictor of sperm fertilizing potential for oligozoospermic men during intrauterine insemination (Huszar et al., 1990). Whether this marker will be more generally applicable (e.g., for idiopathic infertility) remains unknown at this time, but it does show great promise as an additional biochemical test that might be related to sperm functional ability.

Basically, it seems that the spermatozoa containing high levels of CK activity do so because of a relatively large volume of retained (spermatid) cytoplasm. This morphological feature is abnormal, immature, or both and apparently is closely related to these spermatozoa's ability to produce reactive oxygen species (see below).

Glutamic-Oxaloacetic Transaminase

In domesticated species the leakage of intracellular enzymes, notably glutamic-oxaloacetic transaminase (GOT; EC 2.6.1.1), has long been employed as a marker of sperm integrity. Studies on the release of GOT from human spermatozoa indicate that it may also be a useful clinical marker for the loss of sperm integrity (Mortimer and Bramley, 1981; Mortimer et al., 1988).

Hyaluronidase

The enzyme hyaluronidase, which has classically been believed to be involved in facilitating sperm penetration through the cumulus mass (whose matrix consists largely of hyaluronic acid), is also located within the acrosome. Enzymatic methods that measure hyaluronidase activity are based on its hydrolysis of the bond between *N*-acetylhexosamines and D-glucuronate residues (Polakoski and Zaneveld, 1977). Although a modified film lysis test has also been reported, it is apparently far more difficult and much less reliable than that for acrosin (see above).

Lactate Dehydrogenase Isozymes

An isozyme of lactate dehydrogenase, known as LDH-C_4 (or LDH$_X$), is specific to spermatozoa. Measurement of its release from disintegrating dead spermatozoa into semen may be used to assess sperm integrity (Eliasson, 1982).

Nuclear Chromatin Decondensation Test

Principle

Although mammalian sperm chromatin is highly condensed and inactive in mature spermatozoa, human sperm chromatin has an intrinsic ability to decondense when exposed to a combination of detergent (sodium dodecylsulfate, or SDS) to lyse the cell membranes and a chelating agent (EDTA) to remove zinc ions that stabilize the sulfydryl groups on the protamines not involved in disulfide bonds (Kvist et al., 1980; Huret, 1986). Although this nuclear chromatin decondensation (NCD) ability does vary between the ejaculates of fertile and infertile men (Le Lannou and Blanchard, 1988), NCD testing has not been found to be predictive of IVF success (Liu et al., 1987).

Reagents

Tris buffer is prepared by dissolving 7.889 g NaCl (135 mM), 0.373 g KCl (5 mM), and 4.481 g Tris (37 mM) in reagent water to a total volume of 1 liter. The pH is adjusted to 8.0 using 5 N HCl.

Borate buffer is a 50 mM solution of borax prepared by dissolving $Na_2B_4O_7 \cdot H_2O$ at 19.07 g/L in reagent water. The pH is adjusted to 9.0 using 1 N NaOH.

SDS/EDTA solution is 1.0% SDS and 6 mM EDTA in borate buffer. Dissolve 1.0 g SDS and 0.228 g EDTA in borate buffer to a final volume of 100 ml.

Glutaraldehyde fixative is 1% (v/v) glutaraldehyde in borate buffer. It is prepared by mixing 4.0 ml stock (25% v/v) glutaraldehyde and 96 ml borate buffer.

Specimen

Either seminal spermatozoa or a prepared sperm population (e.g., swim-up from semen or Percoll gradient methods) is adjusted to at least 20×10^6 spermatozoa/ml and washed into Tris buffer. Only 400 µl of this sperm suspension is required, so each 200-µl aliquot contains at least 5×10^6 spermatozoa.

If seminal spermatozoa are being used, they must be washed at least one extra time (600 g for 5 minutes) using Tris buffer.

Method

1. Transfer two 200-µl aliquots of the sperm suspension in Tris buffer into 1.5-ml Eppendorf tubes. Mark one CONTROL and the other TEST.
2. Centrifuge at 600 g for 5 minutes at ambient temperature.

3. Discard the supernatant and resuspend the pellets: Use 1.0 ml Tris buffer for the CONTROL tube and 1.0 ml SDS/EDTA for the TEST tube.
4. Incubate at ambient temperature for *exactly* 5 minutes.
5. Add 1.0 ml glutaraldehyde fixative to each tube and mix thoroughly.
6. Allow to stand at least 20 minutes.
7. Centrifuge the tubes at 1000 g for 10 minutes.
8. Discard the supernatants and resuspend the pellets in 200 µl Tris buffer.
9. Using at least two 25-µl aliquots of each resuspended pellet, make smear preparations on clean microscope slides and allow to air-dry.
10. Fix the slides with 75% (v/v) ethanol for 1 minute and stain according to the Shorr method (see Chapter 3).
11. Mount the slides with DPX or equivalent mountant and allow to stand overnight for the mountant to dry.
12. Examine under brightfield optics (Köhler illumination) at 1000× magnification. Slides must be randomized and coded before scoring to eliminate observer bias. Count at least 200 spermatozoa per slide and classify according to the following scheme of assessment of the sperm head.

Normal (N)	not swollen at all
Doubtful (D)	slight swelling changes
Swollen (S)	definitely swollen
Very swollen (S+)	highly swollen with dispersing chromatin

Results

Calculate the percentage incidence of each class on each slide and then break the randomization code. If a pair of slides is not within 10% for major classes (i.e., those including at least 25% of the spermatozoa), a third slide should be coded and scored and the three sets of values averaged to give the final result. Otherwise, calculate the average incidence of each class from the pair of slides. To check that the pairs of values are within 10%, use the formula:

$$\text{(Higher value } - \text{ lower value)} \leq \text{(sum of values} \div 20)$$

Results may be expressed as the proportion of normal cells (class N only) or of swollen cells (combined classes S and S+). A weighted score may also be used to express the results of the NCD test (Huret, 1983). It is calculated from the final scores according to the formula:

$$WS = D + (S \times 2.5) + (S+ \times 4)$$

Reactive Oxygen Species Production

Human spermatozoa are capable of generating reactive oxygen species (ROS), or free radicals, a property that has been implicated in the etiology of male infertility (Aitken and Clarkson, 1987). Although ROS production is an activity normally associated with infiltrating leukocytes present in the semen, it is now known that a specific subpopulation of less dense spermatozoa (when prepared on Percoll density gradients) have the capacity to generate ROS (Aitken and West, 1990).

In addition to the irreversible damage that ROS have on spermatozoa during certain methods for sperm preparation (see Chapter 12), the simple presence of increased numbers of spermatozoa with this capacity in a semen sample is indicative of impaired sperm maturation or morphological abnormality. The basis of this problem is that these spermatozoa have retained excessive amounts of (spermatid) cytoplasm, a defect also detectable using the measurement of CK activity (see above).

Although measurement of ROS production is technically simple, it requires a very sensitive, expensive luminometer that can measure chemiluminescence using a probe that reacts with a variety of ROS including hydrogen peroxide, superoxide, and hydroxyl radicals (e.g., luminol). Treatment with the ionophore A23187 (10 μM) is used to trigger the generation of ROS.

In functional terms, sperm populations exhibiting high ROS-generating capacity have impaired fertilizing ability (Aitken et al., 1989a,b). Unfortunately, prohibitive equipment cost hinders routine application of this assay, which will probably remain of research interest only for the present.

Malonaldehyde Production

The production of malonaldehyde is a measurable endpoint of sperm membrane phospholipid peroxidation (Alvarez et al., 1987). Malonaldehyde exhibits powerful spermicidal properties (Jones et al., 1979). However, a recent study has shown that another end-product of this process, (E)-4-hydroxy-2-nonenal (HNE), is more common and has greater cytotoxic effects (Selley et al., 1991). Furthermore, unlike malonaldehyde, HNE does not diffuse out into the surrounding aqueous phase but accumulates in the membranes.

BIOCHEMISTRY OF SEMINAL PLASMA

Secretory products specific for the human prostate are acid phosphatase, citric acid, zinc, and magnesium. Prostaglandins (PGs) and fructose are specific for the seminal vesicles. Markers that have been proposed for the epididymis include L($-$)-carnitine, glycerophosphocholine, and the enzyme neutral α,1-4 glucosidase or α-glucosidase (Cooper et al., 1988). Precise roles for all these substances have not yet been determined, although fructose certainly serves as a substrate for the glycolytic metabolism of spermatozoa. Zinc is probably involved in protecting the condensed chromatin within the sperm nuclei from becoming "superstabilized" as a result of excessive disulfide bond cross-linking of the protamines (by protecting free thiol side chains), and in seminal plasma much of the zinc is chelated by citrate.

Infection, dysfunction, aplasia, or dysplasia cannot be diagnosed on biochemical grounds alone. Cytological, microbiological, endocrinological, and, most importantly, clinical evaluations are needed as well. The following sections discuss the various markers (see Table 4-1 for normal ranges); and where routine methods exist, assay methods are given.

Acid Phosphatase

Principle

Acid phosphatase is a marker for prostatic function. Its assay is based on the hydrolysis of *p*-nitrophenylphosphate to *p*-nitrophenol at pH 4.8 and 37°C. The acid phosphatase activity is measured kinetically by the increased intensity of the yellow color (read as absorbance at 405 nm) formed during the reaction.

Reagents

Saline is a solution of 9.0 g NaCl in reagent water to a total volume of 1000 ml. Store at 4°C. Discard if there are any signs of contamination or sedimentation.

Citric acid buffer is prepared by dissolving 18.9 g citric acid and 165 ml 1 N NaOH in reagent water to 1000 ml. The resulting pH is 4.8. Store at 4°C. Discard if there are any signs of contamination or sedimentation.

PNPP substrate is Sigma 104 phosphatase substrate (Sigma Cat. No. 104-0) used at 5.5 mM in citric acid buffer. Dissolve 0.051 g in 30 ml; this amount is sufficient for up to 80 determinations.

NaOH 0.1 N is made by dissolving 4.0 g NaOH in reagent water up to 1000 ml. Store at 4°C. Discard if there are any signs of contamination or sedimentation.

Table 4–1   Normal ranges for biochemical constituents of seminal plasma

Substance	Units	Normal Range	Source
Acid phosphatase	U/ejac	≥ 200	WHO (1992)
	kU/l @ 37°C	96–750	Documenta Geigy (1970)
		127–1790	Abyholm et al. (1981)
L-Carnitine (free)	nmol/ejac	390–1830	Soufir et al. (1984)
Citric acid	μmol/ejac	≥ 52	WHO (1987, 1992)
	mmol/l	9.4–43.4	Dondero et al. (1972)
Fructose	μmol/ejac	≥ 13	WHO (1987, 1992)
	mmol/l	6.7–33.0	Eliasson (1977)
α-Glucosidase	mU/ejac	≥ 20	WHO (1992)
Glycerophosphocholine	μmol/ejac	1.2–22.6	Mieusset et al. (1988)
Magnesium	mmol/l	2.9–10.3	Eliasson (1977)
Prostaglandins[a]			
PG_E	μg/ml	73 (2–272)	Templeton
19-OH PG_E	μg/ml	267 (53–1094)	et al.
PG_F	μg/ml	2.1 (0.1–7.0)	(1978)
19-OH PG_F	μg/ml	18.3 (3–62)	
Zinc	μmol/ejac	≥ 2.4	WHO (1987, 1992)
	mmol/l	1.2–3.8	Eliasson (1977)

[a]Values are the mean (range).

Specimen

Cell-free seminal plasma is required for the assay. It is prepared from liquefied semen at exactly 30 minutes after ejaculation as follows.

1. Centrifuge semen at 1000 g for 15 minutes. Because only 20 µl of seminal plasma is required, it is recommended that only 100 µl of semen be centrifuged. Alternatively, the procedure may be combined with that for the preparation of seminal plasma to use in other procedures such as antibody titration.
2. A 20-µl aliquot of cell-free seminal plasma is diluted with 1.98 ml of saline (i.e., diluted 1/100 and stored in 4-ml autoanalyzer cups frozen at −20°C until assayed.

Method

1. Switch on the spectrophotometer and set for absorbance readings at 405 nm. Allow sufficient time for stabilization.
2. Set the waterbath to 37°C.
3. Calibrate the spectrophotometer against a reagent water blank.
4. Prepare pairs of test tubes for each unknown or control sample. Each tube requires 250 µl pH 4.8 citric acid buffer and 250 µl 5.5 mM PNPP substrate in citric acid buffer.
5. Incubate all tubes at 37°C for 5 minutes in the waterbath.
6. Dilute the thawed unknowns and control sample(s) 1 + 99 again with 0.9% NaCl, i.e., 20 µl sample + 1.98 ml saline.
7. Add 50 µl of the diluted seminal plasma samples to the reaction tubes, each sample in duplicate, at 15-second intervals (i.e., sufficient time for each pair of tubes to be read at the end of the assay).
8. Incubate at 37°C for 30 minutes in the waterbath.
9. Stop the reaction by adding 2.5 ml of 0.1 N NaOH at intervals in the same sequence as in step 7. Vortex mix each tube thoroughly.
10. Recheck the reagent water blank.
11. Read each determination and note the absorbance at 405 nm.

N.B. Acid phosphatase loses its activity at room temperature. Consequently, the initial aliquot is taken from the liquefied ejaculate at a standard time. In addition, the preparation of both the initial dilution and the post-thaw dilution at the time of assay must be performed as quickly as possible.

Results

Check that the pairs of values are within 10%, using the formula:

$$\text{(Higher value} - \text{lower value)} \leq \text{(sum of values} \div 20)$$

Samples whose pairs of values do not meet this requirement must be reassayed.

Acid phosphatase activity (in U/ml $\equiv$ kU/l in the original sample) is calculated using the average absorbance readings of the paired determinations in the following formula:

$$(\Delta A/min) \times (V \div v) \times DF \div E \div d = kU/l$$

where: V = total assay volume (3.05 ml)
          DF = dilution factor (10,000)
          E = absorption coefficient of p-nitrophenol at 405 nm (18.5 $cm^2/\mu mol$)
          d = light path (usually 1 cm)
          v = specimen volume (0.05 ml)

This equation condenses to: ΔA (per 30 minutes) $\times$ 1099 = kU/L

The accepted normal range for seminal acid phosphatase activity is ≥200 U per ejaculate (127–1790 kU/l) at 37°C. However, in view of the numerous factors that may influence the acid phosphatase activity present in a semen sample, the significance (if any) of values outside this range *must* be evaluated by a competent physician/andrologist.

Quality Control
No biochemical standards are used in this procedure, as the molar absorption coefficient of the product, p-nitrophenol, is known. Control material consists of a stock seminal plasma pool. Aliquots (100 µl) of this control sample are stored frozen at −70°C and are thawed immediately before the second dilution step in the procedure. This control sample must be run with each set of unknowns: control limits are the mean ± 2 SD from 10 independent determinations.

Values outside these limits are to be treated as follows. Thaw another control aliquot and prepare the dilution; prepare a new batch of PNPP substrate; repeat the assay, testing the new control sample against a standard enzyme control. If acceptable control levels are found, repeat the entire assay of unknowns with a new control sample and PNPP substrate preparation. If the control sample shows decreased activity, repeat the assay of unknowns using another control.

Carnitine

L(−)-Carnitine is primarily of epididymal origin, with only a minor contribution from either the seminal vesicles or the prostate. The most reliable assay for carnitine is enzymatic, using carnitine acetyltransferase, which is unfortunately rather expensive. Consequently, carnitine measurements are likely to remain of only research interest for some time.

Citric Acid

Principle
Citric acid can be an indicator of prostatic gland function. Decreased levels of citric acid may indicate either prostatic dysfunction or a prostatic duct obstruction. This assay method uses a Boehringer enzymatic, NADH-linked, kit.

Reagents

Boehringer Kit No. 130976 (sufficient for 3 × 15 determinations). It contains:

3 × Bottle 1 (mainly NADH), which is reconstituted by adding 12 ml reagent water and shaking well. Solution 1 is stable for 4 weeks at −20°C.

3 × Bottle 2 (citrate-lyase), which is reconstituted by adding 0.3 ml reagent water and shaking well. Solution 2 is stable for 4 weeks at −20°C.

TRA buffer pH 7.7 is prepared by dissolving 14.9 g triethanolamine in 750 ml reagent water and adjusting the pH to 7.6 by adding 1 N HCl. Dissolve 0.027 g $ZnCl_2$ in 250 ml reagent water and add it to the triethanolamine solution. Add 0.5 g of sodium azide and mix thoroughly.

TCA 15% is a solution of 15 g trichloroacetic acid in 100 ml reagent water.

NaOH 6 N is made by dissolving 24 g NaOH pellets in 100 ml reagent water.

Citric acid standard is a simple solution of 0.174 g citric acid in 10 ml reagent water. Make a 1 + 57 dilution of this standard as with the unknowns (25 µl + 1425 µl reagent water).

Specimen

Cell-free, protein-free seminal plasma is required for the assay. It is prepared from liquefied semen at exactly 30 minutes after ejaculation as follows.

1. Centrifuge 250 µl semen in an Eppendorf tube at 1000 *g* for 15 minutes.
2. Add 100 µl of the supernatant to 4.95 ml of 15% trichloroacetic acid in a small capped vial and shake well.
3. Add 0.75 ml 6 N NaOH. The pH must exceed 7.0; check with pH paper, and add more NaOH if necessary. The extract must be clear and should be centrifuged at 2000 *g* for 15 minutes if necessary.
4. Freeze three 0.5-ml aliquots of the extract in Eppendorf tubes at −20°C. (Discard any extra samples once a successful assay has been completed and reported.)

Method

1. Switch on the spectrophotometer, set for absorbance readings at 340 nm, and allow sufficient time for stabilization.
2. Mix the following reagents in disposable cuvettes (e.g., Fisher Scientific No. 14-385-985): 0.5 ml solution 1; 2.3 ml TRA buffer; and 0.2 ml sample, standard, or blank. Prepare duplicate tubes for each determination.
3. Zero the spectrophotometer with a cuvette containing reagent water.
4. For each sample, measure its initial absorbance (A1).
5. Add 20 µl solution 2. Shake, wait exactly 5 minutes, and measure the absorbance again (A2).

N.B.   a. A fresh citric acid standard must be prepared for each assay.

   b. For accurate analysis by this method the concentration of citric acid in a sample must fall between 0.02 and 0.40 mg/ml.

Results

Determine the absorbance differences (A1 − A2) for the blank (A_{BLANK}) and the samples (A_{SAMPLE}) and correct the A_{SAMPLE} values by subtracting the A_{BLANK} to get ΔA. Occasionally, a negative value of A_{BLANK} is obtained, and this value is added to A_{SAMPLE}.

Check that the pairs of values are within 10% using the formula:

$$(\text{Higher value} - \text{lower value}) \leq (\text{sum of values} \div 20)$$

Samples whose pairs of values do not meet this requirement must be reassayed.

The citric acid concentration in the original sample is calculated using the following general formula:

$$\Delta A \times (V \div v) \times DF \times MW \div E \div d \div 1000 = g/l$$

where: DF = specimen dilution factor (58)
           V   = final volume (3.02 ml)
           MW = molecular weight of substance assayed (192.1)
           E   = absorption coefficient of NADH at 340 nm (6.3 cm^2/μol)
           d   = light path (usually 1 cm)
           v   = sample volume (0.2 ml)

This equation condenses to: $\Delta A \times 139.0$ = mmol citric acid/l.

The accepted normal range for seminal citric acid concentrations is ≥52 μmol per ejaculate (9.4–43.4 mmol/l). However, in view of the numerous factors that may influence the concentration of citric acid present in a semen sample the significance (if any) of values outside this range *must* be evaluated by a competent physician/andrologist.

Quality Control

If, upon assay, the absorbance obtained for any determination of the standard falls outside the normal range (mean ± 2 SD obtained by 10 independent determinations), the standard must be discarded, a fresh one prepared, and the assay repeated.

Fructose: Quantitative Analysis

Principle

Fructose is a marker for seminal vesicle function. Its function in the seminal plasma is as a substrate for the glycolytic (anaerobic) metabolism of the spermatozoa. This assay method uses a Boehringer enzymatic, NADPH-linked, UV kit for glucose/fructose analysis.

Reagents

Perchloric acid 0.33 N is made by mixing 1.0 ml of 60% perchloric acid with 26.88 ml reagent water.
Boehringer Kit No. 139106 (sufficient for 18 determinations) contains:

Bottle 1 (NADP and ATP), which is reconstituted by dissolving the contents in 27 ml reagent water. Solution 1 is stable for 4 weeks at 4°C and for 2 months at −20°C.

Bottle 2 (enzymes) is used undiluted. Solution 2 is stable for 1 year at 4°C.

Bottle 3 (enzyme) is used undiluted. Solution 3 is stable for 1 year at 4°C.

Fructose standard is a simple solution of 600 mg fructose in 100 ml reagent water. Make a 60× dilution by adding 50 μl of the above to 2950 μl reagent water.

Specimen

Cell-free, protein-free seminal plasma is required for the assay. It is prepared from liquefied semen at exactly 30 minutes after ejaculation as follows.

1. Add 60 μl semen to 540 μl 0.33 N perchloric acid in a 1.5-ml Eppendorf tube and mix (i.e., 1/10 dilution).
2. Centrifuge at 1000 g for 15 minutes.
3. Freeze the supernatant in 1.5-ml Eppendorf tubes at −20°C as three 150-μl aliquots. Discard any extra samples once a successful assay has been completed and reported.

Method

1. Switch on the spectrophotometer, set for absorbance readings at 334 nm, and allow sufficient time for stabilization.
2. Zero the spectrophotometer with a cuvette containing reagent water.
3. Mix in disposable cuvettes (e.g., Fisher Scientific No. 14-385-985): 1.6 ml solution 1; 10 μl solution 2; and 60 μl sample, standard, or blank.
4. Wait 3 minutes.
5. Measure the initial absorbance (A1).
6. Add 20 μl of solution 3, mix, and wait 10 minutes.
7. Measure the absorbance again (A2).

N.B.   a. A fresh fructose standard *must* be prepared for each assay.

b. For accurate analysis by this method the concentration of fructose present in a sample must fall between 0.03 and 0.5 g/l

---

Results

Determine the absorbance differences (A1 − A2) for the blank, standards, and samples and correct the ΔA values by subtracting the blank. Each standard and patient sample must be run in duplicate and the ΔA values averaged if they are within 10% determined using the formula:

$$\text{(Higher value − lower value)} \leq \text{(sum of values} \div 20)$$

Samples whose pairs of values do not meet this requirement must be reassayed.

Fructose concentration in the original sample is calculated according to the following general formula:

$$\Delta A \times (V \div v) \times DF \times MW \div E \div d \div 1000 = g/l$$

where: DF = specimen dilution factor (10
         V   = final volume (1.69 ml)
         MW = molecular weight of substance assayed (180.16)
         E   = absorption coefficient of NADPH at 334 nm (6.18 cm^2/µmol)
         d   = light path (usually 1 cm)
         v   = sample volume (0.06 ml)

This equation condenses to: $\Delta A \times 45.6$ = mmol fructose/l.

The accepted normal range for seminal fructose is ≥13 µmol per ejaculate (6.7–33.0 mmol/l). However, in view of the numerous factors that may influence the concentration of fructose present in a semen sample, the significance (if any) of values outside this range *must* be evaluated by a competent physician/andrologist.

Quality Control

If the absorbance obtained for any determination made on the standards falls outside the normal range (mean ± 2 SD obtained from 10 independent determinations), the standards must be discarded and fresh ones assayed.

Fructose: Spot Test

Principle

Fructose is a marker for seminal vesicle function. Its function in the seminal plasma is as a substrate for the glycolytic (anaerobic) metabolism of the spermatozoa. The assay is a simple semiquantitative colorimetric test for any ketohexose (Jungreis et al., 1989).

Reagents

Test reagent is prepared by dissolving 0.4 g *p*-methylaminophenol sulfate (metol) in 20 ml 40% sulfuric acid. Use a brown glass bottle and cover in aluminum foil to minimize photooxidation. Store at 4°C when not in use. It remains stable for 2–3 months. Discard if there are any signs of contamination or sedimentation.

Fructose standard. A *stock solution* is made by dissolving 270 mg fructose in 100 ml reagent water (equivalent to 15 mmol fructose/l, an average seminal plasma value). This stock is stored at 4°C when not in use. Discard if there are any signs of contamination or sedimentation. The *working solution* is a 100× dilution using reagent water. Prepare daily and discard any unused portion at the end of the day.

Method

1. Preheat a white porcelain spotting plate to 55°C on an electric hotplate.
2. Dilute the test sample 1:100 with reagent water.
3. Place 20- and 50-µl aliquots of the test sample in separate wells on the spotting plate. In another well place 50 µl reagent water as a blank and 50 µl of the working fructose standard in another.
4. Allow all wells to evaporate to dryness.

5. Add one drop (about 50 μl) of reagent solution to each well.
6. After 10 minutes examine the wells for the development of distinct blue coloration or a blue ring, indicative of the presence of fructose (or any other keto-hexose).

Results

The intensity of the blue coloration is proportional to the ketohexose (fructose) concentration. Aldohexoses such as glucose do not react. Positive reactions in the 20- and 50-μl test sample wells correspond to semen fructose concentration of ≥2700 and ≥1080 μg/ml, respectively (i.e., ≥15 and ≥6 mmol/l, respectively).

The accepted normal range for seminal fructose is ≥13 μmol per ejaculate (6.7–33.0 mmol/l). If both test sample wells are negative, it is indicative of a deficiency of seminal fructose, i.e., < 1080 μg/ml or < 6 mmol/l. If only the 50-μl test well shows blue, the value is in the low normal range. In view of the numerous possible factors that may influence the concentration of fructose present in a semen sample the significance (if any) of values outside this range *must* be evaluated by a competent physician/andrologist.

Quality Control

This assay is a simple semiquantitative assay that does not require elaborate quality control measures. If the working fructose standard fails to show a blue color in the test, both it and the reagent should be discarded and fresh solutions prepared.

α-Glucosidase

Principle

The enzyme neutral α,1-4-glucosidase is secreted exclusively by the epididymis and is therefore considered a specific marker for epididymal function. Activity of the acid isoenzyme, which comes from the prostate, can be inhibited by SDS (Cooper et al., 1990; World Health Organization, 1992).

Reagents

Phosphate buffer (100 mM, pH 6.8) is prepared by mixing 12.0 ml 200 mM K_2HPO_4 and 13.0 ml 200 mM KH_2PO_4, adding about 15 ml reagent water, adjusting the pH to 6.8 using either KH_2PO_4 or K_2HPO_4 (if the pH is > 6.8 or < 6.8, respectively), and finally making up to 50 ml using more reagent water. Store at 4°C. Just before use add 1% (w/v) SDS (e.g., 50 mg SDS per 5 ml) as an inhibitor of acidic α-glucosidase.
PNPG substrate is *p*-nitrophenol glucopyranoside 5 mg/ml in pH 6.8 phosphate buffer. Stir at 50°C for about 10 minutes for complete dissolution.
Castanospermine is an α-glucosidase inhibitor. Prepare a 10 mM stock by dissolving 1 mg in 0.53 ml reagent water and store frozen at −20°C. For use, dilute the stock 1 + 9 (e.g., 100 μl castanospermine stock + 900 μl reagent water) and store at 4°C for use. Store spare aliquots frozen at −20°C.

Sodium carbonate is a 100 mM solution prepared by dissolving 6.20 g $Na_2CO_3 \cdot H_2O$ in 500 ml reagent water.

PNP standards, required for the standard curve, are prepared from a 5 mM stock solution of *p*-nitrophenol. The stock is made by dissolving 0.0695 g PNP in reagent water (with warming if necessary) and making it up to 100 ml. Store at 4°C in a brown glass bottle.

Specimen

Sperm-free seminal plasma is prepared by centrifuging an aliquot of semen at 1000 *g* for 15 minutes. It may be stored frozen at −20°C until assayed.

Method

1. Prepare a waterbath at exactly 37°C for the incubation step (step 5).
2. Thaw out and vortex-mix the specimens to be assayed.
3. Prepare the PNPG substrate solution in Eppendorf tubes (2 × 100 μl for each sample or blank).
4. Using a positive displacement pipette, add duplicate 10-μl specimen aliquots into the Eppendorf tubes. Include water as a blank as well as high and low internal standards and semen blanks (see Quality Control, below).
5. Vortex-mix each tube and incubate for exactly 4 hours at 37°C.
6. *PNP standard curve* is prepared within 1 hour of reading the assay. Dilute 400 μl of the 5 mM stock PNP up to 20 ml in Na_2CO_3 solution to give a 100 μM standard and then dilute this standard volumetrically using Na_2CO_3 to give other standards of 80, 60, 40, 20, and 0 μM. Read the absorbance of all six standards at 405 nm.
7. Stop the reaction by adding 1.0 ml of Na_2CO_3 to each tube and vortexing.
8. Read the absorbance of each sample at 405 nm against a water blank.

Results

Glucosidase activity is expressed in micromolar units, i.e., 1 unit = 1 μmol PNP produced per minute at 37°C. The slope of the standard curve (S) is the absorbance per micromole. Glucosidase activity is calculated from the formula:

$$[(A_{SAMPLE} - A_{BLANK}) \div S] \times [V \div v] \div 240 = mU/ml$$

where: A_{SAMPLE} = absorbance of the sample tube
A_{BLANK} = mean absorbance of the semen blank tubes
S = slope of the standard curve
V = total assay volume (i.e., 1.11 ml)
v = specimen volume (i.e., 0.01 ml)
240 = Duration of the incubation (in minutes)

This equation condenses to: $\Delta A \div S \times 0.46 = mU/ml$.

Multiply this activity by the original ejaculate volume to obtain milliunits per ejaculate. Normal values are ≥ 20 mU/ejaculate.

Each standard and patient sample must be run in duplicate and the ΔA values averaged if they are within 10% determined using the formula:

$$(\text{Higher value} - \text{lower value}) \leq (\text{sum of values} \div 20)$$

Samples whose pairs of values do not meet this requirement must be reassayed.

Quality Control

Internal standards for interassay control should be included in each run. Seminal plasma standards (pools or from a large-volume ejaculate) should be established with high and low α-glucosidase activity. In addition, semen blanks should be run with each assay; the blanks are aliquots of the internal standards with 5 µl of the castanospermine solution added to inhibit α-glucosidase activity. If the absorbance obtained for any determination made on the standards falls outside the normal range (mean $\pm$ 2 SD obtained from 10 independent determinations), the standards must be discarded and fresh ones assayed.

Glycerophosphocholine

Although glycerophosphocholine (GPC) has been proposed as a marker of epididymal function, some also comes from the seminal vesicles, making its biochemical assay rather more uncertain as a clinical application.

Magnesium

Magnesium in seminal plasma, like zinc, is best measured by atomic absorption spectrosocopy, although a colorimetric method does exist (Polakoski and Zaneveld, 1977). The reported normal range for seminal plasma magnesium is 2.9–10.3 mmol/l (Eliasson, 1977).

Prostaglandins

The origins, functions, and classes of prostaglandins (PGs) in semen have long been the subject of debate. Although it is now known that they originate from the seminal vesicles and they are primarily PGEs and 19-OH PGEs, their functional importance remains unknown. Suggested functions include the stimulation of sperm motility at ejaculation and possible roles as ionophores. However, any role in the induction of rapid sperm transport in the female tract now seems unlikely (see Chapter 2).

The most sensitive and reliable technique for the assay of PGs is by gas chromatography with mass spectrometry. Mean concentrations of PGs in the semen of fertile men have been reported as 73 µg PGE/ml, 267 µg 19-OH PGE/ml, 2.1 µg PGF/ml, and 18.3 µg 19-OH PGF/ml, with wide ranges (Templeton et al., 1978). Until the roles of PGs in semen are better understood, however, their routine measurement is of little clinical value.

Zinc

Principle

Zinc is a marker for prostatic function. Although atomic absorption is the preferred method for its analysis, a reliable colorimetric method is available (Johnsen and Eliasson, 1987).

Reagents

The kit of reagents (obtained from Wako Pure Chemical Industries, Osaka, Japan) is stable for several years at temperatures below 25°C. The relationship between absorbance and seminal plasma zinc concentration is linear up to at least 7 mM.

Chromogen solution is prepared by mixing color reagents A and B in proportions of 4:1 (e.g., 20 ml A and 5 ml B). This mixture is stable for 1 week at 2°–10°C and for 2 days at ambient temperature.

Zinc standard is supplied by the kit manufacturer as a 30.6 μmol/l solution.

Specimen

Cell-free seminal plasma is required for the assay. It is prepared from liquefied semen at exactly 30 minutes after ejaculation as follows.

1. Centrifuge semen at 1000 *g* for 15 minutes. Because only 10 μl of neat seminal plasma is required, it is recommended that only 100 μl of semen be centrifuged; alternatively, the procedure can be combined with that for the preparation of seminal plasma for other procedures, such as antibody titration.
2. A 10-μl aliquot of cell-free seminal plasma is diluted with 1.99 ml of saline (i.e., 1/200 dilution) and stored in 4-ml autoanalyzer cups frozen at −20°C until assayed.

N.B. A protein precipitation step is unnecessary because of the high dilution of the seminal plasma before adding the color reagent.

Method

1. Switch on the spectrophotometer, set for absorbance readings at 560 nm, and allow sufficient time for stabilization.
2. Prepare pairs of test tubes with 0.5 ml zinc standard or diluted seminal plasma (use reagent water in one tube as a blank).
3. Add 2.5 ml working chromogen solution to each tube and mix well.
4. Leave at ambient temperature for 5 minutes.
5. Measure the absorbance within 1 hour.

Results

Each standard and patient sample must be run in duplicate and the ΔA values averaged if they are within 10% determined using the formula:

$$(\text{Higher value} - \text{lower value}) \leq (\text{sum of values} \div 20)$$

Samples whose pairs of values do not meet this requirement must be reassayed.

Subtract the absorbance difference of the blank from that of each average value for the standards and samples to obtain the $A_{STANDARD}$ and A_{SAMPLE} absorbance values. Calculate the concentration of zinc in the original seminal plasma using the formula:

$$(A_{SAMPLE} \div A_{STANDARD}) \times \text{STANDARD} \times \text{DF} \div 1000 = \text{mmol/l}$$

where: STANDARD = zinc solution concentration (30.6 mmol/l)
DF = specimen dilution factor (200)

The accepted normal range for seminal zinc is ≥ 2.4 µmol per ejaculate (1.2–3.8 mmol/l). In view of the numerous factors that may influence the concentration of zinc present in a semen sample, the significance (if any) of values outside this range *must* be evaluated by a competent physician/andrologist.

Quality Control
If duplicate absorbance values are not within 10%, the sample must be reassayed.

References and Recommended Reading

Åbyholm, T., Kofstad, J., Molne, K., and Stray-Pedersen, S. (1981). Seminal plasma fructose, zinc, magnesium and acid phosphatase in cases of male infertility. *Int. J. Androl.* **4,** 75.

Aitken, R. J., and Clarkson, J. S. (1987). Cellular basis of defective sperm function and its association with the genesis of reactive oxygen species by human spermatozoa. *J. Reprod. Fertil.* **81,** 459.

Aitken, R. J., and West, K. M. (1990). Analysis of the relationship between reactive oxygen species production and leucocyte infiltration in fractions of human semen separated on Percoll gradients. *Int. J. Androl.* **13,** 433.

Aitken, R. J., Clarkson, J. S., and Fishel, S. (1989a). Generation of reactive oxygen species, lipid peroxidation, and sperm function. *Biol. Reprod.* **41,** 183.

Aitken, R. J., Clarkson, J. S., Hargreave, T. B., Irvine, D. S., and Wu, F. C. W. (1989b). Analysis of the relationship between defective sperm function and the generation of reactive oxygen species in cases of oligozoospermia. *J. Androl.* **10,** 214.

Alvarez, J. G., Touchstone, J. C., Blasco, L., and Storey, B. T. (1987). Spontaneous lipid peroxidation and production of hydrogen peroxide and superoxide in human spermatozoa. Superoxide dismutase as major enzyme protectant against oxygen toxicity. *J. Androl.* **8,** 338.

Auger, J., Mesbah, M., Huber, C., and Dadoune, J. P. (1990). Aniline blue staining as a marker of sperm chromatin defects associated with different semen characteristics discriminates between proven fertile and suspected infertile men. *Int. J. Androl.* **13,** 452.

Comhaire, F., Vermeulen, L., Ghedira, K., Mas, J., Irvine, S., and Callipolitis, G. (1983). Adenosine triphosphate in human semen: a quantitative estimate of fertilizing potential. *Fertil. Steril.* **40,** 500.

Cooper, T. G., Yeung, C.-H., Nashan, D., and Nieschlag, E. (1988). Epididymal markers in human infertility. *J. Androl.* **9,** 91.

Cooper, T. G., Yeung, C.-H., Nashan, D., Jockenhövel, F., and Nieschlag, E. (1990). Improvement in the assessment of human epididymal function by the use of inhibitors in the assay of α-glucosidase in seminal plasma. *Int. J. Androl.* **13,** 297.

Dadoune, J. P., Mayaux, M. J., and Guihard-Moscato, M. L. (1988). Correlation between defects in chromatin condensation of human spermatozoa stained by aniline blue and semen characteristics. *Andrologia* **20,** 211.

Documenta Geigy (1970). *Scientific Tables,* 7th ed. Diem, K., and Lentner, C. (eds). Geigy Pharmaceuticals, Macclesfield, UK.

Dondero, F., Sciaria, F., and Isidori, A. (1972). Evaluation of relationship between plasma testosterone and human seminal citric acid. *Fertil. Steril.* **23,** 168.

Eliasson, R. (1977). Semen analysis and laboratory workup. In Cockett, A. T. K., and Urry, R. L. (eds): *Male Infertility. Workup, Treatment and Research.* Grune & Stratton, Orlando, FL.

Eliasson, R. (1982). Biochemical analysis of human semen. *Int. J. Androl.* **Suppl. 5,** 109.

Evenson, D. P., Jost, L. K., Baer, R. K., Turner, T. W., and Schrader, S. M. (1991). Individuality of DNA denaturation patterns in human sperm as measured by the sperm chromatin structure assay. *Reprod. Toxicol.* **5,** 115.

Ficsor, G., Ginsberg, L. C., Oldford, G. M., Snoke, R. E., and Becker, R. W. (1983). Gelatin-substrate film technique for detection of acrosin in single mammalian sperm. *Fertil. Steril.* **39,** 548.

Harrison, R. A. P. (1983). The acrosome, its hydrolases, and egg penetration. In André, J. (ed): *The Sperm Cell. Fertilizing Power, Surface Properties, Motility, Nucleus and Acrosome, Evolutionary Aspects.* Martinus Nijhoff, The Hague.

Huret, J. L. (1983). Variability of the chromatin decondensation ability test on human sperm. *Arch. Androl.* **11,** 1.

Huret, J. L. (1986). Nuclear chromatin decondensation of human sperm: a review. *Arch. Androl.* **16,** 97.

Huszar, G., Vigue, L., and Corrales, M. (1990). Sperm creatine kinase activity in fertile and infertile oligozoospermic men. *J. Androl.* **11,** 40.

Irvine, D. S., and Aitken, R. J. (1985). The value of adenosine triphosphate (ATP) measurements in assessing the fertilizing ability of human spermatozoa. *Fertil. Steril.* **44,** 806.

Johnsen, O., and Eliasson, R. (1987). Evaluation of a commercially available kit for the colorimetric determination of zinc in human seminal plasma. *Int. J. Androl.* **10,** 435.

Jones, R., Mann, T., and Sherins, R. (1979). Peroxidative breakdown of phospholipids in human spermatozoa, spermicidal properties of fatty acid peroxides, and protective action of seminal plasma. *Fertil. Steril.* **31,** 531.

Jungreis, E., Nechama, M., Paz, G., and Homonnai, T. (1989). A simple spot test for the detection of fructose deficiency in semen. *Int. J. Androl.* **12,** 195.

Kennedy, W. P., Kaminski, J. M., Van der Ven, H. H., Jeyendran, R. S., Reid, D. S., Blackwell, J., Bielfeld, P., and Zaneveld, L. J. D. (1989). A simple, clinical assay to evaluate the acrosin activity of human spermatozoa. *J. Androl* **10,** 221.

Kvist, U., Afzelius, B. A., and Nilsson, L. (1980). The intrinsic mechanism of chromatin decondensation and its activation in human spermatozoa. *Dev. Growth Differ.* **22,** 543.

Le Lannou, D., and Blanchard, Y. (1988). Nuclear maturity and morphology of human spermatozoa selected by Percoll density gradient centrifugation or swim-up procedure. *J. Reprod. Fertil.* **84,** 551

Liu, D. Y., Elton, R. A., Johnston, W. I. H., and Baker, H. W. G. (1987). Spermatozoal nuclear chromatin decondensation *in vitro*: A test for sperm immaturity. Comparison with results of human *in vitro* fertilisation. *Clin. Reprod. Fertil.* **5,** 191.

Mieusset, R., Bujan, L., Mansat, A., Pontonnier, F., Grandjean, H., and Chap, H. (1988). Glycerophosphocholine in seminal plasma of fertile and infertile men. *Int. J. Androl.* **11**, 405.

Mortimer, D., and Bramley, T. A. (1981). Evaluation of the measurement of glutamic-oxalacetic transaminase leakage from human spermatozoa as an indicator of cryodamage. *Arch. Androl.* **6**, 337.

Mortimer, D., Johnson, A. V., and Long-Simpson, L. K. (1988). Glutamic-oxaloacetic transaminase isozymes in human seminal plasma and sperm extracts. *Int. J. Fertil.* **33**, 291.

Polakoski, K. L., and Zaneveld, L. J. D. (1977). Biochemical examination of the human ejaculate. In Hafez, E. S. E. (ed): *Techniques of Human Andrology.* Elsevier/North Holland, Amsterdam.

Royere, D., Hamamah, S., Nicolle, J. C., Barthelemy, C., and Lansac, J. (1988). Freezing and thawing alter chromatin stability of ejaculated human spermatozoa: fluorescence acridine orange staining and Feulgen-DNA cytophotometric studies. *Gamete Res.* **21**, 51.

Selley, M. L., Lacey, M. J., Bartlett, M. R., Copeland, C. M., and Ardlie, N. G. (1991). Content of significant amounts of a cytotoxic end-product of lipid peroxidation in human semen. *J. Reprod. Fertil.* **92**, 291.

Soufir, J. C., Ducot, B., Marson, J., Jouannet, P., Feneux, D., Soumah, A., and Spira, A. (1984). Levels of seminal free L($-$)carnitine in fertile and infertile men. *Int. J. Androl.* **7**, 188.

Templeton, A. A., Cooper, I., and Kelly, R. W. (1978). Prostaglandin concentrations in the semen of fertile men. *J. Reprod. Fertil.* **52**, 147.

Tummon, I. S., Yuzpe, A. A., Daniel, S. A. J., and Deutsch, A. (1991). Total acrosin activity correlates with fertility potential after fertilization in vitro. *Fertil. Steril.* **56**, 933.

World Health Organization (1987). *WHO Laboratory Manual for the Examination of Human Semen and Semen-Cervical Mucus Interaction,* 2nd ed. Cambridge University Press, Cambridge.

World Health Organization (1992). *WHO Laboratory Manual for the Examination of Human Semen and Sperm-Cervical Mucus Interaction,* 3rd ed. Cambridge University Press, Cambridge.

5

Antisperm Antibodies

That postmeiotic male germ cells, spermatozoa, or sperm antigens can induce the production of auto- and isoantibodies that may interfere with fertility has been established since the beginning of the century (see Chapter 11). This chapter provides an overview of the methods for appropriate diagnostic tests to identify antispermatozoal antibodies (ASABs) in various body fluids. A brief overview of the mechanisms whereby ASABs affect spermatozoa is also provided; greater detail may be found in Chapter 11.

MECHANISMS OF ACTION

In extreme cases, male autoimmunity to postmeiotic germ cell antigens can result in the destruction of all spermatogenic cells in the testicular germinal epithelium (e.g., mumps orchitis). However, clinical infertility is more often confronted with less clear-cut problems caused by the presence of circulating ASABs or those present in genital tract secretions.

Traditionally ASABs were termed either spermagglutinating, when they induced the agglutination of motile donor spermatozoa, or spermotoxic, when they induced a complement-dependent loss of vitality. The latter type of ASABs are also often called sperm-immobilizing antibodies because they induce a loss of motility as a consequence of sperm death. The discovery of sperm-specific antibodies that cause neither effect but induce a "shaking" pattern of motility when such antibody-coated spermatozoa are exposed to cervical mucus can cause some confusion with regard to the term "immobilization"—such antibodies are not spermotoxic.

Antisperm antibodies may be suspected in men if the semen analysis shows many motile spermatozoa specifically involved in agglutinates (Fig. 5-1) or a low percentage of live cells (assessed by vital staining, not motility). Agglutinates can usually be distinguished microscopically from aggregates (which are not immunologically mediated) by their involvement of mostly immotile spermatozoa in conjunction with other nonspermatozoal cells and debris. To have such effects the antibodies must be present in the seminal plasma either as a result of transudation from the blood or by local secretory activity within the accessory glands of the male genital tract.

The classic spermagglutinating and spermotoxic antibodies obviously impair a man's fertility potential by reducing the availability of spermatozoa in his ejaculate that are competent to penetrate the cervical mucus, a process that depends on ade-

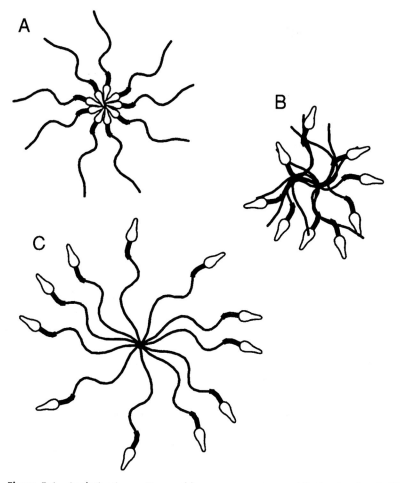

Figure 5-1 Agglutination patterns of human spermatozoa. **(A)** Head-to-head. **(B)** Tail-to-tail. **(C)** Tail tip-to-tail tip.

quate numbers of progressively motile spermatozoa. Other, sperm-coating antibodies are often not apparent at semen analysis but cause negative or poor mucus penetration when evaluated under in vivo (postcoital test) or in vitro (Kremer test) conditions (see Chapter 9).

Circulating antibodies may be transuded into the female genital tract secretions and follicular fluid, and local secretion of antibodies can occur at the cervix. Obviously ASABs in cervical mucus may impair sperm penetration and the initiation of sperm transport, and those present in the higher levels of the female tract could interfere with sperm–egg interaction. The latter mechanism is difficult to establish in vivo, but several studies in conjunction with IVF procedures have demonstrated that female serum containing ASABs can inhibit, and even totally prevent, fertilization when used as a culture medium supplement.

DIAGNOSTIC TESTS FOR ANTISPERM ANTIBODIES

Overview

Sperm agglutination and Sperm immobilization

A comprehensive review of classic tests for sperm agglutination and sperm immobilization is available for detailed consideration of the available techniques (Rose et al., 1976). The methods recommended in this chapter are modifications of the Friberg micro tray agglutination test (TAT) for spermagglutinating antibodies and the Isojima sperm immobilization test (SIT) for complement-dependent spermotoxic antibodies. These tests can be performed on male or female blood serum or seminal plasma. If cervical mucus is liquefied using bromelain, an enzyme extracted from pineapples, it too can be tested.

Antibodies on the Sperm Surface

The mixed antiglobulin reaction (MAR test), a modified Coombs' test, was used to detect the presence of immunoglobulin on the sperm surface (Jager et al., 1978). However, this test suffered from two disadvantages: (1) it required a regular availability of sensitized sheep erythrocytes; and (2) in most centers it was available only for IgG class antibodies.

In recent years the MAR test has largely been replaced by the Immunobead test (IBT), which uses polyacrylamide beads coated with antihuman immunoglobulin antibodies against either the α-, γ-, or μ-chains, i.e., specific for the IgA, IgG, and IgM isotypes, respectively (Clarke, 1990) (Fig. 5-2). Another bead specific for heavy and light chains of human immunoglobulins, and which therefore identifies the IgG, IgA, and IgM simultaneously (hence the name GAM-bead), is also available and can be used as a screening test (Pattinson and Mortimer, 1987). An excellent correspondence exists between GAM-IBT-positive samples and those positive by one or more of the isotype-specific Immunobead tests with no false positives or false negatives.

The IBT can also be used as an indirect test where prepared donor spermatozoa are exposed to test samples (male or female serum, seminal plasma, or bromelain-treated cervical mucus) to allow passive transfer of any ASABs they may contain. These antibody-coated donor spermatozoa are then tested using the IBT in the usual way.

Other screening tests for sperm surface antibodies have appeared in kit form (Hellstrom et al., 1989; McClure et al., 1989):

1. The SpermMAR Test (Ortho Diagnostics: Fertility Technologies, Natick, MA, USA) can be used on unwashed seminal spermatozoa but can detect only IgG class antibodies (although an IgA version is under development). The inability to detect other isotypes of ASABs and the relatively high cost of the kit compared to the Immunobead test outweigh the advantage of being able to use unwashed spermatozoa, except perhaps in a private office practice.
2. The SpermChek Test (Biorad Laboratories, Clinical Division) is a single Immunobead test employing a 40:40:20 mixture of anti-IgG, anti-IgA, and anti-

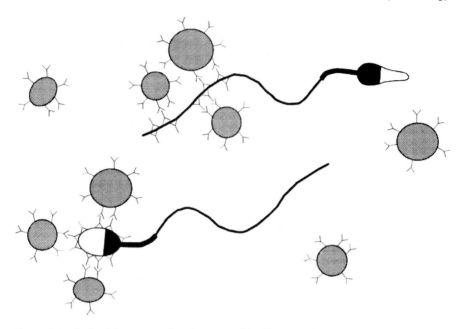

Figure 5-2   Basis of the Immunobead test. (Modified from Clarke, 1990.)

IgM beads. Its benefit over the GAM-bead screening test is unclear, and it is considerably more expensive.

Antibodies in Cervical Mucus

In addition to the assays already discussed, ASABs present in cervical mucus can also be detected by the sperm–cervical mucus contact (SCMC) test, where aliquots of cervical mucus and liquefied semen are mixed and then examined for the development of a characteristic "shaking" pattern of sperm motility. The SCMC test is a direct test of sperm function, and if used in the crossed-hostility format it can isolate the antibody problem to either the spermatozoa or the mucus (or occasionally both). SCMC tests are most powerful if used in combination with the IBT and Kremer-type tests of sperm–mucus interaction (see Chapter 9).

Both IgG and IgA class antibodies are found in cervical mucus, and mucus IgA has a strong correlation with complement-dependent sperm-immobilizing antibodies (SIT assay) in serum. Furthermore, positive IgA-IBT results occur only in mucus samples that show poor penetration by normal spermatozoa. There is also a clear relationship between sperm surface IgA antibodies and impaired sperm penetration, but not for IgG antibodies.

Other Methods for Detecting ASABs

Techniques such as enzyme-linked immunosorbent assays (ELISA) and radioimmunoassays (RIA) have also been developed to identify ASABs. This area is one of active current research, and interested readers should search the recent literature for the latest developments. However, with the interest in avoiding environmentally unfriendly assay techniques such as RIA (due to the large volumes of low-level radioactive waste produced), it is not expected that this method will pass into routine use. A number of ELISA-based kits for screening, quantitating, and typing of ASABs are commercially available, although their acceptance into routine clinical use has been low. Certainly the sensitivity of many such kits to storage and shipment conditions make them less robust and rather unreliable.

Many of the evaluations of these new assays have been by comparing them with older, established assays or with predefined clinical populations. Ideally, all ASAB assays, including the established techniques described below, should be validated in a prospective manner using appropriate clinical endpoints such as in vivo fecundity rates of IVF fertilization rates. Laboratories that are considering use of commercial kits should include this consideration in their selection criteria.

Spermagglutinating Antibody Titration: Friberg Test

Principle

The Friberg micro tray agglutination test (TAT) is designed to detect spermagglutinating antibodies by their ability to cause washed motile spermatozoa from a normal control donor to agglutinate when exposed to serial dilutions of test body fluids.

Reagents

Baker's medium is prepared by dissolving 3.00 g glucose, 0.46 g $Na_2HPO_4 \cdot 7H_2O$, 0.01 g KH_2PO_4, and 0.20 g NaCl in reagent water to 100 ml. The pH of the final solution is 8.1. Filter-sterilize the solution using Millipore Millex-GV 0.22-μm filter units or autoclaved Millipore Swinnex-25 units containing a 0.22-μm Durapore (GVWP) membrane and an AP-25 depth type prefilter in 50-ml lots into sterile plastic culture flasks (e.g., Falcon No. 3013).

Specimens

Seminal Plasma

1. Centrifuge at least 200 μl of semen at 1000 g for 15 minutes in a small (1.5 ml) capped Eppendorf tube.
2. Transfer the supernatant to a clean tube, stopper, and heat-inactivate (to destroy complement) in a waterbath at 56°C for 30 minutes.
3. Store the cell-free seminal plasma at −70°C until assay.

Blood Serum

1. Centrifuge clotted blood at 1000 g for 15 minutes.
2. Transfer 1 ml to a clean, stoppered tube and heat-inactivate at 56°C for 30 minutes.
3. Store frozen at −70°C until assay.

Cervical mucus

1. Cervical mucus is sampled as described in Chapter 9 for the Insler score.
2. Expel the mucus from the suction catheter onto a glass slide and then, using a 1-ml syringe and 18-gauge needle, transfer an appropriate aliquot of the mucus

into a 1.5-ml Eppendorf tube. Estimate the aliquot volume from standard reference tubes.

3. Add an equal volume of PBS (see Direct Immunobead Test, below) containing bromelain (Sigma Cat. No. B-2252) 10 U/ml.

N.B.   Bromelain does not dissolve well; but if thoroughly mixed, most should dissolve within 15–20 minutes.

4. Stir the mucus-bromelain-PBS mixture well with a pipette tip and incubate at ambient temperature for 10 minutes.
5. Check that liquefaction is complete and then centrifuge for 10 minutes at 2000 g.
6. Remove the supernatant and heat-inactivate in a waterbath at 56°C for 30 minutes.
7. Store the solubilized cervical mucus supernatant at -70°C until assay.

N.B.   Remember that the sample has already been diluted 1:1, and correct any titer value accordingly.

Method

1. Prepare a suspension of washed spermatozoa at 25×10^6 to 40×10^6 motile cells/ml using either the Percoll gradient or direct swim-up method as described in Chapter 12 and leave at ambient temperature until needed.
2. For the standards and any positive samples being reassayed, use 96-well Linbro/Titertek trays (V-shaped wells) as 8 rows of 12 wells (1/4 to 1/8096 dilutions). For unknown samples mark the tray so that each half comprises 8 rows of 6 wells (1/4 to 1/128 dilutions).
3. Using a 25-μl repeat dispenser, place 75 μl Baker's medium in the first well of each row and 25 μl in each of the other wells.
4. Add 25 μl of the test or control sample to the first well in each row, which gives an initial 1 in 4 dilution.
5. Using an 8-channel 25-μl multipipette, mix the contents of the first well in each row. Then transfer 25 μl from the first wells into the second well in each row. Mix by repeat pipetting, and then repeat so that each of the wells contains a one-half dilution of the preceding well.
6. Half-fill Lux 60-well HL-A plates with liquid paraffin (about 8 ml, warmed to 37°C before use) so all the wells are full of paraffin, with no air bubbles. Use one tray per 10 tests.
7. Using a microsyringe pipette (model 702: Hamilton Micro-Syringe Co., Anaheim, CA, USA), transfer 5 μl of each dilution of each sample into a well of the HL-A plate. Always work from the highest dilution (usually 1:128) to the 1:4 dilution, using a fresh tip for each set of serial dilutions.
8. Using a positive displacement microsyringe dispenser (Hamilton PB-600-1 with a 50-μl 705-SN syringe), add 1 μl of the sperm suspension to each of the wells in the HL-A plates. Start each tray at 5-minute intervals (this method allows time for scoring them later). Replace the lid on each tray as it is completed and return it to the 37°C incubator.

9. Incubate each tray at 37°C for 120 minutes. Take trays from the incubator at 5-minute intervals.
10. Using an inverted microscope and preferably phase-contrast optics, evaluate the presence of agglutination exhibited by the spermatozoa in each well. Do not confuse any possible aggregation of dead spermatozoa with the specific agglutination of (usually) motile spermatozoa. Note the type of association exhibited by agglutinating spermatozoa.
11. Discard the trays and plates in sealed polythene bags.

Results
The titer of spermagglutinating antibody is expressed as the reciprocal of the highest dilution in which the agglutination was present at the end of the 2-hour incubation (see Appendix IV for a sample report form). For example, if a sample shows agglutination up to and including the 1/64 dilution but not in the 1/128 dilution, the titer is given as 1:64. In addition, the type of agglutination should be stated using the following conventions: head-to-head (H-H), midpiece-to-midpiece (MP-MP), tail-to-tail (T-T), tail tip-to-tail tip (tt-tt); mixed types may be seen as well, e.g., head-to-tail (H-T).

If there is so much agglutination the pattern cannot be identified, report it as undefined. When more than one type of agglutination seems to be present, report it as mixed.

If an unknown sample at first assay is positive all the way to 1:128, it should be reassayed subsequently, but taking the serial dilutions out to 1:8096. Although samples with titers of ≥ 1:8 should be flagged for a repeat test on another sample obtained from the patient, only titers higher than 1:16 are considered genuine positives of biological significance.

Quality Control
Each assay must include serial dilutions of known spermagglutination positive and negative seminal plasma or serum samples (as appropriate). These standards are obtained from patients known to be either positive or negative for spermagglutinating antibodies and are prepared in the same way as the samples for testing (except in larger volumes) and stored frozen at −70°C in 40-µl aliquots in small, capped Eppendorf tubes sealed with Parafilm.

Acceptable interassay limits for the positive control sample should be set, e.g., ± 1 serial dilution ≡ 1 titer value). If the positive control is not within ± 1 titer of its norm or the negative control shows appreciable agglutination (≥ 1:16) the entire assay should be repeated including both the original positive and negative controls as well as new ones (i.e., from different donors).

Spermotoxic Antibody Detection/Titration

Principle
Complement-dependent cytotoxicity is characterized by a rapid decline in sperm vitality after exposure to the body fluid containing the spermotoxic antibodies. The

technique described below (a variant of the Isojima sperm immobilization test, or SIT) is designed to detect such antibodies in blood serum, seminal plasma, or solubilized cervical mucus. It employs the ability of these antibodies to cause washed motile spermatozoa from a normal control donor to become immotile when exposed to serial dilutions of these body fluids in the presence of guinea pig complement.

Reagents

Baker's medium is prepared as described for the spermagglutinating antibody titration, above.

Guinea pig complement is purchased from any immunological product supplier.

Specimens

Blood serum, seminal plasma, or bromelain-solubilized cervical mucus may be used in this assay. For specimen preparation, see Spermagglutinating Antibody Titration, above. All samples must be heat-inactivated prior to the assay.

Method

The method is exactly as described for the sperm-agglutinating antibody titration, above, except that the following instruction should be inserted between steps 9 and 10.

9A. Using a microsyringe dispenser (Hamilton PB-600-1 with a 50-μl 705-SN syringe), add 1 μl of guinea pig complement to each of the wells of the HL-A plate.

Obviously, instruction 10 should now read:

10. Using an inverted microscope and preferably phase-contrast optics, assess the percentage of motile spermatozoa in each well (≥ 100 spermatozoa per well). A well is considered positive when its proportion of motile spermatozoa is < 50% of that in the negative control series.

Results

Spermotoxicity is *rare*. Genuine spermotoxic activity is considered to be present when the proportion of motile spermatozoa in a well is < 50% of that seen in the negative control series (a sample report form in provided in Appendix IV).

If a maximum titer (1:128) is found, the test should be repeated on another day but with 11 dilutions of the initial 1/4 dilution (i.e., 12 wells per test) to enable titrations of up to 1:8096 to be determined.

Sperm Vitality as the Endpoint of Interest

For absolute confirmation that complement-dependent loss of vitality has occurred, the endpoint can be assessed by eosin exclusion. In this situation the serial dilutions are prepared in the V-well trays, and an equal volume (i.e., 25 μl) of the prepared sperm suspension is added to each well. Discard 50 μl of the first (1/4) dilution well before adding the sperm suspension. After incubation at 37°C for 60 minutes, 25–50 μl of eosin-nigrosin stain (see Sperm Vitality in Chapter 2) is added and mixed, and air-dried smears are prepared. Scoring is as for standard sperm vitality assessment, and a sample dilution is considered positive if the vitality is less than half that seen in the negative control series of wells. Again, a control for direct spermotoxicity of the complement must be included.

Measurement of decreased sperm ATP content has also been used to assess spermotoxicity (Vermeulen and Comhaire, 1982). Although this method can provide a spermotoxic index, eliminating the need for a larger series on serial dilutions, it is technically more complex and expensive unless a laboratory is already equipped to measure ATP by luminometry.

Simplified Screening Assay

As a screening assay the spermagglutination titration assay may be extended by adding 1 μl of guinea pig complement to each of the 1/8 dilution wells and then returning the trays to the incubator for another 60 minutes. In this situation, two extra wells containing 6 μl of sperm suspension must be included so 1 μl of guinea pig complement can be added to one of them (to control for any direct spermotoxicity of the complement preparation); the other serves as an untreated control. The assay is read by determining the percentage motility in each of the 1:8 wells. A sample is considered positive if the motility is less than half that seen in the negative control sample well. If there is significant loss of motility in the complement control well, the assay must be repeated with a fresh sperm preparation.

Positive samples should be reassayed using the complete spermotoxicity method, preferably using eosin exclusion vitality staining as the endpoint.

Quality Control

Each assay must include serial dilutions of both positive and negative controls (i.e., known spermotoxic positive and negative blood serum or seminal plasma samples, as appropriate). These standards are obtained from patients known to be either positive or negative for spermotoxic antibodies and are prepared and stored as described for spermagglutinating antibody standards.

If a positive control sample does not show an acceptable spermotoxicity titer ($\pm$ 1 titer of its norm) or the negative control shows detectable spermotoxicity, the entire assay should be repeated. The repeat assay should include the original positive and negative controls as well as new ones.

Direct Immunobead Test

Principle

Antisperm antibodies in the seminal plasma that coat the sperm surface and cause the shaking phenomenon and other disturbances of sperm function, without causing spermagglutination or spermotoxicity, can be detected by incubating washed spermatozoa with Immunobeads (Biorad Laboratories Chemical Division, Richmond, CA, USA).

Reagents

Phosphate-buffered saline (PBS) is prepared by dissolving 8.000 g NaCl, 0.200 g KCl, 1.150 g Na_2HPO_4, 0.200 g KH_2PO_4, 0.132 g $CaCl_2·2H_2O$, and 0.059 g $MgSO_4$ in reagent water and diluting to 1000 ml. Store at 4°C in clean glass or suitable plastic bottles. Discard if there are any signs of contamination or sedimentation.

Buffer I is 0.3% (w/v) BSA (Sigma Cat. No. A-4503) in PBS. Dissolve 300 mg BSA in PBS to a total volume of 100 ml. This solution must be prepared daily and kept at ambient temperature. Discard any unused portion at the end of the day.

Buffer II is 5.0% (w/v) BSA in PBS. Dissolve 5.0 g BSA in PBS to a total volume of 100 ml. This stock Buffer II is stored frozen at −20°C as 1-ml aliquots in Eppendorf tubes. For use it is thawed and warmed to ambient temperature. Discard any unused portion at the end of the day; do not refreeze.

Immunobeads: For screening tests use the GAM bead for whole B-cell labeling (Biorad Cat. No. 170-5106). For specific immunoglobulin class testing use the separate IgA, IgG, and IgM beads (Biorad Cat. Nos. 170-5114, 170-5100, and 170-5120, respectively). These beads can be purchased as a kit (Biorad Cat. No. 170-5198).

1. Take 100 μl of each Immunobead suspension to be used and add it to 900 μl Buffer I in a small Eppendorf tube.
2. Centrifuge at 600 *g* for 10 minutes.
3. Carefully remove and discard the supernatant, and resuspend the pellet of Immunobeads in 100 μl Buffer II.
4. Store at 4°C until required. Do not keep at ambient temperature for prolonged periods or the beads will become inactive.

Specimens

Washed spermatozoa: Take an aliquot of liquefied semen within 2 hours of ejaculation. The volume of semen required (in microliters) is calculated from the estimated sperm concentration (see Chapter 3) as 5000 divided by the motile sperm concentration (in 10^6/ml).

Motile sperm preparations: The direct IBT can also be performed on preparations of motile spermatozoa prepared, for example, for IVF, GIFT, or IUI (see Chapter 12).

Method

1. Add the aliquot of liquefied semen to 2.0 ml Buffer I in a conical-bottom centrifuge tube (e.g., Falcon No. 2095).
2. Centrifuge at 600 *g* for 10 minutes.
3. Discard the supernatant and gently resuspend the sperm pellet in 5.0 ml Buffer I.
4. Centrifuge at 600 *g* for 10 minutes.

5. Discard the supernatant and gently resuspend the sperm pellet in 200 μl Buffer II.
6. On separate clean microscope slides mix 5 μl of the washed sperm suspension with 5 μl of each of the Immunobead types to be tested. Mount with 22 × 22 mm coverslips.
7. Incubate at ambient temperature in a humid chamber for 10–15 minutes.
8. Examine at 400× magnification using phase-contrast optics. Count at least 200 *motile* spermatozoa, differentiating between those with Immunobeads bound and those with no beads bound. Note the localization of any bead binding (i.e., head, midpiece, tail, tail-tip, or combinations thereof).

N.B. a. Because Immunobeads are inactivated at ambient temperature, both stock and "ready-to-use" bead suspensions must be stored at 4°C.
 b. If a lower BSA-containing buffer is used in place of the recommended Buffer II, significant nonspecific attachment (clumping) of spermatozoa and beads may occur.

Results

Calculate the percentage of motile spermatozoa with beads bound. Identify GAM-bead screening tests as such, and specify IgG class "not determined." If a sample is positive in the GAM-bead screen, it should be retested with the three isotype-specific beads as soon as possible. Alternatively, the isotype-specific testing may be performed on a subsequent sample, as the positive IBT result will have to be confirmed anyway.

Express the results according to the number of motile spermatozoa with bound Immunobeads. Originally, IBT results were rated as: 0% = negative; 1–9% = doubtful; 10–90% = positive; and > 90% = strongly positive (i.e., any test showing > 10% Immunobead binding was considered positive). However, studies from a number of laboratories have shown that sperm function *in vitro* and fertility *in vivo* are not significantly impaired unless ≥ 50% of the motile spermatozoa are coated with antibodies (i.e., are Immunobead-positive). Consequently, it is now proposed that IBT results be reported as: < 20% = negative; 20–49% = positive; ≥ 50% = clinically significant positive (Clarke, 1990; World Health Organization, 1992). The latter class should also have at least 2 beads bound per spermatozoon. Furthermore, antibodies directed against the tail tip are not, on their own, associated with impaired sperm function or fertility.

Quality Control

Because it is not possible to store human spermatozoa in a state suitable for subsequent Immunobead testing, no directly equivalent standards are presently available. It is good practice each day to include indirect Immunobead tests (see below) using donor spermatozoa treated with both positive and negative control sera. This method alerts the user to any deterioration in the stock Immunobeads and to possible problems of nonspecific attachment (clumping) of spermatozoa and beads as may occur if the BSA concentration in Buffer II is low).

It has been suggested that inert Immunobeads could be used as a negative control for nonspecific bead attachment. However, unless such beads are treated exactly the same as those conjugated with immunoglobulin (using perhaps BSA), their surface characteristics are substantially different, making them an invalid control.

Indirect Immunobead Test

Principle
Antisperm antibodies able to coat the sperm surface and cause the shaking phenomenon and other disturbances of sperm function, without causing spermagglutination or spermotoxicity, may also be present in the body fluids. These antibodies can be detected by incubating washed motile spermatozoa with the biological fluid to allow passive transfer of the antibodies to the sperm surface where they can then be detected using Immunobeads (Biorad Laboratories Chemical Division).

Reagents
The same reagents as for the direct Immunobead test (see above) are needed.

Specimens
Blood serum, seminal plasma, or bromelain-solubilized cervical mucus may be used in this assay. For specimen preparation, see Spermagglutinating Antibody Titration, above. All samples must be heat-inactivated prior to assay.

Method

1. Prepare a suspension of washed spermatozoa at about 25×10^6 motile cells/ml using either the Percoll gradient or direct swim-up method as described in Chapter 12 and leave at ambient temperature until needed.
2. Dilute 10 µl of each test or control fluid with 40 µl Buffer II in labeled Eppendorf tubes.
3. Add 50 µl sperm suspension to each tube, mix thoroughly but gently, and incubate at 37°C for 60 minutes.
4. Centrifuge all tubes at 500 g for 10 minutes.
5. Discard the supernatants and gently resuspend each of the pellets in 500 µl fresh Buffer I.
6. Centrifuge all tubes at 500 g for 10 minutes.
7. Discard the supernatants and gently resuspend each of the pellets in 100 µl fresh Buffer II.
8. On separate clean microscope slides mix 5 µl of the washed sperm suspension with 5 µl of each of the Immunobead types to be tested. Mount with 22×22 mm coverslips.
9. Incubate at ambient temperature in a humid chamber for 10–15 minutes.
10. Examine at 400× magnification using phase-contrast optics. Count at least 200 *motile* spermatozoa, differentiating between those with Immunobeads bound and those with no beads bound. Note the localization of any bead binding (i.e., head, midpiece, tail, tail-tip).

N.B. a. Because Immunobeads are inactivated at ambient temperature both stock and "ready-to-use" bead suspensions must be stored at 4°C.

b. If a lower BSA-containing buffer is used in place of the recommended Buffer II, significant nonspecific attachment (clumping) of spermatozoa and beads may occur.

Results

Calculate the percentage of motile spermatozoa with beads bound and present the results as described for the direct immunobead test (above). A sample report form is provided in Appendix IV.

Quality Control

Positive and negative controls should be included for each indirect IBT assay. Positive controls should show the same isotype and regional specificity of Immunobead binding each time they are used. If either of these results changes, the assay must be repeated using this same positive control for verification as well as another of comparable biological activity.

If the level of bead binding changes from one clinical category to another, the assay must also be repeated as described above.

N.B. These changes may be due to deterioration of the stock beads. Attention should also be paid to possible problems of nonspecific attachment (clumping) of spermatozoa and beads as may occur if the concentration of BSA in Buffer II is too low.

CLINICAL APPLICATION

A specific but limited role for auto- and iso-ASABs in the etiology of human infertility is incontrovertible (reviews: Menge, 1977; Jones, 1980; Bronson et al., 1984; Haas and Beer, 1986; Anderson, 1987; Haas, 1987; Mortimer, 1991). The specific diagnosis of such a factor during the workup of an infertile couple requires access to a comprehensive series of carefully standardized, appropriately controlled laboratory tests.

Although tests on male serum are less informative than those on the seminal plasma and spermatozoa, the results of TAT and SIT assays do correlate with the presence of ASABs in the male genital tract. A comprehensive semen analysis provides much valuable information relevant to the presence of ASABs in the seminal plasma: spermagglutinins should be suspected if more than 10% of the motile spermatozoa are involved in specific aggregates; and spermimmobilizins would be suspected if more than 75% of the spermatozoa were dead by vital staining.

Both TAT and SIT assays should be performed on female serum, especially if it is to be used to supplement IVF or IUI culture medium. Indirect IBTs can also be used to detect and titer ASABs in serum samples; they are particularly useful for testing serum for culture medium supplementation. The TAT assay can be used to screen for spermotoxic antibodies (see above). Such screening greatly reduces the number of more labor-intensive SIT assays required.

Perhaps the most informative tests are those of sperm–mucus interaction in vitro (see Chapter 9) when used in the crossed-hostility format in combination with a direct IBT. An indirect IBT can also be included to detect (and titer) ASABs in cervical mucus after bromelain-treatment.

The true significance of immunological infertility will continue to elude us so long as ASABs are ignored clinically. Extensive clinical studies, combining a comprehensive laboratory protocol with appropriate follow up and statistical (epidemiological) analysis, are required to establish the prognostic significance of such antibodies. Autoimmunity and isoimmunity to spermatozoa are undoubtedly significant causative factors in some couples' infertility and must therefore be identified during their initial workup. Failure to consider these antibodies may result in some infertile couples suffering the unnecessary frustration of having their problem diagnosed as idiopathic with no real hope of treatment. Worse still, ignorance of significant ASAB titers could be construed as mismanagement in certain IVF situations if they were responsible for failure of fertilization.

Infertility is fraught with multiple contributory factors of variable significance in any given couple; acceptance of all such potentially relevant factors, even if our understanding of them is presently limited, and their etiological consideration are essential for progress to be made in the diagnosis and treatment of this complex clinical problem.

References and Recommended Reading

Alexander, N. J., and Anderson, D. J. (1987). Immunology of semen. *Fertil. Steril.* **47,** 192.

Bronson, R., Cooper, G., and Rosenfeld, D. (1984). Sperm antibodies: their role in infertility. *Fertil. Steril.* **42,** 171.

Bronson, R., Cooper, G., Hjort, T., Ing, R., Jones, W. R., Wang, S. X., Mathur, S., Williamson, H. O., Rust, P. F., Fudenberg, H. H., Mettler, L., Czuppon, A. B., and Sudo, N. (1985). Anti-sperm antibodies, detected by agglutination, immobilization, microcytotoxicity and Immunobead-binding assay. *J. Reprod. Immunol.* **8,** 279.

Clarke, G. N. (1990). Detection of antisperm antibodies using Immunobeads. In Keel, B. A., and Webster, B. W. (eds): *CRC Handbook of the Laboratory Diagnosis and Treatment of Infertility.* CRC Press, Boca Raton, FL.

Haas, G. G., Jr. (1987). How should sperm antibody tests be used clinically? *Am. J. Reprod. Immunol. Microbiol.* **15,** 106.

Haas, G. G., Jr., and Beer, A. E. (1986). Immunologic influences on reproductive biology: sperm gametogenesis and maturation in the male and female genital tracts. *Fertil. Steril.* **46,** 753.

Hellstrom, W. J. G., Samuels, S. J., Waits, A. B., Overstreet, J. W. (1989) A comparison of the usefulness of SpermMar and Immunobead tests for the detection of antisperm antibodies. *Fertil. Steril.* **52,** 1027.

Jager, S., Kremer, J., and van Slochteren-Draaisma, T. (1978). A simple method of screening for antisperm antibodies in the human male. Detection of spermatozoal surface IgG with the direct mixed antiglobulin reaction carried out on untreated fresh human semen. *Int. J. Fertil.* **23,** 12.

Jones, W. R. (1980). Immunologic infertility—fact or fiction? *Fertil. Steril.* **33,** 577.

McClure, R. D., Tom, R. A., Watkins, M., Murthy, S. (1989) SpermChek: a simplified screening assay for immunological infertility. *Fertil. Steril.* **52,** 650.

Menge, A. C. (1977). Immunoandrology. In Hafez, E. S. E. (ed): *Techniques of Human Andrology.* Elsevier/North Holland, Amsterdam.

Mortimer, D. (1991). Clinical significance of antisperm antibodies. *J. Soc. Obstet. Gynecol. Can.* **13,** 69.

Pattinson, H. A., and Mortimer, D. (1987). Prevalence of sperm surface antibodies in the male partners of infertile couples as determined by Immunobead screening. *Fertil. Steril.* **48,** 466.

Rose, N. R., Hjort, T., Rümke, P., Harper, M. J. K., and Vyazov, O. (1976). Techniques for detection of iso- and auto-antibodies to human spermatozoa. *Clin. Exp. Immunol.* **23,** 175.

Vermeulen, L., and Comhaire, F. (1982). Detection of cytotoxic sperm antibodies using ATP-determination: A comparison with other immunological methods. In Serio, M., and Pazzagli, M. (eds): *Luminescent Assays: Perspectives in Endocrinology and Clinical Chemistry.* Raven Press, New York.

World Health Organization (1992). *WHO Laboratory Manual for the Examination of Human Semen and Sperm-Cervical Mucus Interaction.* 3rd ed. Cambridge University Press, Cambridge.

6

Semen Microbiology and Virology

Infections of the male reproductive tract can be contributory, even direct, causes of infertility (Eliasson, 1977; Fowler, 1981). Their investigation requires not only microbiological testing but seminal plasma biochemistry and careful clinical examination (palpation of the testes, epididymides, and prostate).

Infections or inflammatory disorders can affect the secretory function of both the prostate and seminal vesicles. Biochemical assessment of the semen may be informative, but only if markers for both organs are included in the evaluation. Also, only repeated analyses can provide adequate evidence that secretory function has been changed as a result of disease or therapy.

Infections of the prostate, which may be asymptomatic, can cause partial or complete obstruction of the ejaculatory ducts resulting in oligozoospermia and even azoospermia. In addition, men with a prostatic infection produce ejaculates with slightly decreased volume and low zinc content. Infection of the seminal vesicles often causes substantial reduction in ejaculate volume and a low seminal fructose concentration. It should also be noted that bacteriospermia without any clinical evidence of infection is not uncommon.

PYOSPERMIA

Although many infections result in the appearance of significant numbers of leukocytes in the semen, the finding of pyospermia is neither sensitive nor specific for infection. To differentiate between a specific microbiologically induced pyospermia and, for example, another prostatic abnormality, microbiological examination of the semen should be a routine part of infertility investigations.

The concentration of leukocytes in semen must be determined quantitatively and expressed as millions per milliliter. Vague statements of numbers "per high power field" must be avoided, especially in view of the potential variability of the size of a high power field (see Chapter 9). The combined use of a cytochemical peroxidase stain or immunocytochemical method and a Makler chamber of Microcell make it a relatively simple matter (see Chapter 3).

MICROBIOLOGICAL EXAMINATION OF SEMEN

The microbiological culture of semen is confounded by its high pH and its high content of lysozymes and zinc, both of which are bactericidal. Semen that is to be sent for microbiological culture must be fresh. Precise requirements depend on the laboratory performing the cultures, but it is often most practical to prepare transport swabs for sending to the laboratory rather than simply sending a fraction of the ejaculate.

Collection of Semen Specimens

In addition to the instructions described in Chapter 3, further instructions should be provided to patients producing ejaculates for microbiological examination. It is especially important if a repeat sample is being collected to verify a clinical infection or to test for infection in a case of pyospermia. Such instructions must include the following.

1. Hands must be washed thoroughly with antiseptic soap (e.g., PhisoHex, Septisol) for 2 minutes.
2. The penis should be washed using an antiseptic solution (e.g., a preparation containing benzalkonium hydrochloride).
3. Emphasize that the semen specimen must be collected by masturbation directly into the sterile container provided. Contamination of the specimen container is minimized by removing its lid only at the moment of collection of the ejaculate and replacing it immediately after completing the collection.

Examination of Ejaculate

Microbiological evaluation of semen is a highly specialized procedure best left to laboratories expert in the field. Each laboratory has preferred sampling and transportation methods for their various cultures and tests. A detailed discussion of microbiological laboratory services as they relate to andrology is not appropriate to this text. Further information on the microbiological examination of semen, including some recommended culture methods, can be found elsewhere (Derrick 1977; Jequier and Crich 1986; World Health Organization 1987, 1992).

Some simple diagnostic procedures are now becoming available that are amenable for use in an andrology laboratory. These tests are mentioned below in relation to the various organisms that may infect human semen.

ORGANISMS FOUND IN HUMAN SEMEN

Many organisms have been isolated from human semen, not all associated with pyospermia or even necessarily with an infection of the male urogenital tract. Many organisms are contaminants from the patient's skin or from the air at the time of collecting the ejaculate. Caution must be exercised when interpreting positive microbiology reports; one must not assume that an organism cultured in semen is necessarily related either to a patient's pyospermia or to the cause of his infertility (or even contributory to it).

Ureaplasma and Mycoplasma

Ureaplasma urealyticum and to a lesser extent *Mycoplasma hominis* are found relatively often in the semen of infertility patients. Although some authors report that the presence of these organisms is associated with impaired sperm motility, the allegation has been denied by other workers, and their true role in male infertility remains to be established. Their presence is abnormal, however, and most authorities agree that such infections should be treated with an appropriate antibiotic.

Chlamydia

Chlamydia trachomatis is occasionally found in human semen, although its presence in the male reproductive tract can only be diagnosed reliably using urethral swabs. *Chlamydia* may be detected in such swabs either by tissue culture or using monoclonal antibody test kits (e.g., MicroTrak from Syva Diagnostics).

Chlamydia cannot be cultured from semen because a seminal plasma factor is toxic to the cell line used for the culture (it is an intracellular organism). New tests for anti-*Chlamydia* antibodies in seminal plasma are now available but require validation. These antibodies may also be detected in serum.

Not only can *Chlamydia* cause epididymitis, it may be transmitted to the female partner and there cause salpingitis. Indeed, *Chlamydia* is most often diagnosed from cervical swabs from the female partner with the subsequent treatment of both partners. Elimination of this organism from the reproductive tract of both partners simultaneously is a high priority in both fertile and infertile individuals.

Neisseria gonorrhoeae

In general, gonorrhea in men causes severe symptoms and is easily diagnosed. Consequently, its detection in infertility patients (certainly associated with pyospermia) is uncommon, but it should always be tested for in men with pyospermia. As in other body fluids, *Neisseria gonorrhoeae* may be identified in semen as gram-negative intracellular diplococci.

Other Organisms

Other pathogenic bacteria may be found in human semen, including *Trichomonas vaginalis,* although this organism has never been specifically confirmed as causing either pyospermia or male infertility.

Escherichia coli is often found in the semen of men with a history of urinary tract *E. coli* infections. It can colonize the prostate and may induce production of IgA, which can cause spermagglutination. Its presence should be suspected in men with pyospermia and significant spermagglutination.

Numerous other organisms that may be part of the normal flora of the male reproductive tract or skin contaminants are commonly found in semen cultures. They include enterococci such as *Streptococcus faecalis* and staphylococci such as *Staphylococcus epidermidis*.

Although tuberculosis is a rare cause of infertility in Western countries, *Mycobacterium tuberculosis* may be present in the semen even in the absence of pyospermia. This organism should certainly be tested for in countries where tuberculosis is still common.

Candida albicans may also be present in semen, although it usually colonizes only smegma. It does not cause male infertility and must be considered a contaminant.

Viruses

Numerous viruses can be isolated from human semen. Of greatest importance is probably *human immunodeficiency virus* (HIV). HIV-I can be detected by both culture and the polymerase chain reaction, and it may be tested for serologically by testing for circulating anti-HIV-I antibodies; tests are not yet widely available for HIV-II.

Another retrovirus, *human T-cell lymphotrophic virus type I* (HTLV-I), which has been associated with the development of hairy cell leukemias, can also be transmitted in semen and should now be taken into consideration when screening semen donors (see below).

Although it is not considered as dangerous as HIV, *hepatitis B virus* is considerably more infectious and can be transmitted sexually. Hepatitis B virus is usually detected in the patient's serum by antibodies against viral surface and core antigens. Non-A/non-B hepatitis has been subclassified into several new viruses. Of these *hepatitis C virus* may be transmitted sexually and can now be detected serologically.

Genital *herpes virus* is often isolated from semen in infected individuals. Although there is little evidence for any direct deleterious effect on the male urogenital tract, sexual contact is its primary route of infection.

Cytomegalovirus (CMV) and *human papilloma virus* (HPV) can be detected in semen using polymerase chain reaction (PCR) technology, as well as by more traditional culture techniques and by serology. The role of PCR in this area of diagnostics has not yet been established, and great caution must be exercised when interpreting positive PCR findings. Although PCR is an extremely sensitive technique that holds enormous potential to revolutionize microbiological screening in the future, unless an assay is well characterized, there is a great risk of false-positive results.

INFECTION CONTROL AND SEMEN DONORS

Strict attention must be paid to screening semen donors to minimize as far as possible any risk of transmitting an infectious organism through semen (Alexander,

1990). For this reason only cryopreserved semen may be used in therapeutic donor insemination programs. This method allows microbiological testing of each ejaculate before use and permits a quarantine period for seroconversion to occur in individuals infected with viruses such as HIV and hepatitis B.

No standardized management protocol for semen donors exists, but the American Fertility Society has published revised guidelines for the use of donor semen (American Fertility Society, 1990). Similar information is also available from the Canadian Fertility and Andrology Society (1988, 1992). This section describes a management protocol based on the latter guidelines. Readers are also referred to the *Standards for Tissue Banking* published by the American Association of Tissue Banks (1984). Suggested forms for donor screening are provided in Appendix V.

Initial Screening

Before a semen donor candidate may be accepted, in addition to semen quality requirements he must be subjected to thorough microbiological and virological screening.

Serum

1. Serology for antibodies against HIV-I, CMV, hepatitis C, and HTLV-I must be performed.
2. Test for hepatitis B surface antigen (HBsAg). Core antigen testing is not necessary, as any core-antigen-positive individuals are also positive for the surface antigen, and this condition is sufficient for thier rejection.
3. VDRL testing is done for syphilis.

Semen

1. A general culture and sensitivity (C&S) bacteriological screen is performed.
2. Specific cultures for *Ureaplasma urealyticum, Mycoplasma hominis,* and *Neisseria gonorrhoeae* are prepared.

Urethra

Test for *Chlamydia trachomatis* using either culture or a fluorescent monoclonal antibody kit.

Repeat Screening

The serum and urethral tests listed above should be repeated at least every 6 months and preferably every 3 months. During this time the donor's frozen semen specimens remain in quarantine.

Each Ejaculate

Appropriate aliquots could be sent for microbiological testing, as listed above, on a part of the test thaw unit from each specimen provided.

Actions for Positive Tests

If a positive result is found, the following management options are the safest in terms of maximizing recipient safety.

Semen Microbiology

For a positive culture result for *U. urealyticum, M. homonis, N. gonorrhoeae,* or any other organism identified in the C&S screen that may be considered pathogenic:

1. Discard all units of the infected semen specimen.
2. Treat the donor *and* his partner medically for the infection(s).
3. Do not accept any further donations until the donor and his partner have completed treatment *and* the donor tests negative.

Urethral Chlamydia *or Serum VDRL*

1. Discard all banked ejaculates back until the donor's last negative result.
2. Treat the donor and his partner medically.
3. Do not accept any further donations until the donor and his partner have completed treatment *and* the donor tests negative.

Serum CMV Antibody

Many individuals are serologically CMV antibody (CMV-Ab) positive, both donors and recipients. Consequently, it is more practical to only use CMV-Ab-positive donors for recipients who are also CMV-Ab-positive and to reserve the few CMV-Ab-negative donors for similar recipients.

Change the donor's status from CMV-Ab-negative to CMV-Ab-positive effective from the first sample frozen after his most recent negative test.

When we are able to test for CMV in the semen (e.g., using PCR technology), it will probably be best to test for CMV in each ejaculate and then discard all positive specimens. This approach would obviate the need for CMV-Ab status distinctions.

Serum Hepatitis B, Hepatitis C, HIV-I, and HTLV-I

If any of the tests for serum hepatitis B, hepatitis C, HIV-I, or HTLV-I is confirmed positive, the following actions must be taken.

1. The individual must be terminated as a donor and all specimens in the bank destroyed (treat as infected biohazard material).
2. Inform *all* physicians who have used any straws from the donor at any time in the past and provide them with a complete history of the donor's serology.

References and Recommended Reading

Alexander, N. J. (1990). Sexual transmission of human immunodeficiency virus: virus entry into the male and female genital tract. *Fertil Steril.* **54,** 1.

American Association of Tissue Banks (1984). *Standards for Tissue Banking.* AATB, Arlington, VA.

American Fertility Society (1990). New guidelines for the use of donor semen insemination. *Fertil. Steril.* **53(3),** Suppl.

Canadian Fertility and Andrology Society (1988). *Guidelines for Therapeutic Donor Insemination.* CFAS, Montreal.

Canadian Fertility and Andrology Society (1992). *Guidelines for Therapeutic Donor Insemination.* 2nd ed. CFAS, Montreal.

Derrick, F. C., Jr. (1977). Bacteriological examination of the ejaculate. In Hafez, E. S. E. (ed): *Techniques of Human Andrology.* Elsevier/North Holland, Amsterdam.

Derrick, F. C., Jr., and Dahlberg, B. (1976). Male genital tract infections and sperm viability. In Hafez, E. S. E. (ed): *Human Semen and Fertility Regulation in Men.* Mosby, St. Louis.

Eliasson, R. (1977). Seminal plasma, accessory genital glands and infection. In Cockett, A.T.K., and Urry, R. L. (eds): *Male Infertility. Workup, Treatment and Research.* Grune & Stratton, Orlando, FL.

Fowler, J. E., Jr. (1981). Infections of the male reproductive tract and infertility: a selected review. *J. Androl.* **3,** 121.

Jequier, A. M., and Crich, J. P. (1986). *Semen Analysis. A Practical Guide.* Blackwell, Oxford.

Ulstein, M., Capell, P., Holmes, K. K., and Paulsen, C. A. (1976). Nonsymptomatic genital tract infection and male infertility. In Hafez, E.S.E. (ed): *Human Semen and Fertility Regulation in Men.* Mosby, St. Louis.

World Health Organization (1987). *WHO Laboratory Manual for the Examination of Human Semen and Semen-Cervical Mucus Interaction,* 2nd ed. Cambridge University Press, Cambridge.

World Health Organization (1992). *WHO Laboratory Manual for the Examination of Human Semen and Sperm-Cervical Mucus Interaction,* 3rd ed. Cambridge University Press, Cambridge.

7

Computer-Aided Sperm Analysis and Sperm Kinematics

There are several commercial systems using digital image analysis technology for the automated analysis of sperm concentration, sperm motility, and sperm movement characteristics. This new area of andrology has come to be known as computer-aided sperm analysis (CASA) (Boyers et al., 1989). Occasionally, CASA is used to mean computer-assisted semen analysis, or the alternative acronym CASMA (computer-aided/assisted/automated sperm motility analysis) may be seen.

At least six CASA systems are currently available (in alphabetical order of manufacturer).

1. Cryo Resources (Montgomery, NY, USA): CellSoft Systems 2000 and 3000; a new System 4000 was reportedly under development in 1990 but has not been released. Research, Hyperactivation, and Morphologizer (sperm head morphology assessment) Modules are available for use with System 3000.
2. Hamilton-Thorn Research (Beverly, MA, USA): HTM-S (stroboscopic illumination) and HTM-C (clinical) versions of the older HT-M2030 integrated analyzer system. A third-generation system named IVOS (Integrated Visual Optical System) is also now available capable of up to 60 frames/second analysis with internal data storage on hard disk; a system incorporating a fluorescence imaging capability is under development (HTM-SPECTRA).
3. JC Diffusion (La Ferté-Fresnel, France): The Speed-Sperm system was developed at the University of Rennes in France.
4. Motion Analysis Corporation (Santa Rosa, CA, USA): The CellTrack/S (ex model 3060) system operating at image framing rates of up to 60 Hz. A 200 frames/second research orientated system, the CTS-200, is also available. Other systems from this company include a simplified semen analyzer, CellCount, which requires more user input to reliably identify spermatozoa from nonsperm cells, as well as a dedicated, automated sperm morphology system CellForm.
5. Strömberg-Mika (Bad Feilnbach, Germany): The SM-CMA cell motility analyzer system offers improved discrimination of immotile objects as spermatozoa or nonsperm cells by virtue of checking for the presence of a tail. The software incorporates intelligent algorithms to track spermatozoa through collisions, giving this system an advantage over others such as CellSoft, HTM, and CellTrak in this regard.

6. TS Scientific (Perkasie, PA, USA): The Labscan VI system, which is described as having improved methods for setting the digitization threshold, gives better detection of spermatozoa than other commercial systems.

In addition, a system developed by Dr. Dale Hoskins at the Oregon Regional Primate Research Center is intended for commercialization.

Although similar basic principles underlie the operation of all CASA systems, appreciable differences exist in the optical systems used, image capture technology, sperm identification techniques, track reconstruction and collision algorithms, movement analysis algorithms, and data analysis. Obviously, anyone intending to use one of these systems or even use the data produced by one of them must be familiar with the basic principles of sperm movement analysis and the specific system. It is clearly both inappropriate and impossible to provide a detailed description of all facets of operation of any of these systems in this chapter. However, several of the more important characteristics and differences are discussed, although the reader must remember that this technology is rapidly evolving, and significant changes and improvements are continually being made to software and hardware.

LIMITATIONS OF CASA TECHNOLOGY

Fundamental Principles of Digital Image Analysis

Video Image

The image from a video camera is composed of a rectangular array of picture elements, or *pixels*. The strength of the signal from a given pixel is proportional to its brightness or intensity. During formation of the video image standard cameras first scan the even rows in this array and then the odd rows. Each scan of the array (or *video field*) forms only half of the video image. Sequential pairs of video fields are then *interlaced* to produce the complete *video frame*.

In North American NTSC systems a video field is generated every $\frac{1}{60}$ second, so there are 30 video frames per second (i.e., a video frame rate of 30 Hz). Each video frame is composed of 525 lines.

In European and Australian systems (PAL and SECAM), video fields are generated every $\frac{1}{50}$ second to give a video frame rate of 25 Hz, although each frame has 625 lines. The difference between the PAL and SECAM systems (and their variants) is in the encoding of the color information, or chrominance, in the signal, although some other variants also exist (e.g., M-PAL, with a video framing rate of 30 Hz).

Digitization

Digitization (Fig. 7-1) is the process of encoding video pixels as numbers. The simplest monochrome image has only two "colors," black and white, so the pixels are either off or on. This process is *binary digitization*. If a monochrome image includes shades of gray, each pixel has a numerical value on this *gray scale,* which may have as many as 256 levels.

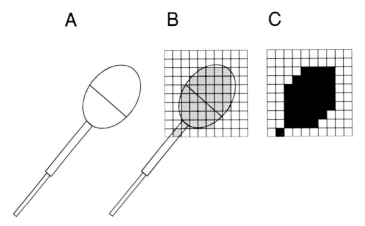

Figure 7-1 Digitization. The spermatozoon (**A**) is considered to lie on a grid representing an array of pixels (**B**). Those pixels that are at least half-covered by the object are shaded to indicate a binary state of 1; squares less than half-covered by the object retain a binary state of 0. (**C**) Appearance of the digitized object.

Many CASA systems use a binary digitized image for analysis, and so a *threshold gray level*, or intensity value, must be selected (usually by the operator) to identify the level that separates the two ranges of intensity, or gray scale values, that become black and white. Clearly, there is ample opportunity for error when setting the optimum threshold to achieve maximum discrimination between sperm heads and the background. If it is set too far one way, many small "hot spots" in the background are digitized as spurious objects; if it is set too far the other way, some less bright sperm heads (perhaps a little out of focus) are lost into the background, or the less bright border of the sperm head is lost, making it a smaller object. Depending on the actual settings of the size criteria or gates used to identify an object of interest (i.e., sperm head), mistakes in object classification may occur. It is easy to see how errors may be made when identifying *all* the sperm heads in a field and, at the same time, identifying *only* the sperm heads.

Most CASA systems use phase-contrast microscope images where the sperm head appears white on a dark background. At digitization it is common to invert the image so black tracks appear on a white background.

Object Detection
The identification of specific objects within the pixel array of each video frame (or field) often uses the technique of *edge detection*. Each object is composed of a contiguous group of pixels that are opposite in value to the background. Having identified one or more edges of an object (depending on the sophistication of the video processor and the tracking algorithms), a simple calculation determines the position of its *centroid* ("average spatial location" or geometric center) (Fig. 7-2). This calculation may involve mathematically weighting each pixel in the group for its intensity.

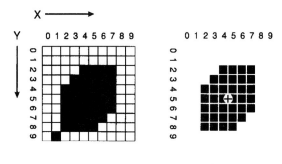

CENTROID COORDINATES: X = 4.5,   Y = 5.0

Figure 7-2 Centroid identification for the digitized object shown in Figure 7-1C. Each square of the pixel array has x,y coordinates, as shown on the left. On the right, the area of pixels describing the object (sperm head) extends from $x = 2$ to $x = 7$ and from $y = 2$ to $y = 8$. Hence the centroid, indicated by the cross, is defined as having the x,y coordinates $4.5,5.0$.

Track Reconstruction

From the series of digitized images, each containing a number of object centroids, the CASA program has to plot the movement of each one that was identified as a sperm head from one frame to the next throughout the entire sequence. This creation of *trajectories* is achieved by defining the maximum distance a spermatozoon could have traveled between one frame and the next. This maximum spatial displacement, which is calculated from a maximum velocity supplied to the program (often by the user), is divided by the frame rate to define the radius of a circle of maximum likelihood that is drawn around the location of the sperm head in one frame and then projected into the next frame (Figs. 7-3 and 7-4). For example, a maximum velocity (VCLmax; see below) of 300 μm/s and an NTSC video standard give a radius of $300 \div 30 = 10$ μm. Any centroid found within this circle is assumed to be the centroid of the cell that was projected from the previous frame. The two centroids are connected, forming a path. This process is continued through the sequence of frames to reconstruct the cell's trajectory.

If more than one centroid is found within the circle (e.g., because another cell was swimming nearby, or the first cell was approaching an immotile cell or other object) (Fig. 7-5), various alternative procedures may be employed to resolve the conflict.

1. Calculations for the present path (and usually also the second object's path) are terminated, sometimes referred to as trajectory truncation.
2. The centroid closest to the center of the circle is used to construct the path.
3. The path is flagged, and the reconstruction continues. After the tracks are complete, the program looks at the confused points and attempts a best-fit reconstruction based on the general direction of movement (vector) and specific pattern of movement (kinematics).

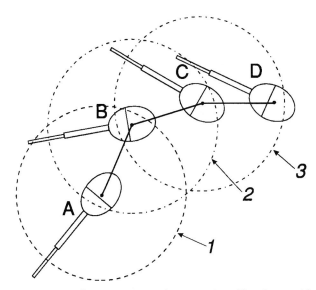

Figure 7-3   Track reconstruction from a series of head centroids in sequential images. In the first frame the circle of maximum likelihood is drawn around the centroid of the sperm head in position A. In the next frame the spermatozoon has moved to position B; and because it lies within the first circle of maximum likelihood, the track is reconstructed as a line joining centroids A and B. A second circle of maximum likelihood is then drawn around centroid B and the sperm head located in the third frame. Again the centroid (position C) lies within the circle, and the track is further reconstructed by joining centroids B and C. A third circle of maximum likelihood is then drawn around centroid C and projected into the fourth frame, where the sperm head is located at position D, and the track is extended by joining centroids C and D. This process is continued throughout the sequence of images to reconstruct the entire track.

Although they are different in their real effect on sperm movement, real and perceived collisions (sometimes referred to as bumps and crosses, respectively) are treated identically by image analysis programs. With a real collision the two cells actually bump into each other, whereas in perceived collisions their paths just cross, usually at different depths within the preparation and perhaps with a temporal separation as well.

If no centroid is found within the circle, again several options are available.

1. The path is terminated (trajectory truncation).
2. The projected circle can be increased in size and the search continued.
3. The circle can be doubled in size and projected into the next frame.

The last approach is termed trajectory interpolation as the cell's path in the missing frame is assumed, or interpolated. Some programs interpolate over two or three frames, a feature that is sometimes user-definable, where the cell is "missing."

If the centroid does not move between successive frames, it is considered

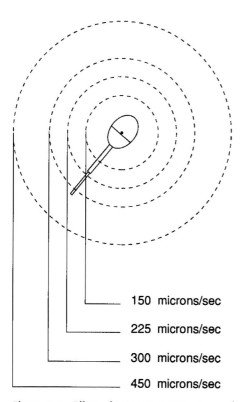

150 microns/sec

225 microns/sec

300 microns/sec

450 microns/sec

Figure 7-4   Effect of increasing VCLmax on the area of the circle of maximum likelihood used for finding the sperm head centroid in the next image. When analyzed at 30 images per second, a VCL of 150 μm/s requires a circle of maximum likelihood of radius 5 μm, while a VCL of 300 μm/s requires a radius of 10 μm. The areas of these two circles are 78.54 and 314.17 μm², respectively, demonstrating that a doubling of radius causes a four-fold increase in area.

immotile. A program usually requires lack of movement over a certain number of frames (e.g., three or four) before a cell is classified as immotile. The path may then be terminated to save processing time.

Once the trajectories have been reconstructed, their shape is analyzed according to certain current concepts to derive movement characteristics describing the motion of each cell. This aspect of CASA is termed *sperm kinematics* and is dealt with later in the chapter.

Sources of Error in CASA Systems

Object Recognition Errors
Depending on the size and sometimes the shape of the (digitized) object, it may be classified as being a sperm head or another object. If two (or more) sperm heads are

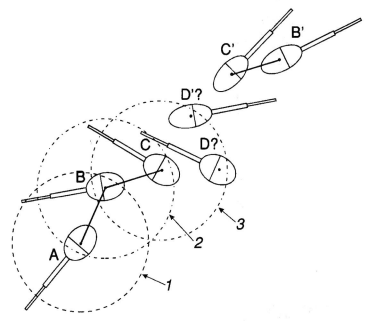

Figure 7-5   Problem of finding two centroids within a circle of maximum likelihood giving rise to a perceived collision. In this case the track being reconstructed in Figure 7-3 has become confused in the fourth frame owing to the presence of a second sperm head within the circle of maximum likelihood drawn around centroid C in the third frame and projected into the fourth frame. The program cannot be sure which cell, D or D', is the correct one to use for further reconstruction of the tract. Furthermore, this second cell is the prolongation of a track that was reconstructed in previous frames as track B'-C'. If the closest head to each previous position were to be taken, correct reconstructions would be achieved *in this case,* but not always, and there is no knowing at this stage just where the two cells would be in relation to each other in the next frame.

touching or even in close proximity (depending on the resolution of the digitizer), they may be digitized as a single contiguous object, which is therefore too large for a sperm head and is rejected from the analysis (Fig. 7-6). This problem is common to all CASA systems currently available.

Obviously refractile debris of similar size and appearance (i.e., intensity) to a sperm head may be erroneously identified as a sperm head. The problem of distinguishing between a single immotile spermatozoon and another immotile object can be at least partially resolved if immotile objects of the appropriate size and shape to be a sperm head are subjected to more detailed morphometry or shape analysis. For example, if the object has a tail it is clearly a sperm head, whereas objects without tails are far more likely to be debris (e.g., as with the Strömberg-Mika SM-CMA System). This level of sophistication requires substantially more intelligent algorithms and certainly greater computing power for it not to delay the analysis seriously.

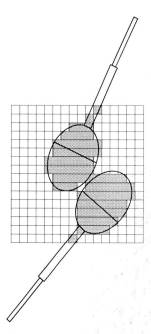

Figure 7-6 Problem of contiguous digitization of two objects in close proximity. It can be seen that even though these two sperm heads are not actually touching, one pixel is occupied by part of each head so that together they occupy more than 50% of its area. This causes it to be digitized as a binary 1, thereby causing the two heads to digitize as a single contiguous group of pixels. The total size of this group is obviously double that for a typical sperm head and would probably cause it to be rejected from analysis because it is too big.

Collisions

Obviously, if two swimming spermatozoa collide, they interfere with each other's movement. A similar problem exists if a swimming spermatozoon collides with an immotile one or with a large piece of debris or another cell (e.g., a leukocyte). In fact, because the beat envelope of a sperm tail is at least as wide as the apparent trajectory width, spermatozoa do not need to actually collide for their movement to be altered. Dealing with this concept has been a difficult problem for all those working on movement analysis.

Systems Using Trajectory Truncation

In CASA systems that drop cells from analysis when they collide or approach the same location (e.g., CellSoft Systems 2000 and 3000), there is a bias in that primarily motile cells are lost. As a consequence of such "collision algorithms," some CASA systems are highly concentration-dependent. Reliable motility analysis and certainly optimum movement analysis can be performed only on samples with up to about 40×10^6 spermatozoa/ml. Higher concentrations result in increased loss of trajectories from movement analysis in a manner that is dependent not only on the sperm concentration but also on the proportion of motile cells and their velocity distribution. Obviously, with higher maximum velocities, such as for washed spermatozoa (usually VCLmax = 300 or 400 µm/s) (Fig. 7-4) or deeper preparations, the maximum analyzable concentration is reduced.

In general terms trajectory truncation causes two problems.

1. Loss of motile cells, especially in high-concentration samples, where collisions are more likely within the first few frames
2. Creation of spuriously motile cells as a result of their being moved hydrodynamically by another cell swimming past or as a result of a direct collision.

These problems exist in addition to digitization problems (see above), whose commonest effect is:

3. Loss of clumped, primarily immotile, cells from analysis as objects too large to be of interest

Put simply, the common effect of a trajectory truncation collision algorithm in a present-generation CASA system is underestimation of the sperm concentration and overestimation of the proportion of motile cells. In addition, because it is the most motile cells that are more likely to be involved in collisions, the reported movement characteristics for a sperm population are biased toward those of the slower cells.

Proximity to other cells also affects how a motile spermatozoon moves, a problem that is more significant in samples with high concentration and motility.

Systems Using Closest Point Reconstruction
In addition to the problems of close proximity causing modified sperm movement described above, another source of error is introduced if the reconstruction of colliding trajectories uses the nearest centroid to the cell's position in the previous field to construct the path (e.g., as in the Hamilton-Thorn and Motion Analysis systems). The probability is that it will be correct in only half of the cases for each time there are two centroids within the same circle. Consequently, depending on the general direction of the colliding cells, there is a variable likelihood of two incorrect part trajectories being joined. This situation may cause sharp changes in the cells' apparent directions (affecting the trajectories' straightness); or if the two cells had rather different kinematics, their "track average" movement characteristics are altered toward the average of the two cells' overall movement.

Systems Using Trajectory Interpolation
If a cell's centroid cannot be found within the circle and its diameter is doubled and projected forward to the second next frame (or tripled and projected forward yet another frame), there is obviously a risk that the centroid ultimately discovered within the circle does not belong to the original cell (e.g., as in the Hamilton-Thorn and Motion Analysis systems). The commonest problems with this approach are either (1) that an erroneous combination trajectory is reconstructed, or (2) that the track of a cell that leaves the area of the field being analyzed is joined onto another cell, which enters it within the spatial and temporal limits of the interpolation.

If no centroid is found within the limit of the interpolation, the trajectory is truncated. However, if the program recognizes new cells in frames after the first, the cell may be picked up again and its trajectory reconstructed in subsequent frames as a different cell. This problem is termed *track breakage* or *track fragmentation*. If the program does not recognize any new cells in frames after the first one, track breakage is not a problem.

Systems Using "Intelligent Tracking" Algorithms
If the partial trajectories of colliding cells are examined after reconstruction is complete to identify the paths with the best matching vector and kinematic characteristics for concatenation, the likelihood of errors is greatly reduced (e.g., as in the Strömberg-Mika system). This solution to the collisions problem is ideal, but it requires substantially greater computing power and streamlined algorithms if it is not to prolong the analysis time substantially.

APPLICATION OF CASA SYSTEMS TO SEMEN ANALYSIS

Validation of CASA Semen Analysis Results

Many of the world's several hundred CASA users are trying to use their systems to standardize semen analysis and obtain more objective, accurate results. Despite this fact, only a few rigorous comparisons of any system with carefully standardized and quality-controlled traditional semen analysis methods have appeared to date. The general opinion is that current CASA systems cannot provide as accurate values for sperm concentration and motility as can be achieved using semen analysis techniques and quality control procedures comparable to those described in the present text (Knuth et al., 1987; Ginsburg et al., 1988; Knuth and Nieschlag, 1988; Mahony et al., 1988; Mortimer et al., 1988b; Vantman et al., 1988; Chan et al., 1989; reviews: Boyers et al., 1989; Mortimer, 1990).

Direct comparisons between different CASA systems are few (e.g., Gill et al., 1988; Mahony et al., 1988) but support the notion that trajectory truncation at real or perceived collisions causes the greatest errors in sperm concentration and motility results. Its concentration dependence also makes this approach the least convenient for the laboratory.

Some of the apparent inaccuracy of CASA results may be attributable to unreliable use of the Makler chamber in routine practice (D. H. Douglas-Hamilton, personal communication; see also Mortimer, 1990). Although the advent of the Microcell chambers may help solve this problem, some semen samples of increased viscosity do not flow into the 20-µm chambers, and the problem is greater with the 12-µm chambers. As a corollary, the increased preparation depth of 20-µm Microcells only exacerbates any problems of concentration dependence.

Consequently, any laboratory that wants to achieve optimum accuracy and reliability in its semen analysis results should continue to use appropriate traditional methodology (e.g., World Health Organization, 1987, 1992). It does not, however, preclude the important application of CASA systems for sperm movement analysis, which is becoming established as an important adjunct to assessments of sperm functional potential. Nor does it mean that CASA systems may not be sufficiently improved to achieve this goal in the near future.

Possible Solutions to Problems of CASA

A modified approach to the way CASA systems are used might improve their performance in routine semen analysis. Coupled with more elegant algorithms for dealing with static objects and collisions (such as those used in the Strömberg-Mika system), it might take us into the era of reliable automation of sperm concentration and motility assessments.

Separation of the analysis of static and moving objects into two procedures that require different preparations would allow the aliquot for static analysis to be treated with a diluent to disaggregate clumped spermatozoa. If this diluent were also able to render all the spermatozoa immotile (i.e., kill them), lyse many of the round cells and residual cytoplasmic masses present in many clinical semen specimens, and dissolve much of the debris, it would greatly facilitate accurate determination of the total sperm concentration.

Subsequently, in the "fresh" aliquot preparation, the system would need to consider only the moving objects, which, properly defined, must be spermatozoa. Collisions would be dealt with using more sophisticated tracking of cells through collisions, incorporating not only the vector and kinematics characteristics of each cell but also perhaps the morphometry and expected shape changes associated with the cell's rotation.

Finally, the problem of collisions could be reduced if samples were diluted so the sperm concentration was always below about 25×10^6/ml (for use in a 20-μm Microcell). Presently, only dilution with cell-free homologous seminal plasma (obtained by centrifuging part of the sample at 1000 g for 15–20 minutes) is considered acceptable. Clearly, it is not always possible with clinical material, especially with donor semen where it would be wasteful. Unfortunately, the use of pooled and frozen cell-free seminal plasma from a large number of ejaculates (obviously excluding samples with abnormal viscosity and antisperm antibodies) has been found unsuitable. Our own preliminary study showed that, although dilution with pooled seminal plasma was acceptable for some ejaculates, in others it caused significant modifications in the proportion of motile spermatozoa and the quality of their motility.

Although it may be tolerable for experimental studies with adequate opportunity for internal controls, dilution with various saline solutions or culture media cannot be used for clinical assessments. Such dilution modifies sperm movement substantially, which is unacceptable as sperm penetration into cervical mucus is known to be strongly dependent on sperm movement in seminal plasma (see Chapter 11). Therefore if a synthetic diluent were available that had rheological properties comparable to those of seminal plasma, routine dilution prior to CASA would become practicable. Unfortunately, little quantitative information is available on the rheology of seminal plasma, and a range of diluents may well be needed. Worse still is that this deficiency in our knowledge is due to the difficulty of measuring semen viscosity objectively, which would be necessary if a particular diluent had to be chosen from a range.

SPERM KINEMATICS

Specific aspects of sperm movement, such as the velocity of progression and the pattern of movement, have been shown to be closely correlated with sperm penetration into cervical mucus, the outcome of the heterologous zona pellucida-free hamster egg penetration test (HEPT), and the results of IVF (see Chapter 11). Specifically, the objective and quantitative measurement of sperm movement characteristics of individual cells was found to be more predictive of functional ability and hence a man's potential fertility. Consequently, increasing attention has been paid to evaluating sperm motility at more than the crude level of determining the proportion of motile spermatozoa.

Sperm Movement Characteristics

Over the years a plethora of terminology has appeared to describe the various movement characteristics of motile spermatozoa. Some terms are synonymous and describe the same characteristic, but sometimes essentially the same term has been used to describe different characteristics. This confusing and unacceptable state of affairs was addressed at a workshop, "Automated Sperm Motility Analysis," held at the American Society of Andrology's Annual Meeting in Houston, Texas (USA) during March 1988. Terminology and abbreviations (and the appropriate numerical precision) were agreed on for the three basic velocity measurements, the three ratios describing progression, and measures of the frequency and amplitude of lateral deviations of the sperm head. This terminology was subsequently accepted at the international symposium "Human Sperm Movement and Its Evaluation" organized by the Fédération CECOS in Montpellier, France in April 1988. The movement characteristics covered by this ASA-CECOS accord are those derived from head centroid analysis (see below) and are of particular current significance because they are those provided by the present generation of CASA systems.

Movement Characteristics Derived from Head Centroid Analysis

Curvilinear Velocity
Curvilinear velocity (VCL) is calculated from the sum of the straight lines joining the sequential positions of the sperm head along the spermatozoon's track (Fig. 7-7). As such, VCL is essentially the two-dimensional projection of the true three-dimensional helical path of the spermatozoon as revealed by the time resolution (i.e., frame rate) of the imaging method used. VCL values are reported in micrometers per second to one decimal place. VCL is still sometimes referred to as the cell's "track speed."

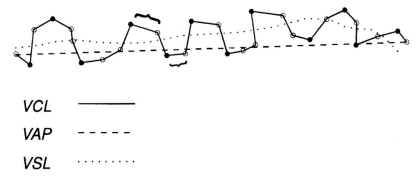

VCL   ——————

VAP   - - - - -

VSL   · · · · · · · ·

Figure 7-7   Derivation of the different sperm velocities from a track reconstructed at 30 frames per second. *Circles* denote head centroid positions (open circles = nonapex points; closed circles = apex points), and the *solid line* joining them is the path followed by the sperm head that is used to calculate the curvilinear velocity (VCL). The average path (in this case visually appraised) used to calculate the average path velocity (VAP) is shown by the *dotted line;* the *broken line* joining the first and last points of the track is the straight-line path used to calculate the straight-line velocity (VSL). One measurement of the instantaneous velocity is shown by the *brace.* (Redrawn from Mortimer, 1990.)

Average Path Velocity

The average path velocity (VAP) is the velocity along the average path of the spermatozoon (Fig. 7-7). Because the average path can be derived in a number of ways, including visual interpolation, various mathematical smoothing techniques, or geometric construction (see below), the precise method used for its derivation must always be stated. VAP values are reported in micrometers per second to one decimal place.

Straight-Line Velocity

The straight-line velocity (VSL) is the linear, or "progression," velocity of the cell. It is calculated from the straight line distance between the start and end of the observed track (Fig. 7-7). VSL values are reported in micrometers per second to one decimal place. It is important to note that many CellSoft CASA systems still use linear velocity to refer to VCL, a major source of confusion for less experienced CASA users.

Progression Ratios

Three progression ratios, expressed as integer percentages, can be calculated from the three velocity measurements described above:

$$\text{Linearity (LIN)} = \text{VSL/VCL} \times 100$$

$$\text{Straightness (STR)} = \text{VSL/VAP} \times 100$$

$$\text{Wobble (WOB} = \text{VAP/VCL} \times 100$$

Older terms include progression ratio (PR), equivalent to linearity, and the curvilinear progression ratio (PRC), equivalent to straightness.

Amplitude of Lateral Head Displacement

The amplitude of the lateral displacement of the sperm head (ALH) is calculated from the amplitudes of its lateral deviations about the cell's axis of progression (average path). Various authors and CASA programs use either an average value (ALHmean) calculated from the individual measurements made over the length of the track, an average calculated from a minimum of three measurements at different places along the track (manual analysis), or the maximum value (ALHmax) of all the measurements made along the track (see below). Traditionally, ALH measurements are expressed as the width across the whole track (i.e., twice the average or maximum measurement) in micrometers to one decimal place. Obviously, to compare results between studies or analysis methods, the derivation of ALH must be stated.

Beat/Cross Frequency

The beat/cross frequency (BCF) is the number of times the curvilinear track crosses the average path per unit time. It is expressed in hertz to one decimal place.

In reality, BCF is a derivation of the true flagellar beat frequency and the frequency of rotation (ROF) of the head. Although it cannot be analyzed by automated CASA systems, the true ROF is the number of times the sperm head rotates through 360 degrees per unit time. A human spermatozoon swimming in seminal plasma usually (but not always) rotates through 180 degrees at the apex of each lateral deviation of the head about the axis of progression (David et al., 1981).

Flagellar Analysis

The most comprehensive description of sperm movement focuses on the detailed kinematics of flagellar beating because it is the generation and propagation of waves along the sperm tail that generate the propulsive force. Although fundamental studies of the flagellar contraction mechanism require this level of analysis, there have been no decisions as yet regarding the most important or most appropriate flagellar parameters to measure.

Although the relationships are complex, analyses of sperm movement derived from following the head can provide a great deal of useful information on sperm movement as well as on flagellar beat characteristics (Serres et al., 1984). Observations on flagellar beating were fundamental to basic descriptions of hyperactivated motility of human spermatozoa in current use (Burkman, 1990; Mortimer and Mortimer, 1990). In view of the limited clinical interest in flagellar motion analysis, this aspect of sperm kinematics is not considered further at this time.

Methods of Measuring Sperm Movement

Although early studies on mammalian sperm movement used primarily microcinematography and various types of time-lapse, multiple-exposure, and timed-exposure photomicrography, these methods must now be considered essentially obsolete and are not considered further here. Over the last few years videomicrography has rapidly become established as the preferred method owing to its relatively low cost and the elimination of film-processing delays (reviews: Boyers et al., 1989; Mortimer, 1990).

The first commercial sperm motility analyzer using a microcomputer to perform digital image analysis of video signals (i.e., CASA instrument) appeared in 1985. Since this time a number of systems have become available, and these machines or their descendants will certainly be of major importance to diagnostic andrology in the future.

Unfortunately, CASA technology has often been embraced uncritically. Although such systems are reliable in terms of their analysis of movement characteristics, critical evaluations of their performance as automated semen analyzers have revealed an essential need for further development and refinement before they can be accepted in andrology laboratories operating to standards such as those recommended by the World Health Organization (see Chapter 16).

Manual Trajectory Analysis

Manually reconstructed trajectories are analyzed by essentially the same methods as those developed for microcinematography, with the measurements being performed by either manual or semiautomated methods (David et al., 1981). This exercise is important for anyone desiring a real understanding of sperm movement analysis. In addition, it is the only way to validate the performance of CASA systems for analysis of sperm kinematics.

Curvilinear and Straight-Line Velocities

Manual measurements of the curvilinear trajectory length are made using a curvimeter or map measurer (e.g., Burnat model 54: Berty, Paris, France). The track is measured starting from each end, and the two values are averaged. A curvimeter can also be used to measure the length of a visually appraised track midline or average path. The straight-line track length is calculated from the distance between the first and last points on the track measured using a rule (Fig. 7-7).

Average Path Velocity

Various methods have been used to derive the average path, including geometric construction and Tukey window running average smoothing (Fig. 7-8). Calculating a five-point running average has been the most widely used, although this method is not always appropriate for every track because VCL is not the same for all cells, not even for all cells with the same VSL or VAP due to variations in BCF and ALH (David et al., 1981; Mortimer et al., 1988a). It is VCL, in conjunction with the frame rate, that determines the spacing and location of the track points.

If equal weight is given to each of the five points, it is termed a rectangular running average (e.g., CellSoft system 3000). Alternatively, variable mathematical weighting may be applied to the points (e.g., Motion Analysis systems, which use a cosine taper). Although five-point smoothing has been found to be the best alternative for human seminal spermatozoa analyzed at a 30-Hz frame rate, it is not for tracks sampled at higher frame rates (e.g., 11 points for 60-Hz trajectories) (Boyers et al., 1989; also see below) or for washed or hyperactivated cells whose VCL val-

A.   Visual appraisal

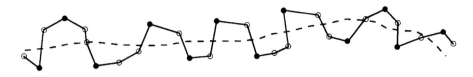

B.   5-point smoothing

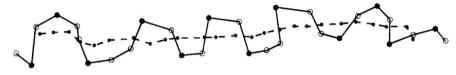

C.   Geometric method

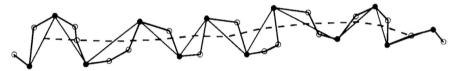

Figure 7-8   Methods for deriving the average path and their effects on its shape—and hence the value of VAP for the track shown in Figure 7-7. (**A**) Visual appraisal. (**B**) Rectangular five-point running average or smoothing. (**C**) Non-frame-rate-dependent geometric method. (Redrawn from Mortimer, 1990.)

ues are much higher than those of seminal spermatozoa (Mortimer and Mortimer, 1990).

Obviously, at least seven track points are needed to provide the simplest five-point-smoothed path. This number is also the minimum requirement for BCF calculations. However, the ASA-CECOS accord has established that at least 0.5 second of reconstructed trajectory should be used (see below). Alternatively, the average path of progressively motile human spermatozoa can be derived using a method based on geometric principles that is neither VCL- nor frame-rate-dependent (Mortimer et al., 1988a,c) (Fig. 7-8).

A common problem with all trajectory-smoothing alorithms is that the first and last two points (assuming a five-point window was used) of the curvilinear path extend beyond the ends of the smoothed path. Several techniques are used to "correct" the smoothed path for the duration of the curvilinear path, this being necessary for calculation of the STR and WOB ratios.

1. The first and last points on the curvilinear path may be used as the equivalent points on the smoothed path with a three-point average being used to determine the second and next to last points on the smoothed path (e.g., Hamilton-Thorn systems).
2. The length of the smoothed path may be increased in proportion to the ratio of its straight-line path and the original curvilinear path's own straight-line path. This rule works reasonably well for typical progressive spermatozoa (e.g., Mortimer et al., 1988a), but it does produce some errors for nonstraight trajectories.
3. The first and last two points on the curvilinear path may be "reflected back" to extend the curvilinear path artificially so that approximate smoothed points may be calculated to correspond to those at the start and end of the curvilinear path (e.g., Motion Analysis systems).

Measurements of Lateral Head Displacement
Measurements of the amplitude of lateral head displacement (ALH) can be made using either parallel rules at, usually, three places along the reconstructed track or by measuring the distance from the apex of a lateral deviation of the sperm head on one side of the average path to the line joining the apices of the lateral deviations immediately before and after it on the opposite side of the average path (Fig. 7-9). This measurement is repeated for every wave along the reconstructed track, and the measurements are then either averaged to provide the ALHmean, or the largest value is taken and used as ALHmax. If ALH values are derived from measurements of the distances between apices of lateral head displacement and the average path, the mean or maximum value is doubled to represent the whole track width.

If ALH is calculated mathematically, a series of straight lines, or risers (RIS) (Boyers et al., 1989), are calculated between each point on the smoothed path and its corresponding point on the curvilinear path (Fig. 7-9). The series is examined, and the peak RIS values are taken as the individual ALH measurements along the track. These peak RIS values can then be averaged and doubled to give the track-average measurement (ALHmean), or the maximum RIS value is taken and doubled to give the track-maximum measurement (ALHmax).

The beat/cross frequency (BCF) is calculated from the number of times that the cell's curvilinear path crosses its average path per unit time. If ALH was calculated mathematically, BCF is derived from the number of peak RIS values.

Advanced Concepts of Trajectory Analysis
Several alternative sperm movement characteristics, or methods for deriving measures of sperm motion, also exist (review: Boyers et al., 1989).

Angular Measures of Sperm Movement
At each point along the reconstructed trajectory the sperm head changes direction. These changes in direction can be computed as angles and used to describe the average shape of the trajectory. The *mean angular displacement* (MAD) is calculated as the time average or track average of the absolute values of the instantaneous turning angle of the sperm head along its curvilinear trajectory. It is usually presented in

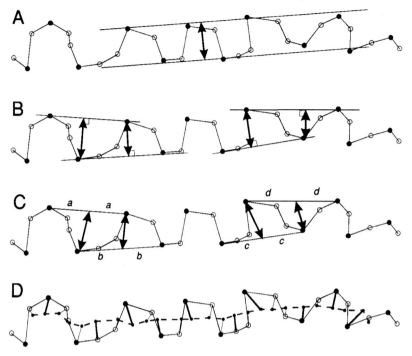

Figure 7-9 Methods for deriving the amplitude of lateral head displacement (ALH, indicated by *double-headed arrows*) for the track shown in Figure 7-7. (**A**) Manual measurements of the "average" track width using parallel rules. (**B**) Measurements on individual "waves" where the perpendicular distance from each apex point to the line joining the previous and next apex points is measured. (**C**) Geometric method that considers the distance from each apex point to the midpoint between the previous and next apex points as the measure of ALH. (**D**) Method using "risers," which are the distances between each point on the curvilinear track an its equivalent point on the smoothed track; local maxima *(thick lines)* are then used to calculate the half ALH value for each "wave." (Modified from Mortimer, 1990.)

degrees. At high frame rates, however, MAD apparently subtends to a value of zero (D. F. Katz, personal communication) perhaps making it of uncertain significance.

Harmonic Analysis of Sperm Movement
Harmonic analysis requires a relatively high image sampling frequency and a relatively long period of observation of the trajectory. No harmonic characteristic of sperm movement has yet been related to physiological function, and this area remains one of specialized research interest.

Fractal Analysis of Sperm Movement
The term fractal geometry was coined by the mathematician Benoit Mandelbrot to describe objects with fractional dimensions. The use of dimensions to describe objects is familiar to all. A point has zero dimensions, a line has one dimension, an

area has two, and a solid has three. Mandelbrot called this last dimension the topo-logical dimension. A fractal object has a quality called a fractal dimension, which is larger than the topological dimension. A nonfractal object has a fractal dimension that equals the topological dimension. The term fractal is used because the fractal dimension is often a fraction.

Almost everything in nature is a fractal: No matter how much it is magnified there is still even more detail. Even brownian motion has a fractal nature. There has been interest in trying to analyze sperm movement using fractals with the idea that it might be possible to describe a cell's movement with a single numerical value. This field is still a young area of research, and no definite results with biological or clinical correlates have been produced. It is potentially an enormously powerful concept that could revolutionize the way we consider sperm movement.

Multiparametric Analysis of Sperm Movement
We are already capable of describing several movement characteristics for each motile spermatozoon; and although many are interrelated, it allows us to select sub-populations using more than one criterion at a time. This type of analysis must be used at the individual cell level; trying to use sample-averaged values is pointless. Not only are many movement characteristics not normally distributed, making the calculation of mean values with standard deviation statistics meaningless, but it conceals the intrinsic variability of the population across movement characteristics.

Cells with a certain range of VCL values have a wide range of VSL values, ALH values, and BCF values; and, even though these four aspects are interrelated, the relationship between them all is complex. Obvious applications of this type of movement analysis include trying to define the subpopulation of ejaculate sperma-tozoa that is best able to penetrate cervical mucus and those that are able to develop hyperactivated motility during capacitation.

Hyperactivation Analysis
An early example of multiparametric sperm movement analysis was the derivation of the CellSoft Hyperactivation Module (Robertson et al., 1988). Here complex movement characteristics were derived from individual cell values and used to define a subpopulation of cells showing what was considered to represent the hyper-activated pattern of motility for human spermatozoa (see Chapter 2). The movement characteristic Dance (DNC) was calculated as the product of VCL and ALHmean, and DNCmean (DNM) was derived as [ALHmean × VCL/VSL].

Subsequently, other workers have used multiparametric definitions for human sperm hyperactivation that require application at the individual cell level (Burkman, 1990; Mortimer and Mortimer, 1990) (Table 7-1). Studies considering only sample-averaged movement characteristics do not allow specific identification of the hyper-activation phenomenon.

Mucus-Penetrating Capacity
It is known that sperm penetration from seminal plasma into cervical mucus is favored by both high VSL or VAP and high ALH (see below; also see Chapter 11); therefore it should also be possible to produce a multiparametric description of a

Table 7–1   Kinematic descriptions of hyperactivated human spermatozoa

Classification	VCL (μm/s)	VSL (μm/s)	LIN (%)	STR (%)	ALH (μm)
Values from Mortimer and Mortimer (1990).					
Forward progressive	—	≥ 40	≥ 60	≥ 95	< 5
All hyperactivated	≥ 100	—	< 60	—	≥ 5
Transition phase	≥ 100	≥ 30	< 60	≥60	≥ 5
True hyperactivated	≥ 100	< 30	< 60	< 60	≥ 5
Values from Burkman (1990)					
All hyperactivated	≥ 100	Not used	≤ 65	Not used	≥ 7.5

subpopulation of spermatozoa ideally suited for penetrating cervical mucus. Although no specific results are available, one might propose a definition as follows: VSL ≥ 25 μm/s AND STR ≥ 90% AND ALH ≥ 2.5 μm. The AND terms are Boolean arguments; that is, each cell must meet all three criteria.

Basic Principles of Sperm Kinematics

Numerous factors, both extrinsic and method-specific, influence the measurement of sperm movement characteristics. The ASA-CECOS accord attempted to resolve many of these confounding factors to achieve maximum comparability among laboratories studying sperm kinematics. The aim was to promote the interchange of information between laboratories and make publications from each laboratory comprehensible to all others. Only in this way was it believed we could facilitate the development of our understanding of the physiological and clinical relevance and this new area of andrology.

Temperature Dependency
Because sperm velocity is highly sensitive to alterations in specimen temperature (e.g., VCL may double between 20° and 37°C), the ASA-CECOS accord requires that all measurements of human sperm kinematics be performed at 37°C. Hence a heated microscope stage, an air-curtain incubator, or a heated microscope enclosure must be used.

Duration of Observation
For reliable kinematic analysis of seminal human spermatozoa, the ASA-CECOS accord requires that only tracks of at least 0.5 second duration be used. Because the images are not themselves of $^1/_{30}$ or $^1/_{25}$ second duration, but are obtained at these time *intervals,* this analysis duration corresponds to 16 track points for 30-Hz systems and 14 frames for 25-Hz systems. Consequently, to reconstruct trajectories that include 15 or 12.5 (i.e., 13) intervals, one more point than half the frame rate is needed.

Numbers of Trajectories Needed for Reliable Analysis
After prolonged discussion, the ASA-CECOS accord established that for sample mean or modal values for the various movement characteristics, at least 100 trajec-

tories must be analyzed. This number refers to *valid* trajectories (i.e., those acceptable for kinematic analysis). Many more cells must be analyzed by the CASA system to yield this number of valid trajectories. For performing subclassifications of the trajectories analyzed, at least 200 should be available per sample.

Effect of Preparation Depth

A preparation depth of 10 μm (e.g., Makler chamber) was accepted by the ASA-CECOS accord as sufficient for analyzing human sperm movement in seminal plasma, but it is not adequate for unimpeded motion of washed, capacitating spermatozoa. Such sperm preparations must be made in chambers of at least 20 μm depth. Studies on human sperm hyperactivation typically use chambers of greater depth, e.g., 32- to 33-μm Chartpak slides (Robertson et al., 1988; Mortimer and Mortimer, 1990); 40-μm (now 50-μm) Microcells; or 50-μm flat glass Microslide capillaries (Burkman, 1990) to achieve reliable data.

Kinematics of Progressive Spermatozoa

Because in semen only progressive spermatozoa are likely to have any functional potential (see Chapter 2), it is only these cells that should be used for movement analysis. Traditional definitions of progressive motility have centered around the concept of space gain, i.e., the absolute translation of a cell across the microscope field. Common definitions are based on the number of head lengths traveled. Sometimes one, usually two, head lengths of space gain are required, corresponding to VSL (and, more or less, VAP) values of 5 or 10 μm/s.

For CASA systems incorporating a user-definable VCL threshold, it should be set at 20 μm/s (Mortimer and Mortimer, 1988); if a selectable VSL or VAP threshold is available, it should be set at 5 or 10 μm/s.

The maximum velocity (which is always VCL) should be set at 200 μm/s for seminal spermatozoa. Although few spermatozoa swim anywhere near this fast, the values seen in the reports are the *track average* values, whereas it is the instantaneous velocity (i.e., VCLmax ÷ frame rate) that is used to determine the radius of the circle of maximum likelihood (see Track Reconstruction, above). Values for the instantaneous velocity can easily exceed 1.5 times the track average value at 30 Hz.

If nonprogressive spermatozoa are included in the population for movement analysis, a substantial bias is introduced into the measurements (Mortimer and Mortimer, 1988). Enforcing a VSL threshold to identify only those cells that are progressive improves the biological relevance of these measurements, especially if only sample mean (or modal) values are used. This reasoning was the basis of the Forward Progression version of the CellSoft System 3000.

In washed or swim-up sperm preparations, the progressive spermatozoa typically show much higher velocities and have a tendency for increased ALH. Consequently, the VCLmax must be increased to at least 300 μm/s and studies on human sperm hyperactivation typically set VCLmax at 400 μm/s. Although a threshold VSL or VAP definition for progressive motility may be enforced on washed sperm populations, any such analysis must be performed *post hoc* because nonprogressive patterns of movement are also of interest in such sperm populations.

Kinematics of Nonprogressive Spermatozoa

Although nonprogressively motile spermatozoa in semen are of no physiological relevance, in populations of washed or swim-up spermatozoa, especially those incubated under capacitating conditions, certains patterns of vigorous, albeit nonprogressive, motility are seen. Many such spermatozoa are showing the hyperactivated pattern of movement known to be essential for eutherian fertilization (see Chapter 2). Consequently, great care should be taken not to accidentally exclude such cells from the population used for movement analysis, which is easily done if the VCLmax is set too low (e.g., 300 μm/s, which might ordinarily be sufficient for progressively motile washed human spermatozoa).

References and Recommended Reading

Boyers, S. P., Davis, R. O., and Katz, D. F. (1989). Automated semen analysis. *Curr. Probl. Obstet. Gynecol. Fertil.* Vol. XII(5). Year Book, Medical Publishers Inc., Chicago.

Burkman, L. J. (1990). Hyperactivated motility of human spermatozoa during in vitro capacitation and implications for fertility. In Gagnon, C. (ed): *Controls of Sperm Motility: Biological and Clinical Aspects.* CRC Press, Boca Raton, FL.

Chan, S. Y. W., Wang, C., Song, B. L., Lo, T., Leung, A., Tsoi, W. L., and Leung, J. (1989). Computer-assisted image analysis of sperm concentration in human semen before and after swim-up separation: comparison with assessment by haemocytometer. *Int. J. Androl.* **12,** 339.

David, G., Serres, C., and Jouannet, P. (1981). Kinematics of human spermatozoa. *Gamete Res.* **4,** 83.

Gill, H. S., Van Arsdalen, K., Hypolite, J., Levin, R. M., and Ruzich, J. V. (1988). Comparative study of two computerized semen motility analyzers. *Andrologia* **20,** 433.

Ginsburg, K. A., Moghissi, K. S., and Abel, E. L. (1988). Computer-assisted human semen analysis: Sampling errors and reproducibility. *J. Androl.* **9,** 82.

Katz, D. F., and Davis, R. O. (1987). Automatic analysis of human sperm motion. *J. Androl.* **8,** 170.

Katz, D. F., Davis, R. O., Delandmeter, B. A., and Overstreet, J. W. (1985). Real-time analysis of sperm motion using automatic video image digitization. *Comput. Meth. Prog. Biomed.* **21,** 173.

Knuth, U. A., and Nieschlag, E. (1988). Comparison of computerized semen analysis with the conventional procedure in 322 patients. *Fertil. Steril.* **49,** 881.

Knuth, U. A., Yeung, C.-H., and Nieschlag, E. (1987). Computerized semen analysis: objective measurement of semen characteristics is biased by subjective parameter setting. *Fertil. Steril.* **48,** 118.

Mahony, M. C., Alexander, N. J., and Swanson, R. J. (1988). Evaluation of semen parameters by means of automated sperm motion analyzers. *Fertil. Steril.* **49,** 876.

Mortimer, D. (1990). Objective analysis of sperm motility and kinematics. In Keel, B. A., and Webster, B. W. (eds): *Handbook of the Laboratory Diagnosis and Treatment of Infertility.* CRC Press, Boca Raton, FL.

Mortimer, D., and Mortimer, S. T. (1988). Influence of system parameter settings on human sperm motility analysis using CellSoft. *Hum. Reprod.* **3,** 621.

Mortimer, D., Curtis, E. F., and Ralston, A. (1988a). Semi-automated analysis of manually-reconstructed tracks of progressively motile human spermatozoa. *Hum. Reprod.* **3,** 303.

Mortimer, D., Goel, N., and Shu, M. A. (1988b). Evaluation of the CellSoft automated semen analysis system in a routine laboratory setting. *Fertil. Steril.* **50,** 960.

Mortimer, D., Serres, C., Mortimer, S. T., and Jouannet, P. (1988c). Influence of image sampling frequency on the perceived movement characteristics of progressively motile human spermatozoa. *Gamete Res.* **20,** 313.

Mortimer, S. T., and Mortimer, D. (1990). Kinematics of human spermatozoa incubated under capacitating conditions. *J. Androl.* **11,** 195.

Robertson, L., Wolf, D. P., and Tash, J. S. (1988). Temporal changes in motility parameters related to acrosomal status: identification and characterization of populations of hyperactivated human sperm, *Biol. Reprod.* **39,** 797.

Serres, C., Feneux, D., Jouannet, P., and David, G. (1984). Influence of the flagellar wave development and propagation on the human sperm movement in seminal plasma, *Gamete Res.* **9,** 183.

Vantman, D., Koukoulis, G., Dennison, L., Zinaman, M., and Sherins, R. J. (1988). Computer-assisted semen analysis: evaluation of method and assessment of the influence of sperm concentration on linear velocity determination. *Fertil. Steril.* **49,** 510.

World Health Organization (1987). *WHO Laboratory Manual for the Examination of Human Semen and Semen-Cervical Mucus Interaction,* 2nd ed. Cambridge University Press, Cambridge.

World Health Organization (1992). *WHO Laboratory Manual for the Examination of Human Semen and Sperm-Cervical Mucus Interaction,* 3rd ed. Cambridge University Press, Cambridge.

8

Ultrastructure of Spermatozoa

Assessment of sperm morphology at the light microscopic level can provide only limited information on the internal structure of the spermatozoa inferred from differential cytochemical reactions and affinities for the various stains. More detailed examination of sperm structure using the transmission electron microscope or scanning electron microscope can reveal major, often unsuspected, abnormalities. Using such a high-resolution technique has revealed that spermatozoa considered to be morphologically abnormal at the light microscopic level possess, in addition, many subtle defects of one or more region of the cell. However, this situation also seems to be true for many of the spermatozoa considered morphologically normal at the light microscopic level.

Consequently, the real value of electron microscopy is emphasized in situations where most of the spermatozoa in an ejaculate have a single predominant abnormality or the same combination of associated defects. In these situations there does seem to be a relationship between specific morphological defects and impairment of sperm function (Dadoune, 1988; Zamboni, 1987, 1991). This situation is comparable to the so-called "sterilizing defects" described for various domesticated species.

ELECTRON MICROSCOPY OF HUMAN SPERMATOZOA

Scanning Electron Microscopy

The scanning electron microscope (SEM) permits examination of the whole spermatozoon at a higher magnification and greater resolution than does light microscopy. Its particular value is that it enables visualization of the cell surface (Fléchon and Hafez, 1976; Liakatas et al., 1982). Although SEM has little to offer in the clinical andrology laboratory, it has been of benefit in research areas.

Transmission Electron Microscopy

The transmission electron microscope (TEM) is the principal technique used for diagnostic purposes. It is generally used with thin sections and enables examination of intracellular structures (Pedersen and Fawcett, 1976; Zamboni, 1987, 1991; Dadoune, 1988) (Figs. 8-1 to 8-3). TEM examination of thin sections allows an experienced morphologist to identify numerous structural defects of the tail that impair, or even prevent, sperm motility. Other defects in the head, particularly of

159

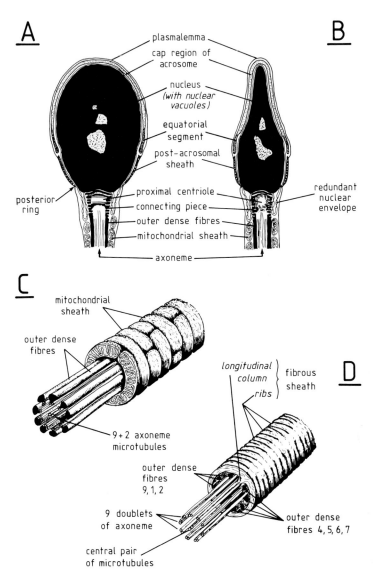

Figure 8-1 Ultrastructure of the human spermatozoon. Longitudinal sections of the human sperm head parallel (**A**) and perpendicular (**B**) to the axis of the proximal centriole. Cutaway drawings show the organization of the midpiece (**C**) and principal piece (**D**) regions of the human sperm tail. (**A–D**, adapted from Pedersen, H., and Fawcett, D. W. Functional anatomy of the human spermatozoon. In Hafez, E.S.E. (ed.): *Human Semen and Fertility Regulation in Men.* Mosby, St. Louis, 1976, p. 65.)

E

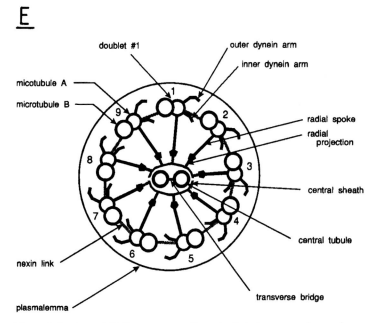

Figure 8-1 *(cont.)* (**E**) Transverse section of a 9 + 2 axonemal complex.

the acrosome and postacrosomal sheath regions, may impair or again prevent fertilization.

At the electron microscope level the human spermatozoon possesses basically the same components as other eutherian spermatozoa, although with a few differences in detail (see Fig. 8-1). From a practical standpoint it is important to note that the existence of structural defects is even more common when spermatozoa are examined at the ultrastructural level.

Although the entire spermatozoon is enclosed within a continuous plasma membrane, many studies have now demonstrated not only that this membrane is highly locally specialized but that these specializations change as the spermatozoon matures, capacitates, and then undergoes the acrosome reaction. Hence membrane fluidity is extremely important for normal sperm function. Because human spermatozoa contain a high proportion of unsaturated fatty acids they are highly sensitive to peroxidative damage. Phospholipid peroxidation makes the membrane less fluid and thereby impairs, and may even completely block, sperm fertilizing ability.

The chromatin of the normal human sperm nucleus is heavily condensed and appears dense and homogeneous in transmission electron micrographs, although small nuclear vacuoles are common (Fig. 8-2A). However, in many human spermatozoa the chromatin shows an "immature" appearance, typified by a coarsely granular nature with more and larger vacuoles. Around the nucleus there is a nuclear envelope that has a double membrane structure. However, unlike somatic cells it

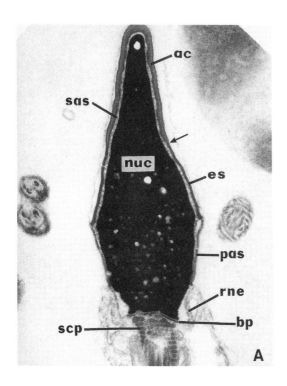

A

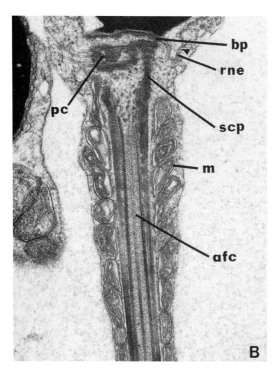

B

Figure 8-2 Ultrastructure of the human spermatozoon. (**A**) Transmission electronmicrograph of a sagittal section through the sperm head (×30.5K). See Figure 8-1 and text for descriptions. **ac** = acrosomal cap region; **es** = equatorial segment; **arrow** = cap-equatorial segment boundary; **pas** = postacrosomal sheath; **sas** = subacrosomal space (cytoplasm); **nuc** = nucleus (condensed chromatin); **rne** = redundant nuclear envelope; **bp** = basal plate; **scp** = striated connecting piece. (**B**) Transmission electronmicrograph of a longitudinal section through the sperm tail (×64K). See Figure 8-1 and text for descriptions. **ren** = redundant nuclear envelope (note nuclear pores, indicated by point of triangle); **bp** = basal plate; **pc** = proximal centriole; **scp** = striated connecting piece; **m** = mitochondrion; **afc** = axial filament complex (axoneme + dense fibres). (Micrographs courtesy of Mr. Ross Boadle, EM Unit, Westmead Hospital, Sydney, Australia.)

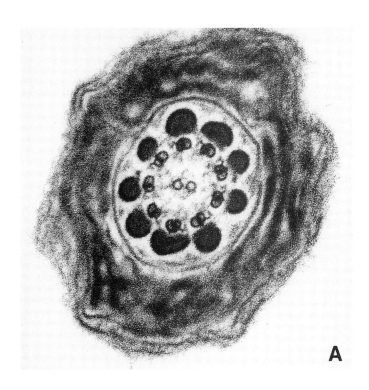

A

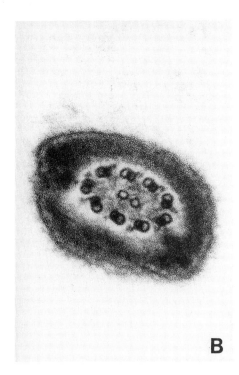

B

Figure 8-3 Ultrastructure of the human sperm tail. Transmission electronmicrographs of transverse sections through the midpiece (**A**) and principal piece (**B**) regions of the tail (both ×140K). See Figure 8-1 and text for descriptions. (Micrographs courtesy of Mr. Ross Boadle, EM Unit, Westmead Hospital, Sydney, Australia.)

does not contain any nuclear pores, except in the limited area over the base of the sperm head between the posterior ring (an O-ring-like structure around the head, posterior to the postacrosomal sheath, which attaches the sperm plasma membrane to the nuclear envelope) and the basal plate, which is a specialization of the nuclear envelope and marks the site of attachment (implantation) of the tail to the head. In this region many spermatozoa show a fold or sleeve of redundant nuclear envelope, perforated regularly by nuclear pores, extending into the proximal neck region.

The anterior half to two-thirds of the human sperm head is covered by the acrosome, a cap-like membrane-bound organelle overlying the nucleus. The anterior part of the acrosome, or cap region, is involved in the acrosome reaction, whereas the posterior part, the equatorial segment, remains intact in acrosome-reacted spermatozoa. An intact equatorial segment is essential as it is the region of initial fusion between the spermatozoon and the oocyte plasma membranes.

The posterior region of the nucleus, between the posterior margin of the equatorial segment of the acrosome and the posterior ring, is overlain by the postacrosomal sheath. Initial contact between the fertilizing spermatozoon and the oolemma is made in this region, perhaps involving a carbohydrate-based attachment mechanism between glycoproteins.

The neck region (Fig. 8-2B) comprises the striated connecting piece of the tail, perhaps equivalent to a ciliary basal body, whose anterior aspect has a cap-like structure (sometimes termed the *capitellum*) that is the site of attachment of the tail to the basal plate of the head. The proximal centriole is embedded transversely within the striated columns of the connecting piece, which are themselves attached to the proximal ends of the 9 dense fibers that surround the typical 9 + 2 axonemal complex of microtubules.

Although there is little residual cytoplasm in the neck region of other eutherian spermatozoa, human spermatozoa often show a substantial amount. The presence of excess residual cytoplasm in this region has recently been associated with a retained ability of these cells to generate reactive oxygen species that cause autoperoxidative damage.

The distal centriole originally present at the base of the flagellum serves as an organizer during formation of the axoneme but disappears later in spermiogenesis concurrently with the formation of the striated connecting piece. The same basic 9 + 2 pattern of microtubules as seen in animal cilia and flagella forms the core of the human sperm tail (Fig. 8-3). Each of the 9 doublets is connected to the central sheath surrounding the central pair of microtubules by a radial link, and adjacent doublets are connected by a nexin link. Each doublet also has a pair of dynein ATPase arms that are essential for normal axonemal motility. Absence of either the outer or inner arms will cause severely impaired sperm motility, whereas the absence of both causes the immotile cilia (Kartagener) syndrome.

In eutherian spermatozoa nine additional dense fibers surround the central axoneme (Fig. 8-3A). The fibers are believed to be elastic elements allowing more efficient flagellar beating in the viscous environments encountered in species with internal fertilization. They taper off toward the distal end of the tail in a differential, but specific, manner. Their progressive reduction in size and number accounts for differences in the sperm tail's rigidity/flexibility along its length. The 9 + 2 axoneme plus the dense fibers comprise the axial filament complex.

In the midpiece region the axial filament complex is surrounded by a sheath of helically arranged mitochondria, although in the principal piece of the sperm tail it is enclosed within a fibrous sheath consisting of two longitudinal columns connected by circumferential ribs that branch and anastomose. At the posterior limit of the midpiece there is an annulus of dense material between the last mitochondrial gyre and the start of the fibrous sheath. Finally, in the terminal segment of the sperm tail there remains only the 9 + 2 axoneme directly covered by the plasma membrane.

Tail Defects

Several studies have described the wide range of structural abnormalities that may exist in the axonemes of human spermatozoa, with the immotile cilia syndrome (Kartagener syndrome) being the best known (Afzelius et al., 1975; Escalier and David, 1984). A typical presentation of this syndrome is a semen analysis that shows normal numbers of spermatozoa with apparently normal (light microscopic) morphology combined with normal levels of sperm vitality but essentially zero motility. In this situation, the absence of the dynein arms (Fig. 8-3) causes the spermatozoa to be immotile, even though their morphology at the light microscopic level appears normal.

Only TEM can confirm the underlying ultrastructural defect in these men (Fig. 8-4) that effectively renders them sterile in terms of achieving conception in vivo. Of interest is a report that if such spermatozoa are induced to undergo the acrosome reaction and then are placed in the perivitelline space by microinjection, normal fertilization can occur (Bongso et al., 1989).

Round-Head Defect

The round-head defect, or globozoospermia, is another morphological abnormality of human spermatozoa that is a sterilizing defect. It is not the situation where the spermatozoa are generally morphologically normal but have a more round than oval head shape; it is a specific defect in which the spermatozoa lack a nuclear envelope, acrosome, and postacrosomal sheath (Tyler et al., 1985) (see Fig. 3–12). Such spermatozoa, which can be recognized reliably by light microscopy, are incapable of fertilization.

Surface Replica Preparations

Metal replicas of either air-dried (or, with slightly better results, critical point-dried) spermatozoa are made by evaporating metal, usually platinum, under high vacuum and then dissolving away the biological material using bleach and acid. These replicas are then viewed by TEM (Fig. 8-5). Although the same aspect of the cells is assessed as with SEM, the higher resolution of the TEM can be advantageous (Mortimer, 1981).

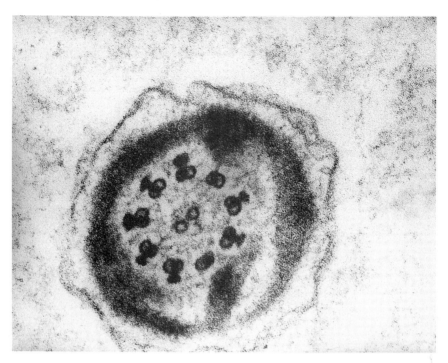

Figure 8-4 Ultrastructure of the human sperm tail in a man with Kartagener syndrome. Note the absence of dynein arms on the outer doublets of the axoneme. (Micrograph courtesy of Mr. Ross Boadle, EM Unit, Westmead Hospital, Sydney, Australia.)

Figure 8-5 Surface replica images of normal and abnormal human spermatozoa. (**A**) Normal form. (**B**) Tapering, pyriform head (note constriction of head just anterior to the neck). (**C**) Two grossly abnormal heads; the upper one is small and shows no acrosomal region, and the lower one is severely tapered and lacks a midpiece. (**D**) Dead spermatozoon (note the absence of the plasma membrane, revealing the intracellular structures of the head and the mitochondria arranged spirally in the midpiece region). (**E**) Essentially normal spermatozoon showing blebbing of the acrosomal cap region, perhaps indicating that the cell is undergoing an acrosome reaction. (**F**) Noninserted tail defect. (**G**) Cytoplasmic droplet extending from the posterior ring of the head over almost the whole midpiece region. (**H**) Coiled tail. (**I**) Midpiece defect note the reduced thickness of the posterior half of the midpiece due to the absence of mitochondria. (Micrograph (A) is from Mortimer, 1981; micrographs (D),(E) and (I) are from Mortimer, 1981. With permission.)

166

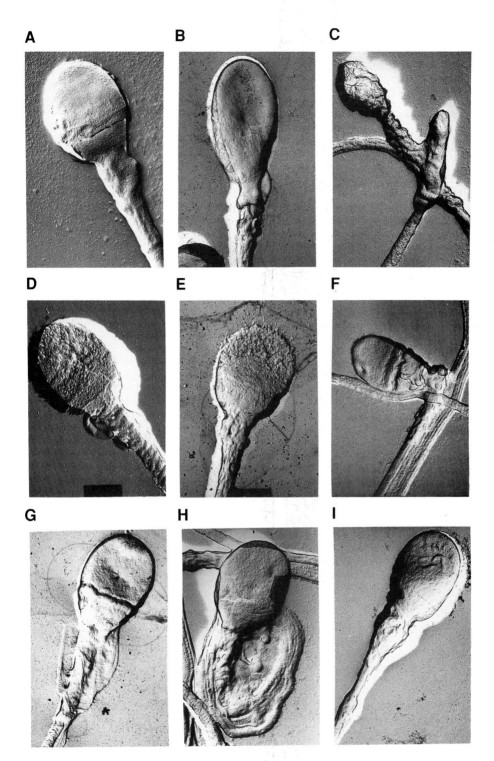

A B C D E F G H I

Figure 8-5

PREPARATION OF HUMAN SPERMATOZOA FOR ELECTRON MICROSCOPY

Transmission Electron Microscopy: Thin Sections

Principle

Thin-section TEM describes the fixation and encapsulation of human spermatozoa, including en bloc staining with uranyl acetate in resin ready for the preparation of thin sections. Much of the method was devised by Dr. Sue Stevens (Westmead Hospital, NSW, Australia, now retired), with some minor modification by the author. However, the method does not describe the making of thin sections or any staining of such sections (e.g., with lead citrate) that may be considered necessary. These methods vary with the electron microscopist's preference and should be left to that individual.

Reagents

N.B. Great caution is advised regarding the correct handling and disposal of the fixatives and other solutions and solvents used when preparing tissues for electron microscopy.

Fix buffer is a 240 mM solution of sodium cacodylate with 4.8% (w/v) sucrose. Dissolve 12.4 g sodium cacodylate (NaCac·3H$_2$O) and 12.0 g sucrose in about 200 ml reagent water. Add 2.07 ml of 1 N HCl and 2.5 ml of a 1% (w/v) solution of CaCl$_2$·6H$_2$O. Mix and bring to a total volume of 250 ml with reagent water. Store at 4°C. Discard if there are any signs of precipitation or contamination.

Rinse buffer is a 200 mM solution of sodium cacodylate with 6.6% (w/v) sucrose. Dissolve 10.7 g NaCac·3H$_2$O and 16.5 g sucrose in about 200 ml reagent water. Add 1.725 ml 1 N HCl and bring to a total volume of 250 ml with reagent water. Store at 4°C. Discard if there are any signs of precipitation or contamination.

Osmium buffer is a 400 mM solution of sodium cacodylate with 13.2% (w/v) sucrose. Dissolve 2.09 g NaCac·3H$_2$O and 3.4 g sucrose in about 20 ml reagent water. Add 0.345 ml of 1 N HCl and bring to a total volume of 25 ml with reagent water. Store at 4°C. Discard if there are any signs of precipitation or contamination.

Fixative is a 4.0% (v/v) solution of glutaraldehyde in 200 mM cacodylate buffer with 4.0% sucrose. It is prepared by mixing five volumes of fix buffer with one volume of a stock 25% (v/v) solution of EM grade glutaraldehyde. Store at 4°C and bring to ambient temperature before use. Use within 24 hours, and discard any unused portion.

Postfixative is 2.0% osmium tetroxide in 200 mM cacodylate buffer with 6.6% sucrose. Mix equal volumes of a 4.0% (w/v) aqueous stock solution of OsO$_4$ and osmium buffer. Only prepare a sufficient amount for immediate use: OsO$_4$ is both expensive and hazardous; it fixes anything with which it comes into contact almost immediately (e.g., skin, cornea, nasal mucosa). Therefore *always* work with OsO$_4$ in a fume hood and wear appropriate protective clothing. When disposing of OsO_4 (usually down the sink, but check local regulations), dilute it with a large volume of cold water before pouring it down the sink with a lot of running cold water. Remember to rinse out pipettes carefully before disposing of them.

Buffered 2.5% glutaraldehyde is made by diluting one volume of stock 25% glutaraldehyde solution with nine volumes of fix buffer. Prepare a sufficient amount for immediate use, and discard any unused portion.

BSA solution is a 10% (w/v) aqueous solution of BSA (Sigma A-4503) prepared by dissolving 0.2 g BSA in 2 ml reagent water.

Uranyl acetate is a 2.0% (w/v) aqueous solution prepared by dissolving 0.1 g uranyl acetate in 5 ml reagent water. Prepare on the day of use and discard any unused portion.

Embedding resins: Do *not* prepare these resins until just before they are to be used. Mix 7.5 ml of Epon (or equivalent), 6.0 ml of Araldite, and 18.0 ml DDSA hardener thoroughly by inversion in a plastic Universal container (e.g., Nunc Cat. No. 364211) to make a total volume of 31.5 ml.

1. Transfer 21.0 ml of this mixture to another plastic Universal container, add 0.21 ml of DMP-30 accelerator, and mix by inversion; this solution is the *embedding resin.*
2. Of the remaining 10.5 ml of resin-hardener mixture, transfer 2.0 ml to a *glass* Universal container and mix with 4.0 ml propylene oxide by shaking; this solution is *impregnation resin No. 1.*
3. Transfer another 4.0 ml of the resin-hardener mixture to a *glass* Universal container and mix with 2.0 ml propylene oxide; this is *impregnation resin No. 2.*
4. The mixture remaining in the plastic Universal container is *impregnation resin No. 3.*

N.B. When using propylene oxide, ensure that there are no rubber liners in the caps of the Universal containers. Glass Universal containers *must* be used with propylene oxide, as it dissolves most plastics. *Always* use propylene oxide in a fume hood as it is highly volatile.

Acetone dehydration series is prepared by the volumetric dilution of analytical grade absolute acetone with reagent water to give 50%, 75%, and 95% (v/v) solutions. Store in well-stoppered glass bottles at ambient temperature.

Method

1. Mix liquefied semen with at least twice its volume of fixative at ambient temperature. Leave for 15–60 minutes.
2. Centrifuge at 600 *g* for 10 minutes at ambient temperature.
3. Remove the supernatant and replace it with an equal volume of rinse buffer. In this and subsequent steps, *gently* resuspend the pellet of cells using a Pasteur pipette.
4. Centrifuge at 600 *g* for 10 minutes at ambient temperature.
5. Remove the supernatant, replace it with an equal volume of rinse buffer, and *gently* resuspend the cells.

6. Centrifuge at 600 *g* for 10 minutes at ambient temperature.
7. Remove the supernatant, replace it with a volume of OsO_4 postfixative equal to the original semen aliquot volume and *gently* resuspend the cells.
8. Allow to postfix for 60 minutes at ambient temperature with *gentle* agitation every 10 minutes.
9. Centrifuge at 600 *g* for 10 minutes at ambient temperature.
10. Remove the OsO_4 postfixative supernatant and *gently* resuspend the pellet in 5 ml of reagent water.
11. Centrifuge at 600 *g* for 10 minutes at ambient temperature.
12. Remove the water supernatant and *gently* resuspend the pellet in another 5 ml of reagent water.
13. Centrifuge at 600 *g* for 10 minutes at ambient temperature.
14. Remove the water supernatant and *gently* resuspend the pellet in reagent water to a total volume of about 0.3 ml.
15. Transfer to a 0.5 ml Eppendorf tube and centrifuge at 600 *g* for 10 minutes at ambient temperature. Use a microfuge if possible.
16. Remove the water supernatant, replace it with about 200 µl of the 10% BSA solution and *gently* resuspend the pellet. Allow to stand for 20–60 minutes at ambient temperature.
17. Centrifuge at 1500 *g* for 15–20 minutes at ambient temperature. Use a microfuge if possible.
18. Remove the supernatant and gently add 200 µl of 2.5% buffered gutaraldehyde over the pellet *without disturbing it. Do NOT try to resuspend this pellet.*
19. Allow to fix for at least 6 hours (even as long as overnight) at 4°C.
20. The pellet is removed by cutting through the Eppendorf tube using a sharp blade. Carefully cut the pellet into pieces of ≤ 1 mm in any dimension on a glass microscope slide. *Do not allow the pieces of the pellet to dry out.* Transfer the pieces of pellet to a small (10 ml) snap-cap glass vial containing 1–2 ml reagent water.
21. Carefully remove all the water from the vial using a Pasteur pipette. Replace it *immediately* with 2–3 ml uranyl acetate solution.
22. Allow to stand at ambient temperature for 60 minutes.
23. Pipette off the uranyl acetate solution and immediately add 2–3 ml 50% acetone.
24. Dehydrate through a graded acetone series a ambient temperature, adding and removing the acetones using Pasteur pipettes as before. Take great care to never allow the material to dry out. The series is:

    50% Acetone for 10–15 minutes
    75% Acetone for 10–15 minutes
    95% Acetone for 10–15 minutes
    100% Acetone for three changes of 10–15 minutes each.

25. Remove the last change of 100% acetone and replace by 2–3 ml of the transition solvent (propylene oxide). Let stand for 10–15 minutes at ambient temperature in a fume hood.

26. Remove the solvent and replace with 2–3 ml fresh propylene oxide for another 10–15 minutes at ambient temperature in a fume hood.
27. Again using Pasteur pipettes (a clean one for each change), transfer the material through the impregnation series at ambient temperature.

    Impregnation resin No. 1 for 20 minutes
    Impregnation resin No. 2 for 20 minutes
    Impregnation resin No. 3 for 60 minutes

28. During the last impregnation step, fill the required number of embedding capsules (e.g., BEEM capsules or gelatin capsules) with the embedding resin. These capsules *must stand upright* (e.g., in a BEEM capsule rack).
29. Using watchmaker's forceps, *very gently* transfer pieces of material from the impregnation resin No. 3 to the capsules. Place only one piece per capsule.
30. Polymerize the resin at 60°C for 48 hours.
31. Carefully mark each block to identify the material it contains.

Note

Samples containing few spermatozoa are difficult to process through all the steps described above unless the spermatozoa are encapsulated in a soft gelatin matrix (either before or after fixation).

Transmission Electron Microscopy: Surface Replicas

Principle

This section describes the preparation of surface replicas of human spermatozoa for examination in the TEM. The air-drying method is used, which although it does cause some surface artifacts is adequate for examining the general morphological appearance and surface topography of human spermatozoa. It is comparable to preparing spermatozoa for SEM but has the advantage of using the TEM, with its wider availability and higher resolution than the SEM.

Critical point drying may be used if the apparatus is available. It produces images of the sperm surface more comparable to SEM but, again, with higher resolution.

Reagents

Fixative is 4.0% (v/v) glutaraldehyde in 200 mM cacodylate buffer (see TEM:Thin Sections, above) but without sucrose.
Buffer is 200 mM cacodylate buffer (prepared as above) but without sucrose.
Bleach is a standard sodium hypochlorite solution (e.g., BDH R07048).
Acid is concentrated sulfuric acid (e.g., BDH B10276).

Method

1. Spermatozoa in seminal plasma are fixed by adding a fivefold volume of fixative at ambient temperature and mixing thoroughly by inversion. Already washed sperm suspensions are fixed by adding an equal volume of fixative.

2. Allow to fix for 1–2 hours at ambient temperature.
3. Centrifuge at 600 g for 10 minutes.
4. Discard the supernatant, and resuspend the pellet in fresh buffer.
5. Centrifuge at 600 g for 10 minutes.
6. Discard the supernatant and resuspend the pellet in fresh buffer.
7. Centrifuge at 600 g for 10 minutes.
8. Discard the supernatant and resuspend the pellet in reagent water.
9. Centrifuge at 600 g for 10 minutes.
10. Discard the supernatant and resuspend the pellet in a small volume of reagent water. Empirically, adjust the sperm concentration so the cells are not over-crowded after drying.
11. Transfer small aliquots of the sperm suspension onto the surface of pieces of freshly split mica and allow to air-dry.
12. Transfer the mica to a high-vacuum evaporator and evacuate to 10^{-4} mm Hg.
13. Shadow with platinum-carbon at 45 degrees to the plane of the mica.
14. Add a "backing" film of carbon at 90 degrees to the plane of the mica.
15. Remove the mica from the evaporator and float the replica(s) off the mica onto the surface of reagent water in a glass petri dish.
16. Using a Pasteur pipette, remove almost all the water and replace it with bleach (pH 13–14).
17. Allow to stand overnight in a dust-free environment.
18. Remove the bleach solution and replace it with fresh water. Repeat until the water in the petri dish reads pH 7.0 using an indicator test strip.
19. Remove almost all the water and replace it with acid.
20. Allow to stand for another day in a dust-free environment.
21. Dilute the acid to water (pH 7.0) by repeatedly removing almost all the volume in the dish and replacing it with reagent water.
22. Once the water reads pH 7.0, pick up fragments of the replica on 200-mesh copper EM grids (without support films). *Carefully* remove residual water from the grid by touching filter paper to its *edge*.
23. Store the grids in a dry, dust-free environment until TEM examination.

Scanning Electron Microscopy

Reagents

Fixative is 2.5% (v/v) glutaraldehyde in 200 mM cacodylate buffer (see TEM: Thin Sections, above), with 4.0% (w/v) sucrose.
Buffer is 200 mM cacodylate buffer (prepared as above) with 4.0% (w/v) sucrose.

Method

Ejaculate spermatozoa are washed three times with PBS or other balanced salt solution (600 g for 10 minutes); already washed spermatozoa may be used directly. Spermatozoa are fixed at 4°C overnight in suspension using at least an equal volume of fixative. The following morning gently resuspend the cells and then proceed according to either of the following protocols.

1. *Membrane filter method:* Filter the fixed sperm suspension through a Nuclepore membrane filter (0.45-μm pores, 35 mm ∅) by gentle suction. The cells collected on the filter are then washed by passing 10 ml fresh buffer through the filter, taking care never to let them dry out. The filter is then removed from its holder and dehydrated through a graded series of ethanols. The filters are either allowed to air-dry or are processed by critical-point drying using liquid CO_2.

2. *Suspension method:* The spermatozoa are washed through three changes of fresh buffer and dehydrated in a graded series of ethanols by repeated centrifugation at 600 *g* for 10 minutes. Transfer drops of the sperm suspension in absolute ethanol onto clean coverslips (perhaps coated with poly-L-lysine to aid cell adhesion) and either allow to air-dry or process by critical-point drying using liquid CO_2.

The specimen is then attached to an SEM stub and sputter-coated with gold before viewing in an SEM.

References and Recommended Reading

Afzelius, B. A., Eliasson, R., Johnson, Ø, and Lindholmer, C. (1975). Lack of dynein arms in immotile human spermatozoa. *J. Cell Biol.* **66,** 225.

Bongso, T. A., Sathananthan, A. H., Wong, P. C., Ratnam, S. S., Ng, S. C., Anandakumar, C., and Ganatra, S. (1989). Human fertilization by microinjection of immotile spermatozoa. *Hum. Reprod.* **4,** 175.

Dadoune, J. P. (1988). Ultrastructural abnormalities of human spermatozoa. *Hum. Reprod.* **3,** 311.

Escalier, D., and David, G. (1984). Pathology of the cytoskeleton of the human sperm flagellum: axonemal and peri-axonemal structures. *Biol. Cell.* **50,** 37.

Fléchon, J.-E., and Hafez, E. S. E. (1976). Scanning electron microscopy of human spermatozoa. In Hafez, E. S. E. (ed): *Human Semen and Fertility Regulation in Men.* Mosby, St. Louis.

Liakatas, J., Williams, A. E., and Hargreave, T. B. (1982). Scoring sperm morphology using the scanning electron microscope. *Fertil. Steril.* **38,** 227.

Mortimer, D. (1981). The assessment of human sperm morphology in surface replica preparations for transmission electron microscopy. *Gamete Res.* **4,** 113.

Mortimer, D., Leslie, E. E., Kelly, R. W., and Templeton, A. A. (1982). Morphological selection of human spermatozoa *in vivo* and *in vitro. J. Reprod. Fertil.* **64,** 391.

Pedersen, H., and Fawcett, D. W. (1976). Functional anatomy of the human spermatozoon. In Hafez, E. S. E. (ed): *Human Semen and Fertility Regulation in Men.* Mosby, St. Louis.

Tyler, J. P. P., Boadle, R. A., and Stevens, S. M. B. (1985). Round-headed spermatozoa: a case report. *Pathology* **17,** 67.

Zamboni, L. (1987). The ultrastructural pathology of the spermatozoon as a cause of infertility: the role of the electron microscope in the evaluation of semen quality. *Fertil. Steril.* **48,** 711.

Zamboni, L. (1991). Physiology and pathophysiology of the human spermatozoon: the role of electron microscopy. *J. Electron Microsc. Tech.* **17,** 412.

9

Assessment of Sperm Transport

Normally, for conception to occur in vivo spermatozoa must be deposited at the site of insemination around the external cervical os at a time when the cervical mucus is receptive to penetration by spermatozoa. This initial process of sperm–cervical mucus interaction is an essential first step in the complex series of events that take place in the relatively inaccessible female tract resulting in the production of a zygote which, hopefully, will implant and develop into a new individual. Consequently, its assessment is an integral part of the diagnostic workup of an infertile couple, and the various techniques available are described in this chapter.

Over the years a number of studies have appeared in the scientific literature reporting investigations of sperm transport through the uterus using uterine lavage techniques and through the fallopian tubes using hysterectomy, salpingectomy, and ampullary aspiration techniques (review: Mortimer, 1983). Sperm transport through the female tract has also considered the presence of spermatozoa in peritoneal fluid, recovered either by culdocentesis or laparoscopy. The most widely used approach as a clinical test has been that of laparoscopic sperm recovery from the peritoneal fluid and the tubal ampulla and fimbria; the technique is described later in the chapter.

CERVICAL MUCUS SAMPLING AND ASSESSMENT

Timing the Procedure

Cervical mucus receptivity to penetration by spermatozoa is cyclic, increasing over a period of about 4 days before ovulation and decreasing rapidly (within 2 days) after. Receptivity is maximal on the day before, or the day of, the LH peak, with ovulation occurring some 36 hours after the start of the rise in serum LH levels. Studies of in vitro sperm penetration into mucus samples collected daily have, however, revealed that the optimum penetrability of the mucus may occur on unpredictable days (Makler, 1976). Consequently, some tests performed on days that would be expected to show optimum results may, in fact, show poor results and could lead to false diagnoses of cervical hostility. Clearly, abnormal tests must be repeated during at least one subsequent cycle to establish that the finding was correct.

Because most variation in cycle length occurs during the follicular phase, the day of ovulation is considered equivalent to day 14 of a "standard" 28-day cycle (where day 1 is the first day of menstrual bleeding). Because of cycle irregularity it is better to calculate day $[14 + (x - 28)]$ where x is calculated as the average length of a minimum of five preceding cycles (Pandya et al., 1986). Obviously, this method for the predictive booking of cervical mucus assessments (for PCTs or SMITs) is not successful for determining the optimum day for every test. However, when incorporated into a logical sequence of management, including the automatic repetition of all abnormal tests, it does represent an efficient method for a busy infertility clinic.

To ensure optimum mucus quality, some workers treat patients with estradiol for several days before sampling (e.g., 80 µg ethinyl estradiol per day for 7 days) (Eggert-Kruse et al., 1989). Although it ensures that the best mucus is obtained for the tests, and the results of such tests *are* predictive of fertility, it might conceal an underlying endocrine disorder that manifests as poor estrogenization of the cervical mucosa. If a patient has repeated abnormal PCT or SMIT results, this approach may be considered. Persistent poor mucus quality would remain a contributory factor to infertility in such couples.

Sampling Cervical Mucus

A warmed speculum is inserted into the vagina, and the cervix is examined for dilation and appearance of the external os, including the amount of mucus present at the os. The external os is gently wiped clean using a clean, dry gauze swab. Collection of mucus into a syringe (e.g., 1-ml tuberculin type) is acceptable for PCTs but does cause a great deal of disruption of the mucus ultrastructure and should not therefore be used when mucus is being collected for in vitro SMIT procedures.

Suitable mucus collection catheters can be purchased commercially (e.g., Kwills: Everett Medical Products, Hinders-Leslies Ltd., London, UK) or made from appropriate tubing and sterilized. A special mucus-collecting syringe (Aspiglaire: BICEF/IMV, L'Aigle, France) is also available, and although it is relatively expensive it is ideal.

The catheter is inserted about 1 cm into the cervical canal and the syringe plunger gently pulled back, drawing mucus into the catheter. Keeping gentle suction applied, the catheter is slowly withdrawn from the cervix. The mucus is then expelled from the catheter onto a clean glass microscope slide. If a Kwill is used, the disposable plastic stirring rod from Sarstedt fits admirably as a plunger. If the mucus is highly elastic (i.e., high spinnbarkeit), it may be necessary to close off the open end of the collection catheter with a pair of forceps to prevent the mucus from pulling out of the catheter as it is withdrawn from the vagina.

Assessment of Cervical Mucus Quality: Insler Score

The Insler score is a semiquantitative method used to assess the quantity and quality of cervical mucus. The mucous secretion of the cervix is under endocrine control and therefore shows cyclic variations during the menstrual cycle. Around the fertile period at midcycle the mucus being secreted is under estrogenic control. It is an abundant, clear, watery secretion (compared to the mucus produced during the luteal and early follicular phases) and is receptive to penetration by spermatozoa. The original score proposed by Insler et al. (1972) has been modified to include a fifth parameter: mucus cellularity. Consequently, there are now five criteria to be scored, each with a value ranging from 0 to 3. This scoring system differs slightly from the mucus quality score described in the 1980 and 1992 editions of the *WHO Laboratory Manual* but is closer to Insler's original definitions. See Appendix VI for suggested laboratory and report forms.

Appearance of the Cervical Os

The criterion based on the appearance of the cervical os considers the degree of dilation and hyperemia of the external cervical os. If the os is tightly closed and the same pink color as the surrounding tissue, the score is 0. If the os is wide open and obviously hyperemic, the score is 3 (the maximum dilation of the os at ovulation is about 6 mm). A score of 1 is assigned if the os is beginning to open and to redden, and a score of 2 is awarded when the condition of the os is better than that for a score of 1 but not good enough for a score of 3.

Mucus Quantity

The second criterion is the quantity of mucus present and is assessed at the same time as the cervical appearance.

0 = No mucus is visible at the external os, and none can be aspirated into the catheter.

1 = No mucus is visible at the external os, but some can be drawn into the sampling catheter (WHO: up to 0.1 ml).

2 = Mucus is visible at the external os and can be drawn into the catheter (WHO: 0.1–0.2 ml).

3 = There is a definite cascade of mucus visible at the external os (WHO: 0.3 ml or more).

Spinnbarkeit

The spinnbarkeit criterion considers the stretchability or elasticity of the mucus, which is measured by placing a small drop of mucus (about 5 mm diameter) on a clean slide. A second slide is then placed across the first in the form of a "+," and the mucus is spread evenly between the two slides. The slides are then pulled gently apart, and the length of the mucus thread is measured in centimeters. This method is preferable to using a coverslip, as the risk of puncturing one's glove or a fingerstick injury are essentially abolished.

0 = Mucus does not stretch at all (< 1 cm).

1 = Mucus stretches 1–4 cm before breaking.

2 = Mucus stretches 5–8 cm before breaking.

3 = Mucus stretches > 8 cm without breaking.

Ferning

The mucus on the slide used for the spinnbarkeit determination is spread evenly, allowed to dry, and the presence and degree of ferning (crystallization pattern) (Fig. 9-1) is assessed as follows.

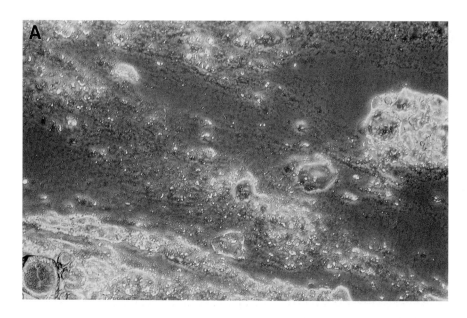

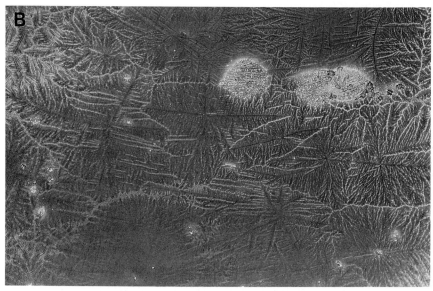

Figure 9-1 Photomicrographs of ferning patterns in dried human cervical mucus. **A, B, C, D** show Insler grades 0, 1, 2, and 3, respectively. (From Mortimer, 1985. With permission.)

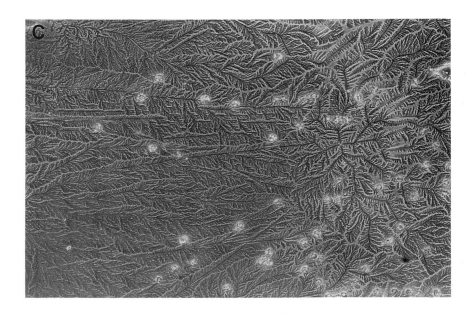

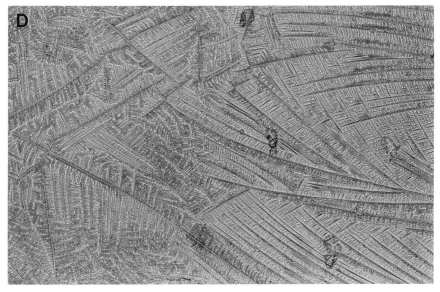

Figure 9-1 (Continued)

179

0 = There is no ferning anywhere on the slide.
1 = Less than half of the mucus is starting to fern.
2 = More than half of the mucus shows good ferning.
3 = All the mucus shows good ferning.

Detailed counting of the numbers of side branches in the crystallization pattern is not useful. It is far more important to ensure that the degree of ferning is assessed over the entire preparation, rather than concentrating on a small area that shows, or does not show, ferning.

Mucus Cellularity

The mucus cellularity criterion considers the number of leukocytes, not erythrocytes or epithelial cells, and is assessed as an inverse score. A 40× objective field (HPF) is considered to be approximately 0.2 mm^2 using a *modern microscope* fitted with widefield high-point oculars (i.e., double that an old-style microscope). However, if glass beads are used to standardize the depth of the mucus preparation (see Appendix II), the number of leukocytes can be expressed per unit volume (i.e., cubic millimeters ≡ per microliter) using a conversion factor of 10 cells/HPF = 500 cells/mm^3.

0 = Mucus is full of leukocytes (> 20/HPF or > 1000/μl).
1 = There are 11–20 leukocytes per HPF (501–1000/μl).
2 = There are 1–10 leukocytes per HPF (1–500/μl).
3 = There are no leukocytes in the mucus.

Calculation of the Insler Score

The five scores awarded, as described above, are added together to give a total Insler score (maximum 15). A score of 12 or more is considered to indicate good ovulatory cervical mucus, and scores of 10 or 11 indicate adequate ovulatory cervical mucus.

Measurement of Cervical Mucus pH

The pH of periovulatory cervical mucus is usually in the range of 8.0–8.4. A pH of 6.0 is incompatible with sperm vitality, and sperm progression seems to be impaired below approximately pH 6.8. Certainly the optimum pH range for sperm migration and survival is between 7.0 and 8.5. Consequently, acidic mucus may be at least a partial explanation for poor sperm–mucus interaction.

Cervical mucus pH is measured using Merck ColorpHast test strips. For general use, the pH 6.5–10.0 strips are ideal; but for mucus samples of pH < 7.0, the pH 4.0–7.0 range strips should also be available.

Storage of Cervical Mucus

Unfortunately, frozen cervical mucus has been found by many workers to be unreliable and unsatisfactory for use in SMIT procedures. It is therefore recommended that donor mucus for use in such procedures be stored for only a few days at 4°C. The ends of the collection catheter should be sealed with an inert material such as hematocrit tube sealant. Plasticine should not be used because it contains substances toxic to the spermatozoa. Before use, the mucus must be allowed to reequilibrate to ambient temperature, and its pH and Insler score should be reassessed. Obviously, only mucus samples of good quality should be used in crossed-hostility testing (see below).

If mucus donors are available, estrogen treatment can ensure optimum mucus quantity and quality (e.g., Eggert-Kruse et al., 1989).

IN VITRO SPERM–MUCUS INTERACTION TESTS

Background

In vitro sperm–mucus interaction tests (SMITs) are derived from two basic techniques: (1) slide tests using apposed drops of semen and mucus under coverslips; and (2) tube (Kremer) tests where mucus-filled capillary tubes are placed with one end in contact with liquefied semen. Penetration in either system is assessed by counting motile spermatozoa at various distances from the semen–mucus interface at certain times after establishment of this contact.

For physiological and clinical relevance, tests must be performed using periovulatory intracervical mucus with an Insler score of $\geq 10/15$ and pH ≥ 7.0. Three days of sexual abstinence should be observed to provide optimum semen characteristics and to minimize any "contamination" of the mucus with spermatozoa from a previous insemination. A complete semen analysis should be performed on the ejaculate used for the test. If the abstinence is not 3 days, some tests may need to be repeated because of abnormal findings of uncertain origin. Sample laboratory and report forms are provided in Appendix VI.

As with all tests of sperm function, SMITs must be commenced as quickly as possible after ejaculation. Normal semen samples are liquefied by 30 minutes after ejaculation, which is an ideal standard starting time. If liquefaction is retarded the tests may be delayed, but mucus-penetrating ability may be reduced with longer exposure of spermatozoa to seminal plasma. Although seminal plasma is important for sperm penetration into cervical mucus, sperm motility and vitality both decline markedly with prolonged exposure.

Kremer-Type Tests

Tests of sperm penetration into and along capillary tubes filled with cervical mucus are generally referred to as Kremer-type tests after their original pioneer in infertility investigations (Kremer, 1965). However, rectangular cross-section glass capillaries are now used almost universally rather than the circular cross-section tubes originally used by Kremer. These "flat" tubes allow much better visualization of the spermatozoa migrating in the mucus inside the tube lumen and make scoring the tests far easier. In addition, the original Kremer "sperm penetration meter" apparatus has been largely superseded by disposable systems (e.g., Pandya et al., 1986).

Slide Tests

The slide test of sperm penetration into cervical mucus, often called the Kurzrok-Miller test after its originators (Kurzrok and Miller, 1928), is the oldest in vitro SMIT method. It involves establishment of an interface between a drop of cervical mucus that has been compressed between a coverslip and an aliquot of liquefied semen (see below). There are great problems in standardizing this test relating to differences in the thickness of the mucus preparation and variations in the contact area of the semen–mucus interface. Consequently, it is difficult to use the test as anything other than a qualitative assessment of sperm–mucus interaction, although some authors do report quantitative results (e.g., World Health Organization, 1987).

Antisperm antibodies in either semen or cervical mucus influence both the penetration of spermatozoa into mucus and their continued survival and migration within it—and hence the ultimate endpoint of fertility (see Chapter 5). The sperm–cervical mucus contact (SCMC) test, which is a simple slide test requiring only the mixing of liquefied semen and cervical mucus (see below), is a valuable screening test for this problem. It is especially useful in the crossed-hostility format in conjunction with Immunobead testing.

The SCMC test is assessed by observing the presence of a highly characteristic "shaking" pattern of sperm movement. High correlations exist between the shaking phenomenon and the failure of sperm penetration into midcycle mucus and between the sperm-agglutinin titers in seminal plasma or cervical mucus and the occurrence of shaking (Kremer and Jager, 1988). It should be noted that antisperm antibodies in mucus are often locally secreted IgA and cannot be detected using more classic test methods on the female serum, although indirect IBTs using solubilized cervical mucus do permit their detection.

Kremer Test

Principle

The Kremer sperm penetration test is an in vitro test of sperm–mucus interaction. A rectangular cross-section glass capillary tube is filled with cervical mucus, sealed at one end, and its open end placed in contact with a reservoir of semen. Penetration of motile spermatozoa into the mucus is assessed by counting their numbers at various distances from the semen–mucus interface.

The outcome of the test is strongly influenced by the concentration of progressively motile spermatozoa at the semen–mucus interface (i.e., in the semen sample) and has been considered as a test of the proportion of successful collisions between spermatozoa capable of mucus penetration and the interface (Katz et al., 1980). Consequently, oligozoospermic samples most likely produce average to poor results, whereas oligoasthenozoospermic samples usually produce abnormal test results. It does not, however, obviate the need for performing the test in any but the most extreme male factor cases.

Reagents

DTT solution: Prepare a solution of dithiothreitol (Sigma D-0632) 10 mg/ml in reagent water. Prepare fresh daily and maintain at ambient temperature. Discard any unused portion.

Specimens

Semen: A 50-µl aliquot of liquefied semen is required for each test. It must be taken from a well-mixed ejaculate specimen within 1 hour of collection and preferably at a standard time, such as 30 minutes.

Mucus: The test must be performed using periovulatory mucus. Intracervical mucus is collected and assessed in terms of its Insler score and pH (see Cervical Mucus Sampling and Assessment, above). Use of condoms during the week before the test would facilitate interpretation of the findings by ensuring that the mucus used for the test is sperm-free, although this method is unlikely to be well received by infertility patients.

Method

N.B. Objective performance of this test requires that microscope objective fields be calibrated so numbers of spermatozoa per field may be converted to numbers per unit area (i.e., per square millimeter $\equiv$ per 10^6 square micrometers (see Appendix II). No dependable method for determining sperm numbers per unit volume within capillary tubes amenable to routine use yet exists.

1. A flat capillary tube (100 × 3 × 0.3 mm rectangular Microslide) (Vitro Dynamics, Rockaway, NJ, USA) is calibrated at 10-mm intervals using a fine-pointed indelible (spirit-based) marker pen (Fig. 9-2).

2. Mucus from the collection catheter is expelled onto a clean glass slide. Trailing mucus from the catheter is cut with iris scissors.

3. Mucus is aspirated from the slide into the capillary tube using suction with a loading manifold (World Health Organization, 1992). The mucus meniscus should be 20–30 mm from the top of the tube, creating a mucus column of 70–80 mm (exact length is noted to the nearest millimeter). Trailing mucus is cut with iris scissors at the lower end of the tube, the loading manifold removed, and the upper end of the tube sealed with hematocrit tube sealant. After sealing, the mucus should protrude slightly from the open end of the tube.

4. Before setting up the test, the mucus-filled capillary tube is checked under the microscope (400× magnification, phase-contrast optics) for the presence of spermatozoa. If any spermatozoa are seen, 10 random fields along the length of the mucus column should be scored, counting the number of spermatozoa and classifying their motility. The average "contamination" per field should be noted

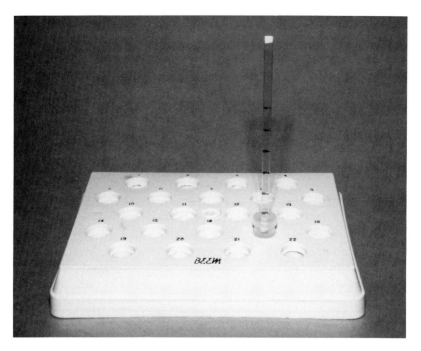

Figure 9-2 Kremer in vitro test of sperm–mucus interaction using a rectangular cross-section glass capillary and disposable BEEM capsule as the sperm reservoir.

and used for correction of the assessment of sperm penetration scores (see Results, below).

5. At 30 minutes after ejaculation, a 50-μl aliquot of the mixed liquefied semen is taken for the test. A No. 00 BEEM capsule is used as the semen reservoir, a slit or small hole being made in its cap to take the capillary tube. The semen is deposited carefully in the bottom of the capsule (which is held upright in a special BEEM capsule rack) and the cap closed.

6. The open end of the mucus-filled capillary tube is inserted through the BEEM capsule's lid until its corners rest on the tapered base of the capsule. The mucus interface is immersed 1–2 mm into the semen. The capsule is replaced in the BEEM capsule rack and incubated at 37°C for 60 minutes (Fig. 9-2).

7. After incubation the capillary tube is removed from the BEEM capsule and the open end of the tube rinsed thoroughly with a freshly prepared solution of DTT to remove residual spermatozoa from the mucus interface and surface of the tube. It is advisable to stand the open end of the tube in the DTT solution for 30–60 seconds to ensure complete removal of any contaminating semen.

8. The depth and degree of sperm penetration into the mucus column is assessed microscopically. Using a magnification of 400× (i.e., a 40× objective, note the combination of optics used), count the number of *in focus* spermatozoa present in each of three microscope fields at the 10-, 40-, and 70-mm marks along the tube. Only count those spermatozoa in focus *without* adjusting the microscope

Table 9–1   Sperm penetration test scores[a]

No. Spermatozoa/mm²	Score	Vanguard Spermatozoa (mm)
0	0	< 30
1–30	1	30–39
31–60	2	40–49
61–120	3	50–59
121–200	4	61–69
> 200	5	≥ 70

Source: Pandya et al. (1986).

[a]These scores are used for assessing the modified Kremer-type migration test of human sperm–cervical mucus interaction using rectangular cross-section capillary tubes.

focus, as adjustment would induce variations in the third dimension of the microscope field being scored.

Results

1. The average number of spermatozoa present in the three fields at each distance along the tube is calculated.
2. Correct the average number of spermatozoa per field for any "contaminating" spermatozoa present in the mucus at the start of the test.
3. Convert the corrected number into per unit area (i.e., 10^6 square micrometers equivalent to 1 square millimeter) using the appropriate microscope calibration factor (see Appendix II).
4. Use these numbers to calculate the Sperm Penetration Test score, an empirically derived scheme used to create a semiquantitative score for this test (Pandya et al., 1986; World Health Organization, 1992). The maximum score is 20, derived from the numbers of spermatozoa per square millimeter 10, 40, and 70 mm from the semen–mucus interface (assessed on a scale of 0–5 each) plus the distance traveled by the vanguard spermatozoa (also assessed on a 0–5 scale) calculated according to the ratings shown in Table 9-1.
5. The test result is derived from the calculated score as shown in Table 9-2.

N.B.   Kremer described an alternative scoring scheme for these tests, although it is rather more complicated and less objective (World Health Organization, 1987).

Quality Control

The Kremer test is a straightforward observational procedure. Quality control aspects relating to the semen analysis and mucus quality assessment are dealt with under the appropriate tests.

   The field area of each combination of microscope objective, intermediate magnification, and oculars must be calibrated to allow calculation of sperm numbers per unit area (see Appendix II). To achieve optimum standardization only a 40× objective should be used so as to eliminate variability in the microscope's depth of focus and hence the third dimension of the microscope field being scored.

Table 9–2 Interpreting the test result
from the sperm penetration test scoring
system[a]

Total Score	Test Result	Rank
0	Negative	0
1–8	Poor	1
9–11	Average	2
12–15	Good	3
16–20	Excellent	4

Source: Pandya et al. (1986).

[a]The system is used to score the modified Kremer-
type migration test of human sperm–cervical mucus
interaction using rectangular cross-section capillary
tubes.

    Changing the incubation time or temperature also alters the quantitative extent of
sperm penetration along the mucus column. Consequently, tests *must* be run at 37°C
for the expected 60 minutes; shorter times require completely redefined criteria for
deriving the score.

Kurzrok-Miller Test

Principle
The Kurzrok-Miller (K-M) in vitro test of sperm–mucus interaction consists simply
of establishing an interface between a drop of endocervical mucus and fresh
liquefied semen (Kurzrok and Miller, 1928).

Reagents
A mixture of glass beads in silicone grease is used to make the 100-μm fixed-depth
preparations (see Appendix II).

Specimens
Semen and cervical mucus samples are required (see Kremer Test, above).

Method

1. Prepare a cleaned microscope slide with four "posts" of the glass beads-silicone
   grease mixture arranged in a square pattern with sides of about 20 mm. Place a
   drop (*ca.* 3 mm ∅) of endocervical mucus in the center of this square and cover it
   with a 22 × 22 mm coverslip. Press down gently on the coverslip so the posts are
   flattened and the coverslip is fixed with a single layer of beads between it and the
   slide. The mucus drop spreads toward the edges of the coverslip; if it extrudes
   from under the coverslip, another preparation must be made using less mucus.
2. Place a drop (about 25 μl) of semen next to the edge of the coverslip. The semen
   then flows under the coverslip and establishes a contact interface with the mucus
   (Fig. 9-3).

3. Incubate the test in a humidified chamber at 37°C for 20–30 minutes.
4. Examine the preparation at a magnification of 200× to 250× using phase-contrast optics.

Subjective Interpretation

Because of the problems of standardizing the semen–mucus interface many laboratories use the K-M test only as a qualitative assessment of sperm–mucus interaction. Useful observations from such tests are as follows.

1. A negative test requires that spermatozoa congregate along the semen side of the interface but that none penetrate the semen–mucus interface. Phalanges may or may not be formed.
2. Spermatozoa penetrate the mucus phase but rapidly become either immotile or show the "shaking" pattern of movement (abnormal results).
3. Although spermatozoa penetrate the mucus phase, most do not progress farther than 500 μm (i.e., about 10 sperm lengths) from the semen–mucus interface (poor result).
4. Spermatozoa penetrate the mucus phase, and most (> 90%) are motile with definite progression (normal result).

Quantitative Assessment

Semiquantitative assessments of the K-M test considered the numbers of spermatozoa seen in the first and second "high power fields" (HPF1 and HPF2) on the mucus side of the semen–mucus interface (Belsey et al., 1980; World Health Organization,

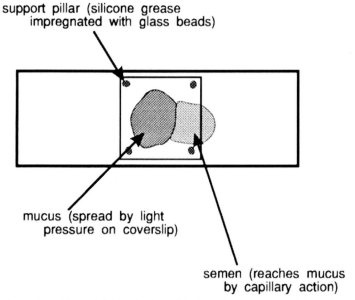

Figure 9-3 Kurzrok-Miller in vitro slide test of sperm–mucus interaction.

1987). However, because of the inability to standardize the test, this approach cannot be recommended as a primary method in an expert andrology laboratory. Although the quantitative scoring system described above (World Health Organization, 1992) does allow sperm numbers to be presented per unit volume, no clinical data are available that correlate such results with outcome. Consequently, it is not recommended that quantitative results of the K-M test be reported until a suitable objective scoring system has been established and its interpretation validated.

Results

The test is reported as either normal, poor, abnormal, or negative according to the subjective observations made in method step 4, above.

Quality Control

Although the K-M test remains an observational technique subject to uncontrollable factors such as the geometry of the semen–mucus interface, the objective method described above achieves the maximum practicable standardization and provides the best quantitative results for the test.

Sperm–Cervical Mucus Contact Test

Principle

The sperm–cervical mucus contact (SCMC) test is a slide test whereby spermatozoa and cervical mucus are mixed to establish the presence of any spermimmobilizing antisperm antibodies in either the seminal plasma or the cervical mucus. The test is performed by mixing drops of mucus and semen (Kremer and Jager, 1976).

Reagents

No reagents are required.

Specimens

Semen and cervical mucus samples are prepared as for the Kremer test (see above).

Method

1. Place equal drops (3–5 mm ∅: about 25 µl) of endocervical mucus and liquefied semen side by side on a clean slide and mix gently using a disposable plastic stirring rod or disposable pipettor tip (Fig. 9-4).
2. Cover with a 22 × 22 mm coverslip and press gently to spread the preparation to the edges of the coverslip.

N.B. Because the SCMC test considers only relative proportions of sperm subpopulations, not their concentrations, the method described here is recommended for its simplicity. Fixed-depth preparations (see Appendix II) are not required.

3. Examine immediately under phase-contrast optics at 250× to 500× magnification for a period of 5–10 minutes. Note the development of any "shaking" pattern of the movement of the motile spermatozoa.

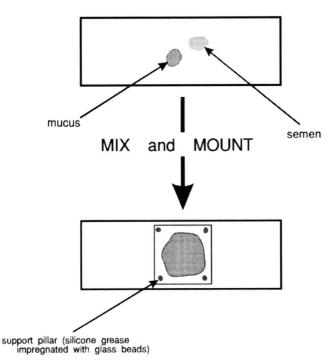

mucus

MIX and MOUNT

semen

support pillar (silicone grease
impregnated with glass beads)

Figure 9-4 In vitro sperm–cervical mucus contact (SCMC) test.

4. Counting at least 100 *actively motile* spermatozoa, determine the percentage of shaking spermatozoa. *Shaking* describes a specific pattern of movement whereby the spermatozoa are actively motile but nonprogressive; they appear to be stuck to some invisible structure within the mucus (as indeed they are).

Results

The result of the SCMC test is reported according to the guidelines shown in Table 9-3.

Quality Control

The SCMC test is a rather subjective observational technique. If the individual performing the SCMC test has seen the shaking pattern of motility before and the

Table 9–3 Interpretation of the sperm–cervical mucus contact test

% Shaking Sperm	Test Result	Rank
0–25	Negative (−)	0
26–50	Positive (+)	1
51–75	Positive (+ +)	2
76–100	Highly positive (+ + +)	3

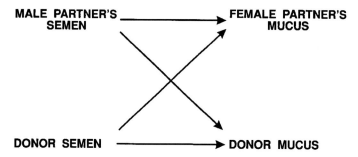

Figure 9-5 Crossed-hostility in vitro sperm–mucus interaction testing.

results are reported as described above the test has achieved its maximum practicable standardization.

Crossed-Hostility Testing

Principle

When a homologous sperm–mucus interaction test has produced a result of average or worse (score of < 12/20), in a subsequent cycle a crossed-hostility test (XHT) should be performed to verify the previous cycle's finding and to evaluate the origin of the problem (i.e., semen or mucus). The four-way cross (Fig. 9-5) also ascertains that the interaction of the donor materials used is normal (Ulstein and Fjällbrant, 1976).

Reagents

Reagents are as per the requirements for the Kremer test (above).

Specimens

Patient semen and mucus are obtained as described for the Kremer test (above).

Donor semen is usually a straw of cryopreserved donor semen with known good mucus-penetrating ability.

Donor mucus is obtained from a patient receiving artificial insemination treatment. Mucus samples are taken and assessed as per standard procedures (see Cervical Mucus Sampling and Assessment, above). Suitable mucus must have an Insler score of ≥ 12/15 and pH ≥ 7.0. Donor mucus may be stored at 4°C for up to 4 days before being used; ensure that stored mucus has reequilibrated to ambient temperature before use.

Method

1. Whenever sufficient material is available, the Kremer test method should be used as the basic test. However, if only a limited amount of the patient's mucus is available, the K-M test may be used instead.

2. An SCMC test (see above) should also be performed on at least the homologous (i.e., patients') sperm–mucus interaction, mucus quantity permitting. If possible, SCMC tests should be performed on all four combinations.

Results

The results of each test combination are provided to the physician requesting the XHT procedure, who is solely responsible for its interpretation. General guidelines may be established, however, (assuming that the interaction of the donor materials was normal).

1. If the patient's spermatozoa penetrate neither his partner's mucus nor the donor mucus, there is probably a male factor problem (e.g., abnormal sperm motility, antisperm antibodies on the sperm surface).
2. If neither the patient's nor the donor's spermatozoa penetrate the patient's mucus, there is probably a female factor problem (e.g., abnormal mucus quality, antisperm antibodies in the mucus).
3. In some cases both of the above problems may be seen simultaneously, indicating the likely presence of both male and female factors.

Clearly, inclusion of a direct IBT on the man's spermatozoa and an indirect IBT on his partner's mucus would greatly facilitate the interpretation of abnormal XHT findings. Kinematic analysis of sperm movement may also help understand the possible origin of a male factor problem.

Mucus Substitutes

There is much interest in mucus substitutes for use in SMITs to eliminate the problem of variability of human cervical mucus quality. Proposed synthetic substitutes have included polyethylene glycol bisacrylate (Bissett, 1980) and polyacrylamide (Lorton et al., 1981). Biological materials that have been suggested for use in Kremer-type tests include a certain fraction of the white of hens' eggs (Hargreave and Nilsson, 1983) and bovine cervical mucus (BCM) (review: Mortimer, 1985).

Of these proposed mucus substitutes, only BCM is available commercially (Penetrak: Serono Diagnostics). However, although BCM seems useful for in vitro tests, it is still a biological product subject to cyclical and interindividual variations. Also, BCM is not absolutely equivalent to human cervical mucus, either in terms of rheology (Tam et al., 1980) or in its practical application: Test methods for human and bovine mucus are different.

A major cause for concern is that when BCM tests are run for 90 minutes normal penetration is defined as a vanguard sperm migration of > 15 mm. Yet when human cervical mucus is used, a penetration of at least 50 mm in 60 minutes is expected, with most normal tests showing at least 70 mm vanguard migration distances. Furthermore, one study has demonstrated that the results of BCM Kremer-type tests are not predictive of subsequent fertility, whereas those from tests with human cervical mucus were (Eggert-Kruse et al., 1989).

High-molecular-weight hyaluronate (Sperm Select: Select Medical Systems, Williston, VT, USA) has also been used as a sperm migration medium. Variations of this molecule show great potential as a hyaluronate migration test for use in conjunction with SMIT procedures and the Immunobead test (see Chapter 10).

The use of any mucus substitute must never replace homologous SMIT evaluations in clinical infertility investigation. After all, it is into his partner's cervical mucus that a man's spermatozoa must be able to migrate to achieve conception.

IN VIVO SPERM–MUCUS INTERACTION TESTING

Background

The postcoital test (PCT) allows assessment of sperm–cervical mucus interaction under in vivo conditions. All PCT attempts must be made during the periovulatory period for optimum mucus quality. Three days of sexual abstinence should be observed to provide optimum semen characteristics and to minimize any contamination of the mucus with spermatozoa from a previous insemination. Motile spermatozoa are counted in randomly selected fields, and these numbers are used to calculate the test result (Belsey et al., 1980; Mortimer, 1985; World Health Organization, 1987, 1992). The method described here uses sperm concentrations and is the most objective currently available (World Health Organization, 1992).

The PCT evaluates the penetration of spermatozoa from liquefied semen into cervical mucus and their survival within that environment. However, debate continues as to the true clinical value and significance of the PCT (see Chapter 11). If sexual dysfunction is suspected, a positive PCT may be taken as evidence of an adequate coital technique. Although antisperm antibodies in cervical mucus may cause poor PCTs, technical problems may also be responsible, and caution is urged when attributing poor PCTs to immunologically hostile mucus.

Notwithstanding these problems, many clinicians still consider the PCT to be an essential part of the infertile couple's workup, and diagnostic laboratories must continue to offer the procedure.

Fractional PCT

The fractional PCT was a suggested method wherein mucus was sampled as a column from the external os to the internal os to allow consideration of the dynamics of sperm migration through the cervix. Although this test had strong proponents for a number of years, other workers showed that the final distribution of the mucus and spermatozoa in the sampling catheter was not truly representative of their original distribution within the cervix. Consequently, any clinical or physiological relevance of the fractional PCT must now be doubted (review: Mortimer, 1983).

Postcoital Test

Principle

The PCT consists of sampling the cervical mucus several hours after intercourse and examining it for the presence of spermatozoa. A PCT must be performed during the periovulatory period, and 3 days of sexual abstinence prior to the "test intercourse" is strongly recommended. Although the use of sheaths/condoms during the follicular phase of the test cycle may facilitate interpretation of the findings, it is unlikely to be well received by infertility patients.

Reagents
A mixture of glass beads in silicone grease is used to make the 100-μm fixed-depth preparations (see Appendix II).

Specimen
Intracervical mucus is obtained, its quality assessed, and pH measured as described in Cervical Mucus Sampling and Assessment, above. Ideally, the sample should be taken within 12 hours after intercourse.

Method

N.B. Objective performance of this test requires that microscope objective fields be calibrated so numbers of spermatozoa per field can be converted to numbers per unit area (i.e., per square millimeter $\equiv$ per 10^6 square micrometers), and that glass beads are used to standardize the preparation depth, allowing sperm numbers to be expressed per unit volume (i.e., per cubic millimeter $\equiv$ per microliter) (see Appendix II). The conversion factor between sperm numbers per traditional high power field and the modern volumetric unit is 10 sperm/HPF = 500 sperm/mm^3.

1. Prepare a cleaned microscope slide with four posts of the glass beads-silicone grease mixture arranged in a square pattern with sides of about 20 mm. Place a drop (*ca.* 3 mm ø) of endocervical mucus in the center of this square and cover it with a 22 × 22 mm coverslip. Press down gently on the coverslip so the posts are flattened and the coverslip is fixed with a single layer of beads between it and the slide. The mucus drop spreads toward the edges of the coverslip; if it extrudes from under the coverslip another preparation must be made using less mucus. If required, a sealed preparation may be made using silicone oil (see Appendix II).
2. Microscopic screening of the mucus is performed under a 40× objective using phase-contrast optics. Briefly scan the slide to check that the sperm distribution in the mucus sample is more or less uniform.
3. In each of 10 *randomly selected* fields away from the coverslip edge (although fields with air bubbles or large patches of epithelium may be rejected) score the number of spermatozoa according to their motility.
   a. Count the number of progressively motile spermatozoa.
   b. Count all the other spermatozoa present in the same field of view, classifying each as immotile, nonprogressively motile, or shaking (see SCMC Test, above).

N.B. If there are large numbers of spermatozoa per field, a part of the field, delimited by an eyepiece graticule, may be used. Ensure that the microscope calibration factor allows for the reduced sample area (see Appendix II).

4. Calculate the average per field incidence of each type of spermatozoa over the 10 fields.
5. Use the appropriate microscope calibration factor (see Appendix II) to convert these averages to numbers per unit area (or per unit volume).

Results

Many gynecologists may disagree with the objective assessment criteria described below, but they are based on recalculation from historic clinical series allowing for modern microscope optics and quantitative laboratory methods.

1. According to the latest WHO criteria (World Health Organization, 1992), under normal clinical conditions > 50 progressively motile spermatozoa are usually seen per HPF (400×), i.e., > 2500/mm^3 or per microliter, in the endocervical specimen at 9–24 hours after coitus. Therefore ≥ 20 spermatozoa with directional motility (WHO class *a*) per HPF (≥ 1000/μl) may be considered satisfactory. The presence of < 10/HPF (< 500/μl), particularly when associated with diminished motility (e.g., WHO class *b*) indicates decreased sperm penetration or abnormal cervical mucus. Therefore according to the average numbers of *progressively motile* spermatozoa per unit volume, the test may be rated as follows.

    Negative = no spermatozoa present
    Poor   = spermatozoa present but < 500/μl
    Average = 500–999 spermatozoa/μl
    Good   = 1000–2500 spermatozoa/μl
    Excellent = > 2500 spermatozoa/μl

2. If ≥ 20% of the spermatozoa are shaking, it should be noted on the report. If > 50% of the spermatozoa show shaking, the PCT is always classified as "poor."
3. With increasing periods of time postcoitum, the motility of spermatozoa in the cervical mucus decreases. Therefore after long postcoital delays, a test that shows many nonprogressive spermatozoa (as distinct from shaking spermatozoa) may be classified more highly than the number of progressive spermatozoa alone would indicate.
4. An Insler score of < 10/15 may be at least a partial explanation of a poor PCT.
5. Acidic mucus may also be at least a partial explanation of a poor PCT.
6. Low sperm count and particularly poor sperm motility (especially if combined with poor sperm morphology) significantly reduce the quantitative penetration of spermatozoa into mucus.

N.B. Interpretation of the clinical significance of a PCT must be the responsibility of the physician requesting the test. Such interpretation should always take into account the mucus quality and partner's semen characteristics (and adequacy of coital technique).

Quality Control

The PCT is a straightforward observational procedure. Aspects relating to the mucus quality assessment and the appraisal of shaking are dealt with elsewhere (see

Cervical Mucus Sampling and Assessment, above). The field area of each combination of microscope objective, intermediate magnification, and oculars must be calibrated to allow calculation of sperm numbers per unit area (see Appendix II).

SPERM TRANSPORT IN VIVO

Background

After the initial reports that spermatozoa could be recovered in peritoneal fluid, obtained preferably as an extension of a routine diagnostic laparoscopy, a number of early studies demonstrated that this parameter could be used as a clinical test of sperm migration through the female tract in vivo and that it was predictive of subsequent fertility (review: Mortimer, 1983).

Although a number of centers have attempted the laparoscopic sperm recovery (LSR) technique, few have published studies reporting their results. Because there is still interest in the clinical application of the LSR procedure, details of the laboratory method are provided below. In fact, the method for handling the peritoneal fluid aspirates could be applied equally to other studies on sperm transport in vivo (e.g., culdocentesis) with minor modifications.

The design of clinical studies using this method are not relevant to the present text and are not considered (see Templeton and Mortimer, 1982; Mortimer, 1985). One report, however, disagreed with the early studies, although there may have been many differences in the patient populations (Ramsewak et al., 1990). Of particular significance is the markedly improved accuracy of timing the LSR procedures, as all patients had the treatment cycle synchronized by progestogen withdrawal. Such pharmacological modification of the cycle could also diminish the clinical relevance of the test in relation to predicting spontaneous pregnancy, an aspect not considered in the more recent study.

Laparoscopic Sperm Recovery

Principle

Because the fimbriated end of the human fallopian tube or oviduct is open, some of the spermatozoa that reach the site of fertilization in the tubal ampulla may pass out into the peritoneal cavity. LSR was developed as a clinical test of sperm migration in vivo with peritoneal fluid being aspirated at a diagnostic laparoscopy scheduled for the immediate periovulatory period, insemination (either coital or artificial) having occurred some 6–17 hours previously (Templeton and Mortimer, 1982).

Reagents

Rinse medium is any balanced salt solution, (e.g., PBS, Hanks', or Earle's) or tissue culture medium, e.g., Medium 199, Ham's F10, or Quinn's HTF medium (see Chapter 12). It must be prepared using tissue culture grade water, as it is used internally to rinse the fimbria and the pouch of Douglas (PoD) or cul-de-sac of the peritoneal cavity.

Saponin solution is a 0.01% (w/v) solution of saponin, a detergent extracted from the soapwort plant, in reagent water.

Glycerine jelly (or glycerol jelly) is used as a semipermanent mountant for phase-contrast microscopy. It is purchased already prepared.

Specimens

Peritoneal fluid is the initial aspirate from the PoD. It is usually a rather bloody fluid.

Rinses are usually obtained by squirting the rinse medium over the fimbria and allowing the medium to flow down into the PoD from where it is aspirated. Additional rinses of the PoD may also be provided.

Method

N.B. If peritoneal fluid is required for subsequent assays of hormones or other substances, it should be kept separate from the rinses until after the first centrifugation step where it can be obtained as a pure supernatant. If not, the PoD fluid and rinses may be mixed from the outset of the processing method described below.

1. Transfer the PoD fluid and rinses into conical bottom plastic centrifuge tubes (e.g., Falcon 2095, 2096, or 2097).
2. Centrifuge at 1000 g for 10 minutes.
3. Remove the supernatants, and resuspend the pellets in small volumes of fresh rinse medium. Combine all the pellets in one tube.
4. Measure the total volume of the washed and resuspended pellets. Mix thoroughly by inversion and take a suitable aliquot for subsequent processing. The aliquot may be $\frac{1}{20}$ to $\frac{1}{5}$ of the total volume, depending on the level of blood contamination. Transfer this aliquot to a clean, capped centrifuge tube.
5. Add a 10× volume of the saponin solution. Mix thoroughly, but gently, by inversion.

N.B. The specimen must not be left for more than 5 minutes before centrifugation otherwise some of the spermatozoa themselves may begin to lyse.

6. Centrifuge at 1000 g for 10 minutes.
7. Carefully aspirate and discard the supernatant and resuspend the pellet in 1.0 ml reagent water. If there is still a relatively large amount of cellular material remaining, the lysing process may be repeated once more. Otherwise go to step 8.
8. Transfer the lysed material to a 1.5-ml Eppendorf tube and centrifuge at 1000 g for 10 minutes.
9. Carefully aspirate the supernatant and resuspend the pellet (which may be almost invisible by this stage) in about 15–20 µl reagent water. Use a larger volume (e.g., 30 µl) if there is an appreciable pellet.
10. Mix this suspension thoroughly by repeat pipetting using a micropipette with disposable plastic tips. Apply 5-µl aliquots of the suspension to a 15-well culture slide (Flow Laboratories, Cat. No. 60-415-05).

11. Allow to air-dry either at ambient temperature or on a slide warmer.
12. Fix the slide by gently rinsing its surface with absolute ethanol. Allow to air-dry.
13. Mount with glyerine jelly that has been warmed to about 60°C and a 50 × 22 mm coverslip.
14. Slides are scored by the systematic scanning of each droplet using phase-contrast microscopy at a final magnification of 200× to 600×, depending on the amount of residual background material. Count only definite spermatozoa, including free heads but not free tails. Disregard *all* doubtful objects. An eyepiece graticule is useful for defining the width of a field to be scanned that is less than the total width of the microscope field of view.

N.B. At step 4 the remaining washed PoD material may be recentrifuged (1000 *g* for 10 minutes), the supernatant discarded, and the pellet resuspended in about 0.5 ml total volume. Drops of this material may then be examined as wet preparations under phase-contrast microscopy (200× to 300× magnification) for the presence of motile spermatozoa.

Results
The only clinical result from this test considered to date has been a simple positive or negative, based on whether any spermatozoa were found in the lysed or wet preparations.

Quality Control
It is essential that the preparations are scanned meticulously to ensure that no area is missed. Provided that only definite spermatozoa are counted, there should be no false-positive results, although there is always the risk of false negatives.

References and Recommended Reading

Belsey, M. A., Eliasson, R., Gallegos, A. J., Moghissi, K. S., Paulsen, C. A., and Prasad, M. R. N. (1980). *Laboratory Manual for the Examination of Human Semen and Semen-Cervical Mucus Interaction.* Press Concern, Singapore.

Bissett, D. L. (1980). Development of a model of human cervical mucus. *Fertil. Steril.* **33,** 211.

Eggert-Kruse, W., Leinhos, G., Gerhard, I., Tilgen, W., and Runnebaum, B. (1989). Prognostic value of in vitro sperm penetration into hormonally standardized human cervical mucus. *Fertil. Steril.* **51,** 317.

Hargreave, T. B., and Nilsson, S. (1983). Seminology. In Hargreave, T. B. (ed): *Male Infertility.* Springer-Verlag, Berlin.

Insler, V., Melmed, H., Eichenbrenner, I., Serr, D. M., and Lunenfeld, B. (1972). The cervical score: a simple semiquantitative method for monitoring of the menstrual cycle. *Int. J. Gynaecol. Obstet.* **10,** 223.

Katz, D. F., Overstreet, J. W., and Hanson, F. W. (1980). A new quantitative test for sperm penetration into cervical mucus. *Fertil. Steril.* **33,** 179.

Kremer, J. (1965). A simple sperm penetration test. *Int. J. Fertil.* **10,** 209.

Kremer, J., and Jager, S. (1976). The sperm-cervical mucus contact test: a preliminary report. *Fertil. Steril.* **27**, 335.

Kremer, J., and Jager, S. (1988). Sperm-cervical mucus interaction, in particular in the presence of antispermatozoal antibodies. *Hum. Reprod.* **3**, 69.

Kurzrok, R., and Miller, E. G. (1928). Biochemical studies of human semen and its relation to mucus of the cervix uteri. *Am. J. Obstet. Gynecol.* **15**, 56.

Lorton, S. P., Kummerfeld, H. L., and Foote, R. H. (1981). Polyacrylamide as a substitute for cervical mucus in sperm migration tests. *Fertil. Steril.* **35**, 222.

Makler, A. (1976). A new method for evaluating cervical penetrability using daily aspirated and stored cervical mucus. *Fertil. Steril.* **27**, 533.

Moghissi, K. S. (1986). Evaluation and management of cervical hostility. *Semin. Reprod. Endocrinol.* **4**, 343.

Mortimer, D. (1983). Sperm transport in the human female reproductive tract. In Finn, C. A. (ed): *Oxford Reviews of Reproductive Biology,* Vol. 5. Oxford University Press, Oxford.

Mortimer, D. (1985). The male factor in infertility Part II. Sperm function testing. *Curr. Probl. Obstet. Gynecol. Fertil.* Vol. VIII (8), 75 pp. Year Book Medical Publishers Inc., Chicago.

Pandya, I. J., Mortimer, D., and Sawers, R. S. (1986). A standardized approach for evaluating the penetration of human spermatozoa into cervical mucus *in vitro. Fertil. Steril.* **45**, 357.

Ramsewak, S. S., Barratt, C. L. R., Li, T.-C., Gooch, H., and Cooke, I. D. (1990). Peritoneal sperm recovery can be consistently demonstrated in women with unexplained infertility. *Fertil. Steril.* **53**, 1106.

Tam, P. Y., Katz, D. F., and Berger, S. A. (1980). Non-linear viscoelastic properties of cervical mucus. *Biorheology* **17**, 465.

Templeton, A. A., and Mortimer, D. (1982). The development of a clinical test of sperm migration to the site of fertilization. *Fertil. Steril.* **37**, 410.

Ulstein, M., and Fjällbrant, B. (1976). In-vitro tests of sperm penetration in cervical mucus. In Hafez, E.S.E. (ed): *Human Semen and Fertility Regulation in Men.* Mosby, St. Louis.

World Health Organization (1987). *WHO Laboratory Manual for the Examination of Human Semen and Semen-Cervical Mucus Interaction,* 2nd ed. Cambridge University Press, Cambridge.

World Health Organization (1992). *WHO Laboratory Manual for the Examination of Human Semen and Sperm-Cervical Mucus Interaction,* 3rd ed. Cambridge University Press, Cambridge.

10

Sperm Fertilizing Ability Testing

Approximately 10–15% of couples trying to get pregnant fail to do so and seek medical advice. Infertility has been diagnosed as being due to a male factor in 25–33% of cases, often combined with a female factor; but 15–20% of couples have otherwise unexplained or "idiopathic" infertility (Templeton and Penney, 1982; Spira, 1986; Collins, 1987; World Health Organization, 1990). About 34% of couples who have never been pregnant (primary infertility), and 21% of those who have previously conceived (secondary infertility) remain infertile after 9 years (Templeton and Penney, 1982). However, most pregnancies resulting from successful medical intervention are due to treatments for female endocrine disorders and surgical treatments of either partner; few are due to any specific medical treatment of a male factor. Indeed, rigorous placebo-controlled trials have revealed many of the supposed treatments for male infertility to be ineffective (Hargreave, 1983). At the same time, numerous instances of fertility despite one or more abnormal semen characteristics and the many occasions where semen analysis and all other factors seem normal yet the couple remains infertile testify to the inadequacy of the traditional "descriptive" approach for predicting an individual's fertility potential.

Because the major part of the spermatozoon's functional life is spent in the female reproductive tract, descriptive semen analysis clearly cannot be expected to provide all the answers. Clear evidence exists for some idiopathic infertility being due to specific defects of sperm function, originating in defective spermatogenesis or spermiogenesis and resulting in failures of gamete approximation or interaction. Although considerable progress has been made in understanding the processes of gamete transport in vivo and fertilization (primarily in vitro) in animal models (see Chapter 2), their regulation in humans remains poorly understood. Nevertheless, assessment of a possibly infertile man's reproductive potential must incorporate some evaluation of the various processes that take place between ejaculation and conception in the relative inaccessibility of the female tract. Current routine clinical testing goes no further than semen analysis and sperm–cervical mucus interaction, and the accepted criteria for a "normal" semen analysis are arbitrary values for concentration, motility, and normal morphology based on statistical correlations (see Chapter 11). Better knowledge of the defects in sperm function should permit more accurate assessment of fertility for the individual man, irrespective of the results of his semen analysis.

This chapter discusses the availability, limitations, and relevance of current laboratory procedures for the assessment of human sperm fertilizing ability.

199

SPERM MIGRATION TESTING

Although this chapter focuses on sperm fertilizing ability, it must not be forgotten that, at least in vivo, spermatozoa must also be transported between the site of insemination and the site of fertilization in the tubal ampulla. Sperm transport, including both sperm–cervical mucus interaction and migration/transport through the female reproductive tract, are considered in Chapter 9. Tests of in vitro sperm migration ability unrelated to the female tract are described here. Although such tests assess aspects of sperm function equivalent to those on which sperm transport depends in vitro migration tests using synthetic media are more amenable as routine laboratory assessments of sperm functional potential not perforce intrinsic to a clinical infertility workup.

Many of these tests employ the substances developed, or at least used, as substitutes for cervical mucus in attempts to standardize infertility diagnostic evaluations. Such materials include polyethylene glycol bisacrylate (Bissett, 1980), polyacrylamide (Lorton et al., 1981), and high-molecular-weight sodium hyaluronate (Sperm Select: Select Medical Systems, Williston, VT, USA) (Wikland et al., 1987). Whereas polyacrylamide has been found difficult to standardize in practice, variations of the sodium hyaluronate molecule seem to show great potential as a hyaluronate migration test (HMT) (Mortimer et al., 1990b), especially when used in combination with SMIT procedures and the Immunobead test. Further studies have also reported that hyaluronate-based migration tests are standardized and are able to assess sperm functional competence (Neuwinger et al., 1991; Aitken et al., 1992).

Hyaluronate Migration Test

Background
Direct comparisons of human sperm migration Kremer tests (HMTs) using a solution of sodium hyaluronate (average molecular weight 2,000,000, 5 mg/ml in a phosphate-buffered medium) showed these two tests to be highly significantly correlated and dependent on similar sperm characteristics. These sperm characteristics were essentially those reflecting sperm progressive ability (including the specific movement characteristic of lateral head displacement amplitude), morphological normality, and cellular vitality as well as the concentration of these more functional cells in the semen. In conjunction with the mucus quality measures of Insler score and pH, the HMT result allowed 92.2% correct prediction of the Kremer test outcome (90.9% of normal tests and 93.1% of abnormal tests). The HMT is therefore likely to be a useful adjunct to routine semen analysis, sperm movement analysis, and the more traditional in vitro SMIT procedures in the diagnostic workup of infertile couples. It effectively assesses the mucus-penetrating ability of a semen sample without the need for relatively large quantities of midcycle cervical mucus. Consequently, the HMT augments, although does not necessarily replace, the homologous Kremer test and reduces the need for donor mucus for crossed-hostility format testing.

Subsequent studies (unpublished data) have resulted in a modified hyaluronate-based medium optimized for use in a human sperm migration test situation. This material will shortly be commercialized in a Hyaluronate Migration Test kit (Select Medical Systems, Williston, VT, USA). The method for this HMT is provided below.

Principle

Sperm penetration into, and migration along, a capillary tube filled with a special synthetic medium containing high-molecular-weight sodium hyaluronate depends on sperm characteristics similar to those needed for migration along a column of human periovulatory cervical mucus.

Reagents

The hyaluronate test medium is a modified Sperm Select medium (Select Medical Systems). It is aspirated into rectangular cross-section glass capillaries (2.0 × 0.2 × 50 mm) that are then sealed using hematocrit tube sealant.

Specimen

Semen: A 50-μl aliquot of liquefied semen is required for each test. It must be taken from a well-mixed ejaculate specimen at 30 minutes after ejaculation.

Method

N.B.   As for SMIT procedures (see Chapter 9), the objective performance of this test requires that microscope objective fields be calibrated so numbers of spermatozoa per field may be converted to numbers per unit area (i.e., per square millimeter $\equiv$ per 10^6 square micrometers) (see Appendix II).

N.B.   It is recommended that HMT procedures be run at least in duplicate.

1. A BEEM capsule (designed for embedding tissue for electron microscopy) (see Chapter 8) is used as the semen reservoir (as for the Kremer SMIT) (see Chapter 9) with a slit or hole (e.g., using a punch plier) being made in the capsule's cap to take the capillary tube. The 50-μl semen aliquot is deposited carefully in the bottom of the reservoir (which is held upright in a special rack) and the cap closed.
2. The open end of the hyaluronate capillary tube is inserted into the semen reservoir so its open end is immersed in the semen.
3. Incubate the test at 37°C for 60 minutes.
4. After exactly 60 minutes the capillary tube is removed from the sperm reservoir, wiped clean of any residual semen at its open end, and transferred to slide for counting. The depth and degree of sperm penetration into the hyaluronate column is assessed microscopically using a magnification of 200× to 250× (i.e., a 20× objective). Note on the laboratory form the combination of optics used.
5. Count the number of spermatozoa present in each of *two* microscope fields at each of the upper and lower glass faces of the tube at each of the 10-, 20-, 30-, and 40-mm distances. If there are few spermatozoa in the first 20 mm of the tube, count at the 5-, 10-, 15-, 20-, and 25-mm distances. If there are many sper-

matozoa in any particular field, the field size may be reduced using an eyepiece graticule or by increasing the intermediate magnification; do *not* use a 40× objective. Count only those spermatozoa *in focus* without adjusting the microscope's focus, as adjustment induces variations in the third dimension of the field's size.

Results

1. The average number of spermatozoa present per field at each distance along the hyaluronate column is calculated and then corrected to give the number per unit area using the known microscope field area (see Appendix II).
2. Perform a log-linear regression using the millimeter distances along the hyaluronate capillary as the *x*-axis values and the log-transformed numbers of spermatozoa as the *y*-axis values. The *r* value should be negative and highly significant (at least $P < 0.01$); if not, the test should be discarded.
3. Calculate the vanguard sperm migration distance (x'mm) for each tube using the fitted straight-line equation for the *y* intercept (i.e., where $y = 0$, equivalent to one spermatozoon per unit area).
4. Provided the two vanguard distances are within 10% (i.e., the equation shown below is true), find the average vanguard distance as the final result of the test. If not, take the higher vanguard distance as the result.

$$\text{(High value} - \text{low value)} \leq [\text{(high value} + \text{low value)} \div 20]$$

Quality Control
The hyaluronate migration test is a straightforward observational procedure. Quality control aspects relating to the semen analysis and mucus quality assessment are dealt with under the appropriate tests.

The field area of each combination of microscope objective, intermediate magnification, and oculars must be calibrated to allow calculation of sperm numbers per unit area (see Appendix II). To achieve optimum standardization, only 20× (or 25×) objectives should be used to eliminate variability in the microscope's depth of focus and hence the third dimension of the microscope field being scored.

Changing the incubation time also alters the quantitative extent of sperm penetration along the mucus column. Consequently, tests must be run for the expected 60 minutes; shorter times require completely redefined interpretation criteria.

Interpretation
Normal semen samples show a vanguard migration distance of at least 20 mm (Mortimer et al., 1990b). Additional studies on the correlation of HMT results with clinical endpoints (e.g., in vivo conception or IVF outcome) (see Chapter 11) are not yet available.

ASSESSMENT OF CAPACITATION

Capacitation is the final stage of maturation by which eutherian spermatozoa acquire the capacity to undergo the acrosome reaction and fertilize eggs (see Chapter 2). It is essential for fertilization both in vivo and in vitro, in the homologous in vitro test of sperm–zona binding, and even in the heterologous test of sperm fertilizing ability using zona-free hamster oocytes (see below). Although capacitation starts with separation of spermatozoa from the seminal plasma, it is more than just liberation from inhibition: A further period of time, usually spent within the female tract, is required for spermatozoa to achieve the capacitated state.

Morphological concomitants of capacitation that might form the basis of laboratory tests are difficult to define, although changes in chlortetracycline fluorescence and modifications of sperm surface glycoproteins have been described (see below).

Sperm Surface Lectin Labeling

Modifications of sperm surface glycoproteins related to capacitation have been monitored using lectins (Ahuja, 1985; Cross and Overstreet, 1987). A method for Concanavalin A labeling of human spermatozoa is provided below.

Reagents

Concanavalin A (ConA) lectin is purchased conjugated with fluorescein (FITC) or rhodamine (TRITC). If FITC-conjugated peanut agglutinin (PNA) is to be used for acrosome reaction assessments on the same sperm population, TRITC-ConA should be used (e.g., Intermedico Cat. No. R-1104) 2 mg/2 ml, OD $\geq$ 0.5 to ensure high fluorescence of the lectin). It should be stored at $-20°C$ until required, with the vials covered in foil to protect them from light, which inactivates the TRITC. For use it is diluted $1 + 9$ with reagent water and kept in a foil-covered container, e.g., Coplin jar for slide staining.

Phosphate-buffered saline (PBS) is prepared as described for the direct Immunobead test (see Chapter 5).

Maunsbach's phosphate buffer is prepared as described for lectin labeling assessment of the acrosome reaction (see below).

Paraformaldehyde fixative is prepared as described for lectin labeling assessment of the acrosome reaction (see below).

A special mountant is used to minimize fading of the fluorochrome during observation under UV light. The two available alternatives are described for lectin labeling assessment of the acrosome reaction, below.

Specimen

Populations of capacitating spermatozoa at $5 \times$ to 10^6 to 10×10^6/ml can be used, but they are ideally concentrated to about 20×10^6/ml before making the smears (see below).

Method

1. About 20 µl of the sperm suspension is spread over one end of a clean microscope slide and allowed to air dry. Multiple smears (at least three) should be prepared in case of problems with labeling or reading.

2. Fix the smears by immersion in 95% ethanol for 5 minutes and allow to air-dry.
3. Immerse the slides in TRITC-ConA solution for 15 minutes at ambient temperature. The staining should be performed in the dark, e.g., a foil-covered Coplin jar.
4. Rinse the slides by gently dipping them into a beaker of PBS.
5. Repeat step 4.
6. Fix the slides by immersion in the paraformaldehyde fixative for 15 minutes at ambient temperature. This step must be performed in the dark.
7. Rinse the slides by gently dipping them into a beaker of PBS.
8. Repeat step 7.
9. The slides are then allowed to air-dry and stored in the dark until scoring, which should be completed within 48 hours of staining.
10. Score two slides, randomized and coded, under epifluorescence, (see Appendix III, Table 1 for suitable filter sets) counting 250 spermatozoa per slide. Each spermatozoon is classified as either *heterogeneous,* in that ConA labeling was dispersed over the whole cell surface, or *acrosome rim,* in that there was a bright crescent of increased fluorescence at the anterior margin of the sperm head. The incidence of the latter class increases with incubation under capacitating conditions.

Results
Calculate the percentage incidence of the "acrosome rim" labeled class for each slide. If the pair of slides is not within 10%, a third slide should be labeled, scored, and the three sets of values averaged to give the final result.

Quality Control
To eliminate observer bias slides should be scored blind, in batches, after randomization and coding.

Chlortetracycline Fluorescence

Changes in chlortetracycline (CTC) fluorescence associated with the time sequence of capacitation and the acrosome reaction have been described in both mouse and human spermatozoa. A protocol for using the CTC fluorescence technique with human spermatozoa (Lee et al., 1987) is provided below.

Reagents

CTC solution comprises a mixture of 5 mM CTC, 20 mM Tris, 5 mM cysteine, and 130 mM NaCl. It is prepared by dissolving 10 mg Tris, 3 mg cysteine, and 30 mg NaCl in reagent water, adding 40 μl of a 500 mM aqueous stock solution of CTC, and bringing to a total volume of 4.0 ml. The pH is adjusted to 7.8 ± 0.5 using 1 N HCl, and the solution is kept cool. The final CTC solution should be used only on the day of preparation.

Glutaraldehyde fixative is a 3% (v/v) solution of glutaraldehyde in 20 mM Tris buffer pH 8.0. The Tris buffer is prepared by dissolving NaCl 7.889 g/l (135 mM), KCl 0.373 g/l (5 mM), and Tris 4.481 g/l (37 mM) in reagent water and adjusting to pH 8.0 with 5 N HCl. The fixative is prepared by mixing 125 µl stock (25% v/v) glutaraldehyde and 875 µl Tris buffer. The final pH should be 7.8 ± 0.5. Keep the fixative cool and use only on the day of preparation. Discard the fixative if it develops a slight yellow tinge and prepare a fresh solution.

Specimen
Populations of capacitating spermatozoa at 5×10^6 to 10×10^6/ml can be used.

Method

1. Place 2.5 µl of the sperm suspension on a clean microscope slide at 37°C and quickly add 2.5 µl CTC solution. Multiple slides (at least three) should be prepared in case of problems with labeling or reading.
2. Within 10 seconds add 0.25 µl glutaraldehyde fixative (using a Hamilton No. 7101NWG microsyringe dispenser with a Teflon tubing tip) and mix using the tip of the microsyringe dispenser.
3. Keep the slides at ambient temperature in a light-shielded humid chamber until ready to score.
4. Score two slides, randomized and coded, under epifluorescence, (see Appendix III, Table 1 for suitable filter sets) counting 250 spermatozoa per slide. Each spermatozoon is classified according to the distribution of fluorescence.

   B = back of the head (postacrosomal region)
   F = front of the head (acrosomal region
   A = all of the head
   N = none

   In categories B, F, and A the midpiece also shows bright fluorescence.

Results
Calculate the percentage incidence of each class for each slide. If the pair of slides is not within 10% for major classes (i.e., those including more than 50 spermatozoa), a third slide should be labeled and scored, and the three sets of values are averaged to give the final result.

Quality Control
To eliminate observer bias slides should be scored blind, in batches, after randomization and coding.

Hyperactivated Motility

Hyperactivated motility is a highly active, but nonprogressive pattern of motility that is characteristic of capacitated eutherian spermatozoa (see Chapter 2). It is essential for the fertilization of intact oocyte–cumulus complexes in vitro and in vivo. Although expression of hyperactivated motility by human spermatozoa was doubted for many years, extensive observations of human spermatozoa under capacitating conditions have permitted the identification and kinematic description of human sperm hyperactivation (see Table 7-1).

No optimized assay for human sperm hyperactivation has yet been described, but certain basic conditions are prerequisites.

1. A CASA-based method is used for sperm kinematic analysis, with established optimized criteria for specifically identifying hyperactivated spermatozoa (see Chapter 7). If the system is not capable of sorting individual cells' track values internally, the data should be exported to an external computer where a spreadsheet or statistical program can be used for *post hoc* analysis (track sorting).
2. A selected motile sperm population must be prepared using a technique known not to cause any damage to the spermatozoa while minimizing contamination with seminal plasma (see Chapter 12).
3. A culture medium known to support human sperm capacitation and, ideally, IVF. The composition of this medium should include about 5 µM free Ca^{2+} ions, 20 mM bicarbonate ions, glucose as a metabolic substrate for the spermatozoa, and albumin to maintain sperm viability and support capacitation.
4. Sperm preincubation must be at 37°C, although the optimum duration of this period is uncertain and may well be subject to interindividual variation. Early reports indicate that within 3 hours after initiation of sperm separation from seminal plasma is optimal. An atmosphere containing 5% CO_2 is essential for maintaining the bicarbonate ions in solution.
5. Preparations for kinematic analysis must be made in chambers of at least 30 µm depth (ideally 40 or 50 µm) and maintained at 37°C. Negative phase-contrast optics are better than the typical positive phase for tracking hyperactivated spermatozoa to minimize track breakage (see Chapter 7).
6. Suggested kinematic criteria to discriminate hyperactivated human spermatozoa are provided in Table 7-1.

ASSESSMENT OF THE ACROSOME REACTION

On completion of capacitation a spermatozoon is, by definition, in a state ready to undergo the acrosome reaction. The acrosomal cap of some mammalian spermatozoa is sufficiently large to be visualized by phase-contrast microscopy but in others, unfortunately including humans, it is too small to be seen directly. Consequently, indirect methods using fluorescein-labeled lectins, monoclonal antibodies, and staining techniques have been developed to visualize the presence or absence of the human sperm acrosome.

Although interpretation of investigations based on acrosome reaction scoring have not yet attracted widespread clinical interest in infertility management, it is a research area of great current interest, and an increasing number of laboratories are establishing methods for monitoring the acrosome status of human sperm populations.

Triple-Stain Technique

The triple-stain technique described by Talbot and Chacon (1981) combines Bismarck brown and rose bengal dyes to differentially stain the sperm head to show the presence or absence of acrosomal material with trypan blue as a vital stain. Four categories of spermatozoa are therefore scored based on vitality and acrosomal status.

Live unreacted cells are unstained by trypan blue with pink acrosomal region and brown postacrosomal region.

Live reacted cells are also unstained by trypan blue, but the acrosome region is unstained and the postacrosomal region remains brown.

Dead reacted cells are stained with trypan blue so the postacrosomal region is a dark blue-black and the acrosomal region is unstained.

Dead unreacted cells have an acrosomal region that appears a slightly darker pink than the live unreacted cells, and the postacrosomal region stains dark blue-black. These cells are often seen at a more or less constant low incidence; they are of unknown physiological significance and may be artifactual.

The triple-stain technique is notoriously capricious, and laboratories are advised to establish their own optimal staining conditions, which will probably vary among batches of stain and even within a batch as the staining solutions age (Talbot and Dudenhausen, 1981). A suggested starting protocol is given below.

Reagents

Culture medium is whatever medium is used for the experiment (see Chapter 12).

Phosphate-buffered saline (PBS) is prepared as described for the direct Immunobead test (see Chapter 5).

Glutaraldehyde fixative is a 3.0% (v/v) solution of glutaraldehyde in 0.1 M cacodylate buffer pH 7.4–7.5. The cacodylate buffer is prepared at 114 mM strength by dissolving 24.45 g sodium cacodylate ($NaCac·3H_2O$) and 3.94 ml 1 N HC1 in reagent water to 1000 ml. For use, mix 10 ml stock (25% v/v) glutaraldehyde solution and 73.3 ml cacodylate buffer. Adjust with 1 N HCl or NaOH to pH 7.4–7.5.

Trypan blue (C.I. 23850) is prepared as a 0.5% (w/v) solution in albumin-free culture medium.

Bismarck brown stain is a 2.0% (w/v) solution of Bismarck brown Y (C.I. 21000) in reagent water with its pH adjusted to 1.8 using 1 N HCl. Establish the pH prior to adding the stain in order to protect the pH electrode.

Rose bengal stain is a 0.8% (w/v) solution of rose bengal (C.I. 45440) in 100 mM pH 5.3 Tris buffer. Establish the pH of the buffer prior to adding the stain in order to protect the pH electrode.

Ethanol dehydration series comprises volumetric dilutions of absolute ethanol in reagent water to give 50%, 75%, 90%, and 95% (v/v). These alcohols are stored in well-stoppered glass bottles at ambient temperature. Absolute ethanol (100% v/v) is also required.

Xylene is used as the clearing agent.

Specimen

Populations of human spermatozoa at 5×10^6 to 20×10^6/ml in culture medium can be used. Ejaculate spermatozoa must be either washed first or prepared by swim-up migration or Percoll gradient centrifugation into culture medium or PBS to reduce the protein concentration. A minimum of 5×10^6 spermatozoa are required for the staining procedure.

Method

1. Dilute the sperm suspension aliquot with an equal volume of trypan blue solution and incubate at 37°C for 15 minutes.
2. Add 10 ml of PBS and centrifuge at 600 g for 8 minutes.
3. Discard the supernatant and resuspend the pellet in 10 ml fresh PBS
4. Centrifuge again at 600 g for 8 minutes.
5. Discard the supernatant, and resuspend the pellet in 1 ml fresh PBS.
6. If the supernatant is clear or pale blue, proceed to step 7, otherwise add another 9 ml of fresh PBS and repeat steps 4 and 5.
7. Add 2 ml of glutaraldehyde solution to fix the spermatozoa for 20 minutes at ambient temperature.
8. Add 10 ml reagent water and centrifuge at 600 g for 8 minutes.
9. Discard supernatant and resuspend the pellet in 10 ml fresh reagent water.
10. Centrifuge at 600 g for 8 minutes.
11. Discard the supernatant and resuspend the pellet in reagent water to a total volume of approximately 100 μl.
12. Prepare at least three slides by allowing 10-μl aliquots of the sperm suspension to dry onto clean microscope slides. Multiwell slides (Flow Laboratories Cat. No. 60-415-05) can be used, allowing up to 15 sperm drops to be stained per slide.
13. Later, when convenient, stain the slides with the Bismark brown solution for 5 minutes at 40°C.
14. Rinse the slides in reagent water for several seconds.
15. Stain the slides with the rose bengal solution for 27.5 minutes at ambient temperature.
16. Rinse the slides in reagent water for several seconds.
17. Dehydrate by passing through a graded alcohol series: 50%, 75%, 90%, 95%, 100%, 100%, 100%. Allow 5 minutes in each at ambient temperature. (The final 100% ethanol step may be replaced by a 100% methanol step to achieve better dehydration.)
18. Clear in two xylene washes for 5 minutes each at ambient temperature in a fume hood.
19. Mount using DPX or equivalent mountant and allow the mountant to dry overnight.
20. Examine at a magnification of at least 1000× (i.e., a 100× oil immersion objective) using correctly aligned brightfield illumination. Count at least 200

spermatozoa per slide (or well) and classify into the four categories described above.

Results

Calculate the percentage incidence of each class for each slide. If the pair of slides is not within 10% for major classes (i.e., those including more than 50 spermatozoa), a third slide should be stained, scored, and the three sets of values averaged to give the final result.

Quality Control

Obviously to eliminate observer bias, slides should be scored blind, in batches, after randomization and coding.

Fluorescent Lectin Labeling

Of the many techniques now available for assessing the acrosomal status of human spermatozoa, those using fluorescent lectins are more widely used than indirect immunofluorescence techniques requiring monoclonal antibodies.

The first lectin-based method used *Ricinus communis* agglutinin I (RCA-60 or simply RCA) (Talbot and Chacon, 1980) but was never popular because of the toxicity of this lectin. Subsequently, three other lectins have been found useful in this application.

Peanut agglutinin (PNA) from *Arachis hypogea* has a specificity for ß-D-galactose residues (the same as RCA; see above) and labels the outer acrosomal membrane (Mortimer et al., 1987).

Pisum sativum agglutinin (PSA) has a specificity for α-methylmannose residues and labels the acrosomal contents (Cross et al., 1986).

Concanavalin A (ConA) binds to D-mannose residues located on the inner acrosomal membrane (Holden et al., 1990).

Both the PNA and PSA methods have been combined with the Hoechst 33258 fluorochrome acting as a vital stain. A method for H33258/FITC-PNA labeling of human sperm populations is provided below.

In addition to their assessment by fluorescence microscopy, lectin-labeled spermatozoa can also be counted using flow cytometry (e.g., PNA-labeled cells) (Purvis et al., 1990).

Reagents

Hoechst 33258 (bis-benzimide, e.g. Sigma B-2883) is prepared as a $1000\times$ stock solution by dissolving 1 mg H33258 in 1 ml reagent water. The stock should be frozen at $-20°C$ in 5- and 10-μl aliquots in small foil-covered Eppendorf tubes to protect the H33258 from light.

FITC-PNA is purchased commercially (e.g., E.Y Labs, Inc., San Mateo, CA, USA; Cat. No. F-2301; 5 mg/ 5 ml. An OD ≥ 2.0 may be needed to ensure good fluorescence of the lectin). Store the stock FITC-PNA frozen at $-20°C$ in 600-μl aliquots in foil-covered Eppendorf tubes to protect the FITC from light.

PVP-40 is a 2.0% (w/v) solution of 40,000 MW polyvinylpyrrolidone (Sigma PVP-40) in PBS.

Phosphate-buffered saline (PBS) is prepared as described for the direct Immunobead test (see Chapter 5).

Maunsbach's phosphate buffer is a mixed aqueous solution of sodium dihydrogen orthophosphate and disodium hydrogen orthophosphate: NaH_2PO_4 2.6 g/l and $Na_2HPO_4·7H_2O$ 30.4 g/l in reagent water. The pH is adjusted to 7.5–7.6 using the appropriate phosphate solution.

Paraformaldehyde fixative is prepared by adding 20 g paraformaldehyde to 50.0 ml of reagent water in a 100-ml beaker in a fume hood. With constant stirring (use a heated magnetic stirrer), the mixture is heated to 65°C. A watch glass is placed over the beaker to minimize evaporative loss during heating. At 65°C, add 10 Pasteur pipette drops (approximately 300 μl) of 40% (w/v) NaOH to clear the paraformaldehyde solution. Filter the final solution through a Whatman No. 1 filter paper and add 20.0 ml to 208.6 ml of Maunsbach's phosphate buffer. Adjust to pH 7.5 and store in a foil-covered conical flask until needed or it may crystallize.

Fluorescence mountant denotes a special mountant that minimizes fading of the fluorochrome during observation under UV light (see Appendix III).

Specimen

Populations of capacitating spermatozoa at $5 \times$ to 10^6 to 10×10^6/ml can be used. Washed ejaculate sperm suspensions may be studied using the same protocol.

Method

1. H33258 is used at a final concentration of 1 μg/ml. Stock H33258 solution is added to culture medium, at 1 μl/ml, in a foil-covered tube, mixed well, and stored in the dark. It is used within 24 hours of preparation.

2. Add an equal volume of H33258 solution to the sperm suspension to be stained and leave for 7 minutes at ambient temperature in the dark.

N.B. *All* the following steps should be carried out in the dark.

3. After 7 minutes, layer the stained sample on a 4.0 ml column of PVP-40 (maximum 1.5 ml sample per PVP-40 column) and centrifuge at 900 g for 5 minutes.

4. Discard the supernatant and resuspend the spermatozoa to about 20×10^6/ml in fresh medium.

5. About 20 μl of the sperm suspension is spread over one end of a clean microscope slide and allowed to air-dry. Multiple smears (at least three) should be prepared in case of problems with labeling or reading.

6. Fix the smears by immersion in 95% ethanol for 5 minutes and allow to air-dry.

7. For use, dilute a 600-μl aliquot of stock FITC-PNA in 15.4 ml reagent water in a foil-covered Coplin jar.

8. When the ethanol-fixed H33258 slides (from step 6) have dried, immerse them in the FITC-PNA for 15 minutes at ambient temperature.
9. Rinse the slides by gently dipping them into a beaker of PBS.
10. Repeat step 9.
11. Fix the slides by immersion in the paraformaldehyde fixative in another foil-covered Coplin jar for 15 minutes at ambient temperature.
12. Rinse the slides by gently dipping them into a beaker of PBS.
13. Repeat step 12.
14. The slides are then allowed to air-dry and stored in the dark until scoring, which should be completed within 48 hours of staining.
15. Score two slides, randomized and coded, under epifluorescence using appropriate filter sets for H33258 and FITC (see Appendix III). Count 250 spermatozoa per slide, classifying the vitality of each spermatozoon according to the H33258 labeling and its acrosome status according to the PNA labeling.

H33258: **Dead** spermatozoa show bright blue-white fluorescence, and **live** spermatozoa show a pale blue fluorescence.

PNA: Four classes of PNA labeling are distinguished (Fig. 10-1).

I *Whole acrosome* labeling denoting an intact outer acrosomal membrane (i.e., acrosome intact).

II *Patchy acrosome* labeling suggestive of a transition stage where the outer acrosomal membrane is fenestrating (see Chapter 2), although this pattern may also be produced as a result of incomplete permeabilization of the plasma membrane during air-drying and ethanol fixation. To be counted in this class, at least 20% of the total acrosomal cap area should be dark.

III *Equatorial segment only* labeling denoting a normally acrosome-reacted spermatozoon that has lost the outer acrosomal membrane over the anterior cap portion of the acrosome but has retained the equatorial segment of the acrosome intact (see Chapter 2).

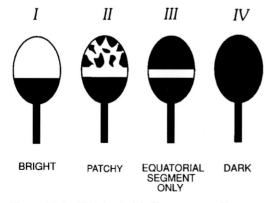

Figure 10-1   PNA lectin-labeling patterns of human spermatozoa.

IV *Dark* or no labeling denoting a spermatozoon with no outer acrosomal membrane either as a result of total acrosome loss or a morphological defect in which the spermatozoon had lacked an acrosome.

Consequently, a total of eight classes are counted:

1 = live, acrosome intact
2 = live, patchy acrosome
3 = live, acrosome-reacted
4 = live, no acrosome (uncommon finding)
5 = dead, acrosome intact (uncommon finding)
6 = dead, patchy acrosome
7 = dead, acrosome-reacted
8 = dead, no acrosome

Results
Calculate the percentage incidence of each class for each slide. If the pair of slides is not within 10% for major classes (i.e., those including more than 50 spermatozoa), a third slide should be labeled and scored and the three sets of values averaged to give the final result.

Depending on circumstances, it may be appropriate, and certainly more reliable, to count only those spermatozoa that have essentially normal head morphology.

Quality Control
To eliminate observer bias, slides should be scored blind, in batches, after randomization and coding.

Acrosome Reaction Induction Protocols

Spontaneous acrosome reactions occur in small proportions of human spermatozoa, although over prolonged incubation high levels of acrosome loss may be seen in the semen of some men. Although it has been reported that biological or biochemical agonists such as follicular fluid, cumulus, and progesterone can stimulate the acrosome reaction in human sperm populations in vitro, the physiological acrosome reaction (i.e., that of spermatozoa which actually fertilize eggs) probably occurs on the zona pellucida after sperm–zona binding, induced by a specific sperm receptor molecule (see Chapter 2).

Although biological materials such as follicular fluid or cumulus can induce the occurrence of acrosome reactions above their background spontaneous rate, the inherent variability of such materials make them poorly suited for establishing standardized test protocols. Consequently, the development of a valid bioassay remains difficult, although the induction of acrosome reactions in populations of usually capacitated spermatozoa by the calcium ionophore A23187 can be used to assess the competence of sperm populations to respond to the calcium influx that initiates a normal acrosome reaction. One publication has related an acrosome reaction after ionophore challenge (ARIC) test to IVF success (Cummins et al., 1991; see also Chapter 12).

The high concentrations of A23187 used in early studies (e.g., 50 µM suspensions of the Ca,Mg salt (e.g., Aitken et al., 1984; Mortimer et al., 1989) were rather toxic to spermatozoa and may have induced artifacts due to significant loss of vitality. More moderate concentrations of the order of 10 µM using dimethylsulfoxide (DMSO) as a carrier molecule (e.g., Mortimer and Camenzind, 1989; Cummins et al., 1991) are substantially less deleterious. Finally, the new reduced-dosage A23187 protocol ($\leq$ 2.5 µM) (World Health Organization, 1992) may prove even better for use as a sperm function test assessing the ability to undergo the acrosome reaction.

Ionomycin, another ionophore with a greater specificity for Ca^{2+} ions compared to A23187, has also been evaluated as an acrosome reaction agonist. Although several workers have suggested that ionomycin has a lower cytotoxic effect on human spermatozoa than A23187 and might therefore be a better agonist for diagnostic studies, we found it to be of no benefit over the less expensive A23187 (D. Mortimer and A. R. Camenzind, unpublished results). Several workers have mentioned in conversation that A23187 from Calbiochem seems to produce more reliable results than the Sigma product.

The carrier molecule DMSO is normally used with ionophores that are essentially insoluble in water. DMSO is known to have toxic effects on many cell types, including human spermatozoa. Studies using an alternative carrier, dimethylformamide (DMF), which is believed to be less toxic, showed no benefit over DMSO when short-exposure protocols were employed (D. Mortimer and A. R. Camenzind, unpublished results).

ARmax Concept

The idea of using A23187 to induce a maximal acrosome reaction (ARmax) response in a capacitated sperm population has been around for some time (e.g., Mortimer and Camenzind, 1989; Mortimer et al., 1989). As yet unpublished studies have also employed this approach as a test of sperm function related to clinical endpoints (see Chapter 11).

The present suggested protocol uses a final A23187 concentration of 10 µM but could perhaps be revised in accordance with the recently described ability to use only 1.25 or 2.50 µM A23187 (World Health Organization, 1992; see also Zona-Free Hamster Egg Penetration Test, below).

1. Prepare a stock solution by dissolving 1.0 mg A23187 free acid in 382 µl DMSO to give a 5 mM (i.e., 500× strength) solution, which should be stored frozen at $-20°C$ in small (e.g., 5- or 10-µl) aliquots.
2. Prepare a day-of-use solution by adding 10 µl of the 500× stock to 4.99 ml of culture medium and mix thoroughly by inversion.
3. The prepared sperm suspension (see Chapter 12) is preincubated for 5 hours under capacitating conditions.

4. Remove a 500-µl aliquot of the sperm suspension and centrifuge at 600 g for 6 minutes.
5. Discard the supernatant, and resuspend the sperm pellet in 500 µl A23187 solution.
6. Incubate at 37°C for 20 minutes.
7. After incubation, centrifuge the sperm suspension at 600 g for 6 minutes.
8. Discard the supernatant, and resuspend the sperm pellet in 500 µl fresh medium.
9. Incubate for another 2 hours under 5% CO_2 in air at 37°C.
10. Prepare slides for acrosome status assessments (see above).
11. The incidence of live acrosome-reacted spermatozoa present in the ionophore-treated population may be corrected for background—spontaneous acrosome reactions observed in a parallel aliquot of the sperm suspension incubated in isolation for an equivalent period of time. A DMSO control has not typically been included, as we have not found that it significantly altered the dynamics of spontaneous acrosome reactions under the conditions used for the test.

ARIC Test

Cummins et al. (1991) described the following protocol using a 10 µM A23187 challenge in a modified Hepes-buffered Tyrode's medium to induce acrosome reactions. It seems unlikely that this specific medium is essential, and probably any suitable Hepes-buffered medium (e.g., HTF) (see Chapter 12) could be used.

1. Prepare a 5 mM stock solution of A23187 free acid in DMSO and store frozen in 300-µl aliquots at $-20°C$.
2. For use, prepare the stock A23187 in a dilution of 1:10 with protein-free medium. Also prepare a 10% (v/v) solution of DMSO as control.
3. Two 0.5-ml aliquots of the prepared sperm population (1×10^6 to 5×10^6 motile spermatozoa/ml) are taken for the test after 3 hours of preincubation. To the test aliquot add 10 µl A23187 solution (i.e., 10 µM final ionophore concentration), and to the control aliquot add 10 µl of the 10% DMSO solution.
4. Incubate at 37°C for 60 minutes.
5. Wash by centrifugation through a 300-µl column of 70% (v/v) Percoll in a 1.5-ml Eppendorf centrifuge tube at 600 g for 12 minutes.
6. Discard the supernatant and gradient material, then resuspend the sperm pellets in 50 µl of 96% ethanol at 4°C.
7. Transfer the ethanol-fixed spermatozoa to clean microscope slides and allow to air-dry.
8. Label the spermatozoa using FITC-conjugated lectin (see above).
9. Score the slides for acrosome status.
10. Calculate the result for each of the test and control samples as the incidence of cells showing equatorial-segment-only fluorescence expressed as a percentage of the total incidence of all classes showing acrosomal labeling (i.e., excluding the "dark" cells showing no lectin labeling).
11. The incidence of ARIC cells is the difference between the test and control val-

ues. If there are more acrosome-reacted spermatozoa in the control aliquot than in the test, the ARIC is taken as zero, not negative.

Although the ARIC test does not consider cellular vitality, it does identify most cells undergoing the acrosome reaction in response to the ionophore challenge. By controlling for spontaneous and DMSO-induced changes it provides a simple assay that should be amenable to routine application.

ASSESSMENT OF SPERM–ZONA PELLUCIDA BINDING

Because much of the species specificity of the human fertilization process occurs at the level of sperm–zona pellucida interaction, which may well include induction of the physiological acrosome reaction, there has been great interest in the development and validation of tests to assess the binding of human spermatozoa to the human zona pellucida (ZP). Further impetus has been provided by the realization that the inability to assess this step during fertilization represents the major weakness of the zona-free hamster egg penetration test (see below).

Sperm–zona binding tests (ZBTs) make use of nonviable, nonfertilizable human eggs from pathological specimens or "spare" eggs from an IVF program. A common prerequisite for this application is that there must be no opportunity for inadvertent fertilization, and hence the oocyte contained within the zona must be rendered incapable of being fertilized. These eggs can either be cryostored using a crude freezing protocol that does not preserve the functional capacity of the oocyte or kept in high salt solutions that denature the ooplasm (Yanagimachi et al., 1979). Bisection of zonae for the hemizona assay (HZA) coincidentally destroys the oocytes, although zonae for this purpose have usually been cryopreserved or salt-stored previously.

The other important consideration for valid ZBT assessments is incorporation of an adequate control. If patient and control (known fertile) donor sperm populations are prepared in parallel and tested on separate groups of zonae, at least four or five zonae are required for each sperm population. With the HZA, patient and control sperm populations are tested on identical halves of the same zonae, requiring only one or two eggs per test. Alternatively, patient and donor sperm populations can be labeled with fluorochromes and then mixed for simultaneous testing in a competitive, or heterospermic, assay system (see Competitive Zona Binding Test, below).

Hemizona Assay

Originally described by Burkman et al. (1988), the HZA involves microdissecting a zona pellucida into equal halves so the binding of patient (or experimentally treated) and control sperm populations can be assessed on matching halves. Usual assay conditions are to prepare selected motile sperm populations over a period of about 60 minutes and then coincubate them with the hemizonae for 4 hours at 250,000 motile spermatozoa/ml in a droplet under oil.

A detailed description of the HZA method is not presented here as the competitive ZBT (CZBT) described below is a technically simpler procedure not requiring access to micromanipulation facilities. It is therefore more amenable for routine use in an andrology laboratory. Interested readers are referred to the review by Burkman et al. (1990).

Competitive Zona Binding Test

In the CZBT, patient and donor sperm populations are labeled with fluorochromes and mixed at equal concentrations of motile spermatozoa for simultaneous testing on the same zona in a competitive, or heterospermic, format assay. When using zonae that have not previously been inseminated, it is necessary to label only the donor spermatozoa (e.g., using fluorescein—FITC) to distinguish them from the patient's spermatozoa. If the zonae have been inseminated previously (i.e., IVF failed fertilization eggs), the two sperm populations must be labeled but with different fluorochromes (e.g., FITC and rhodamine—TRITC) to make them distinguishable from any spermatozoa that might be already attached to the zonae.

Typically, 100,000 motile spermatozoa/ml from the patient and from the donor are mixed either as 50-μl droplets under oil or in a 1.0-ml NUNC-well tray for coincubation with the zonae.

This use of fluorochrome labeling to distinguish sperm populations comes from studies on boar and rabbit spermatozoa that were conducted more than two decades ago. It was first used with human spermatozoa by Overstreet's group (e.g., Overstreet and Hembree, 1976; Blazak et al., 1982). Most recently it has been employed by Liu et al. (1988) working in Melbourne, Australia. In addition to FITC and TRITC, other fluorochromes have been used to label human spermatozoa, such as thiolyte (monobromobimane).

Fluorochrome Labeling of Living Human Spermatozoa

Fluorochrome labeling is fundamental to the CZBT, and it has various other applications when studying mixed sperm populations under competitive or heterospermic conditions. Although the technique is essentially the same for FITC or TRITC labeling, extra care must be taken when using TRITC to ensure no carryover of tiny crystals of TRITC. It is essentially the method described by Liu et al. (1988), which is itself a modification of that reported by Parrish and Foote (1985).

Reagents

FITC solution is prepared by dissolving 1.5 mg fluorescein isothiocyanate (ICN Biomedicals, Costa Mesa, CA, USA, Cat. No. 100276; or Sigma F7250) in 100 μl of 100 mM KOH and then diluting it, within 15 seconds, to 5.0 ml with PBS containing 55.5 mM (i.e., 1.0% w/v) glucose. This solution can be stored at 4°C in a foil-covered plastic tube for up to 7 days.

TRITC solution is prepared by dissolving 1.0 mg tetramethyl rhodamine isothiocyanate (Sigma, TRITC isomer R, T2016) in 100 μl 100 mM KOH and then diluting it, within 15 seconds, to 5.0 ml with PBS containing 55.5 mM (i.e., 1.0%

w/v) glucose. This solution is then centrifuged at 1000 *g* for 20 minutes and the supernatant stored at 4°C in a foil-covered plastic tube for up to 7 days.

N.B. The ability of these fluorochromes to label 100% of the spermatozoa varies considerably among manufacturers and different batches or lots. It may be necessary to try several lots to find one acceptable for this application.

Specimen
The FITC or TRITC labeling can be performed on spermatozoa still in seminal plasma. Liquefied semen should be obtained for labeling the spermatozoa as soon as liquefaction has been completed.

Method

1. Mix equal volumes of semen and FITC or TRITC solution and leave in the dark at ambient temperature for 15 minutes.

N.B. *All* steps involving the fluorochrome labeling of spermatozoa or the subsequent handling of labeled sperm populations *must* be performed in foil-covered tubes and preferably under subdued incandescent lighting.

2. Prepare a motile sperm population by centrifugation on discontinuous Percoll gradients (see Chapter 12).
3. After the post-Percoll washing step, adjust the sperm suspension to 100,000 motile spermatozoa/ml in the required culture medium.

Competitive Sperm-Zona Binding Test Procedure

This section describes the protocol for the CZBT. Fluorochrome-labeled sperm populations are prepared as described above. Whether only the control donor spermatozoa or both the patient and donor spermatozoa need to be labeled depends on the source of the zonae being used (see above).

Any suitable culture medium may be used for this assay (see Chapter 12), e.g., appropriately supplemented HTF, Ham's F-10, or STF.

1. Prepare the required number of zonae for the test, allowing three or four zonae per patient being evaluated. Details for handling salt-stored zonae are provided below (see Salt Storage of Human Zonae Pellucidae). This process may need to be started the day before a test is planned.
2. Into disposable plastic petri dishes (e.g., Falcon 3001) dispense 25-µl droplets of each patient's sperm preparation, one droplet per zona.
3. To each droplet of patient sperm suspension add 25 µl of the labeled donor sperm suspension.
4. Cover the droplets with warmed light paraffin oil (e.g., BDH B29434) and then add one zona pellucida to each drop.
5. Incubate the dishes under an atmosphere of 5% CO_2 in air for 4 hours at 37°C.

6. After incubation, each zona is removed and loosely adherent spermatozoa dislodged by transfer through three wash dishes containing fresh medium and using a finely drawn glass pipette.
7. Each zona is then transferred to a clean microscope slide and mounted under a 22 × 22 mm coverslip supported by four pillars of high vacuum silicone grease at its corners (see Reading the HEPT, below). These preparations are examined first under appropriate epifluorescence for the label(s) used for the spermatozoa (see Appendix III for suitable filter sets) and the number(s) of labeled spermatozoa bound to the zona counted. The total number of bound spermatozoa are then counted under visible light using phase-contrast optics.
8. The numbers of patient, donor, and (if present) previously contaminating spermatozoa are then calculated and the mean values per zona averaged over the different zonae used for the test.

Expression of Zona Binding Test Results

The ZBT results for a patient's spermatozoa are usually expressed relative to the binding seen for the control sperm population.

$$\frac{\text{Average number of patient sperm bound per ZP}}{\text{Average number of donor sperm bound per ZP}} \times 100$$

This value has been variously termed the HZA index (expressed as a percentage) or the sperm-ZP binding ratio (expressed as a decimal value). Because the same concept is applicable to either type of ZBT assay, perhaps this result should be more generically termed the zona binding index (ZBI) and is best presented as a percentage with integer precision.

Results from both the HZA and CZBT methods have been shown to correlate with results of success of in vitro fertilization (see Chapter 11). The results must be validated in a larger number of laboratories around the world, however, before they can be accepted as established sperm function tests. Regrettably, wide implementation of these tests is likely to be limited by the availability of nonviable and nonfertilized human oocytes.

Recovering Zonae Pellucidae from Human Ovarian Tissue

Some laboratories have access to "spare" unfertilized (and preferably uninseminated) oocytes from a clinical IVF program, but such material is often difficult to obtain. Furthermore, with the advent of embryo cryopreservation, most IVF programs now have few spare oocytes. Consequently, increasing numbers of workers resort to extracting zonae from ovarian tissue obtained either during gynecological surgery or postmortem. The following protocol can be used with either source of ovarian tissue.

Reagents

Phosphate-buffered saline (PBS) is prepared as described for the direct
   Immunobead test (see Chapter 5).
Collagenase solution is prepared as 100 µg/ml (e.g., Sigma C9407) in PBS.

Specimen

Human ovarian tissue, removed surgically or postmortem, is placed in sterile PBS
and transported to the laboratory, preferably at 4°C. Provided the specimen is kept
at 4°C, processing may be delayed up to 48 hours after removal or death.

Method

1. Cut the ovarian tissue into small pieces using a sharp scalpel so no piece is
   larger than 5 mm in any dimension. This step is performed in cold, sterile PBS.
2. Transfer to a small blender (e.g., Black & Decker "Handy Chopper") and blend
   for 20–30 seconds.
3. Filter the blended material through a 200-µm nylon mesh (e.g., N200 cloth
   from Henry Simon, Cheshire, UK), collecting the filtrate (Fig. 10-2).
4. Rinse the blender using 20 ml of fresh PBS, and use this rinse to wash the
   material remaining on the N200 filter. Again collect the filtrate.
5. Repeat step 4.
6. Transfer the material remaining on the N200 filter into a small volume of fresh
   PBS in a clean screw-top tube. Back-flush the N200 filter using PBS so no
   material remains on the filter. This material is put aside until step 11.
7. Pass the N200 filtrate through an 80-µm mesh nylon filter (e.g., Henry Simon
   N80 cloth). Discard the filtrate but collect all the material from the N80 filter by

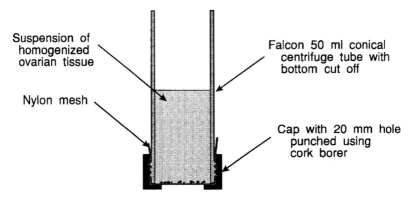

Figure 10-2 Construction of a filter system used for extraction of zonae pellucidae from
homogenized ovarian tissue.

    back-flushing with collagenase solution into a large petri dish (e.g., Falcon 3002). Do not allow the material to dry out on the filter.

8. Stir the N80 material in the collagenase solution at 37°C for about 2 hours.
9. Examine the incubated material under a dissecting microscope and transfer the zonae to a fresh dish of PBS.
10. Salt-store the zonae as described below.
11. After removing all the zonae, pour the collagenase solution into the tube containing the N200 material saved from step 6 and incubate overnight at 37°C.
12. Repeat steps 3–9 (twice if there is residual solid material). Any additional zonae are salt-stored as described below.

Salt Storage of Human Zonae Pellucidae

Zonae pellucidae can be stored until required using either a crude cryopreservation method, which does not preserve the oocyte (Overstreet and Hembree, 1976; Overstreet et al., 1980), or more simply in a high-concentration salt solution (Yanagimachi et al., 1979), which kills the oocyte. Both methods preserve the functional capacity of the zona pellucida to bind spermatozoa. The method described here is a variation of the salt storage approach that has given good results with both IVF "spare eggs" and eggs recovered from ovarian tissue.

Reagents

Zona preservative is an aqueous solution of 20 mM Tris, 0.5% (w/v) 200- to 275-kD dextran, and 2 M ammonium sulfate. It is prepared by dissolving 2.425 g Tris, 5.0 g dextran (e.g., BDH 38014), and 264.26 g $(NH_4)_2SO_4$ in reagent water to a total volume of 1 liter. Adjust the pH to 7.2–7.6 with 1 N HCl.

Culture medium is whatever medium is to be used for the sperm–zona binding test (e.g., HTF) (see Chapter 12).

Specimen

Zonae pellucidae, free of all cumulus oophorus and corona radiata cells, are used. For ethical reasons, great care should be taken to ensure that normally fertilized (i.e., two pronuclei stage) zygotes are not used.

Method

Preservation

1. The zona preservative solution is prepared as 0.5-ml aliquots in small, round-bottom, capped tubes (e.g., Falcon 2003).
2. One zona pellucida is transferred in minimal volume to each tube.
3. Tightly capped tubes are stored at 4°C until required.

Preparation for Use

1. On the day before the zonae are required for a test, using a Pasteur pipette aspirate from the bottom of the storage tube and transfer almost all the salt storage solution into a small petri dish (e.g., Falcon 3001).
2. Examine under a dissecting microscope to find the zona pellucida, and transfer it to a dish of culture medium.
3. If the zona has been found, proceed to step 5; if not, transfer a small volume of the salt solution back into the storage tube and pipette up and down to dislodge the zona pellucida.
4. Repeat steps 1 and 2.
5. Repeat steps 1–4, as necessary, to obtain the required number of zonae for the test.
6. Transfer all the preserved zonae to be used for the test into a single dish of fresh medium. Allow to stand at ambient temperature for 20 minutes.
7. Wash the zonae by transfer through three dishes of fresh medium, 20 minutes per dish.
8. After transfer into the final (fifth) wash dish, place the dish in the refrigerator at 4°C overnight.
9. The following morning (i.e., the day of the test), transfer the zonae into a final wash dish of fresh culture medium. Keep at ambient temperature until required.

ZONA-FREE HAMSTER EGG PENETRATION TEST

Overview

Since its original description by Yanagimachi and colleagues in 1976, the HEPT has been the subject of a plethora of publications in the scientific and medical literature (review to 1984: Yanagimachi, 1984). Although many important studies on human sperm function have used the HEPT, clinically it remains an expensive test subject to both biological and methodological variability. At least partially because many laboratories continue to use procedures that can result in both false-negative and false-positive results, debate continues as to the reliability, accuracy, and physiological relevance of the HEPT (review: Muller et al., 1990; also see Chapter 11).

Because spermatozoa must be acrosome-reacted to penetrate zona-free hamster oocytes, successful capacitation can be presumed. The HEPT therefore evaluates sperm longevity, capacitation, and a spontaneous acrosome reaction. Applications of the HEPT can be categorized into six principal areas.

1. Attempts to describe populations of men classified as "infertile" or "fertile" using previous, often poorly defined and etiologically confused clinical measures such as oligozoospermia, i.e., infertility diagnosis
2. Attempts to use HEPT results to predict the likelihood of a given man achieving a spontaneous pregnancy in vivo, i.e., in vivo fertility prognosis or fecundity determination

3. Attempts to use HEPT results to predict the likelihood of a given man success-fully fertilizing human oocytes in vitro, i.e., in vitro fertilizing ability prognosis
4. Attempts to assess the cryosurvival of spermatozoa in terms of their retention of fertilizing capacity, including possible applications in determining relative donor fecundity
5. Evaluations of experimental treatments aimed at inhibiting or improving the fer-tilizing potential of particular sperm populations, e.g., assessment of potential contraceptive agents or treatment regimens, attempts at pharmacological sperm stimulation, and possible protocols to synchronize capacitation or induce the acrosome reaction
6. Attempts to improve the sensitivity and specificity of the HEPT itself or simplify test procedures

Sperm Preparation Protocols

Variations in sperm preparation and preincubation (capacitation) methods can pro-duce significant alterations in HEPT outcome. A brief overview of some pertinent publications in this area is provided below.

First, spermatozoa must be prepared from liquefied semen rapidly because pro-longed exposure to seminal plasma can drastically impair HEPT results (Rogers et al., 1983). Furthermore, a highly efficient method must be used because even mini-mal contamination with seminal plasma causes a marked reduction in HEPT pene-tration (Kanwar et al., 1979).

Sperm populations prepared by selective methods such as "swim-up" migration or Percoll gradient centrifugation usually produce high HEPT penetration rates, whereas sperm preparation techniques that involve the centrifugal pelleting of unse-lected spermatozoa (e.g., swim-up from a washed pellet) may significantly impair the functional potential of the "good" spermatozoa subsequently selected by migra-tion due to peroxidation of membrane lipids by reactive oxygen (review: Mortimer, 1991). Although such damage may not greatly diminish the functional competence of a normal man's spermatozoa, those from borderline or male factor cases may be rendered incapable of fertilization (see Chapter 12 for detailed methods).

The optimum capacitation incubation time varies considerably among men. Some men show best HEPT success after a short preincubation period, whereas others show optimum penetration after a long period (Perreault and Rogers, 1982). This concept of fast and slow capacitators is important if a laboratory uses only one (sup-posedly standardized) preincubation period for all tests.

Protein source can be a major cause of variation among laboratories performing the HEPT. Differences have been demonstrated between different suppliers of crys-talline HSA and between different patients' sera (Bronson and Rogers, 1988). Also, the serum used to supplement culture media for sperm preincubation can influence the results of the HEPT, dependent on whether it was obtained during the luteal, fol-licular, or preovulatory phase of the cycle, with the luteal phase producing the high-est penetration rates (Margalioth et al., 1988). This effect may be attributable to progesterone content and can also be achieved using follicular fluid (Yee and Cum-mings, 1988).

Several improved sperm incubation methods have been developed in attempts to reduce the interindividual variability of optimum capacitation conditions (see below). In addition, caffeine has been reported to stimulate the HEPT penetration capacity of sperm populations, especially cryopreserved spermatozoa with reduced motility (Aitken et al., 1983a).

Current Types of HEPT Assay Protocols

At the most basic level, HEPT protocols in current use may be considered to fall into three groups:

I. Those that rely on spontaneous acrosome reactions and hence spontaneous capacitation
II. Those in which the acrosome reaction is induced artificially in more-or-less capacitated sperm populations
III. Those that rely on sperm membrane modification and acrosome reaction induction by a combination of cold-shock and fusogenic substances.

In the first two groups, sperm populations free of seminal plasma are prepared by various means (see Chapter 12) and incubated in one of several suitable culture media in the presence of a survival- and capacitation-supporting macromolecule such as albumin (supplied either as pure human serum albumin or as a constituent of serum or follicular fluid). The preincubated sperm population is then tested directly, assessing spontaneously occurring acrosome reactions (type I protocols), or after treatment with an acrosome reaction-inducing substance, or ARIS (type II protocols).

Because not only different men but also sperm populations prepared from different ejaculates are heterogeneous in their temporal requirements for achieving the capacitated state, as well as in their susceptibility to undergoing spontaneous acrosome loss, type I HEPT protocols often produce different results depending on the duration of the preincubation period. For this reason, many workers have struggled to develop alternative test protocols that eliminate this inter- and intraindividual variability. These efforts have given rise to the wide range of type II protocols now in existence, as well as the type III protocols.

With type II protocols, preincubated, and therefore presumed capacitated, sperm populations are exposed to known or putative ARIS treatments. Alternatively, the culture medium is modified in some way to try to synchronize capacitation (e.g., by stimulation) or allow variable spontaneous capacitation to proceed while inhibiting the occurrence of acrosome reactions. Probably the commonest approach has been to trigger the acrosome reaction using calcium ionophore (see below), although hypertonic treatment (Aitken et al., 1983b) and calcium deprivation (Mortimer et al., 1986) have also been reported.

A23187 has been the most commonly used calcium ionophore in HEPT protocols (e.g., Aitken et al., 1984). These protocols have been found to be much better than type I protocols for identifying men with impaired sperm function and for predicting the occurrence of human fertilization in vitro or in vivo conception in infertility clinic patients (Aitken et al., 1983b, 1987, 1991). Furthermore, the quantity of ionophore used has been decreasing, thereby reducing the problem of treatment-induced loss of motility and even sperm death. The latest protocols use only 2.5 μM or less in conjunction with DMSO as a carrier molecule, compared to 50 μM solutions of the Ca,Mg salt of A23187 (see Acrosome Reaction Induction Protocols, above).

Although calcium deprivation in isolation usually causes irreversible loss of motility, substitution of calcium by the divalent strontium cation during the capacitation preincubation induces significant improvements (on average, fourfold) in human sperm fertilizing ability when assessed using the HEPT after washing into calcium-containing medium, an effect that was magnified when EGTA was also added during the capacitation preincubation to chelate any residual free calcium ions (average tenfold penetration rates) (Mortimer et al., 1986). However, although it was originally suggested that this stimulatory effect might be mediated via a synchronization of capacitation so a larger cohort of spermatozoa underwent the acrosome reaction together upon exposure to extracellular calcium, studies on the acrosomal status of sperm populations incubated in calcium- and strontium-EGTA-based media revealed this suggestion to be incorrect (Mortimer et al., 1988). Consequently, stimulation of human sperm fertilizing ability in the HEPT using this technique must be based on a more subtle, as yet unidentified, effect.

Other ARIS compounds employed in the HEPT include human follicular fluid (Yee and Cummings, 1988; McClure et al., 1990), which although it does reduce the prevalence of false-negative results in the HEPT remains a biological material prone to interbatch variability. However, because the acrosome reaction-inducing ability of follicular fluid may well be attributable to its progesterone content (Osman et al., 1989) and sera with high progesterone concentrations also induce higher HEPT penetration rates (Margalioth et al., 1988), the incorporation of this steroid into a defined sperm preincubation medium may achieve the same purpose.

Type III protocols are based on the refrigeration of human spermatozoa in a zwitterion-buffered medium containing egg yolk (Bolanos et al., 1983). Storage in TEST-yolk buffer at 4°C allows spermatozoa to be held (e.g., during transportation) for up to 48 hours prior to testing in the HEPT. This treatment also results in higher HEPT penetration rates (Johnson et al., 1984) as a result of rather drastic effects on the spermatozoa.

Because the intracellular free calcium ion concentration ($[Ca^{2+}]_i$) is substantially lower than the extracellular concentration, Ca^{2+} ions are continually entering the sperm cell and being pumped back out by a Ca^{2+}-dependent membrane ATPase or calcium pump. When the temperature is reduced from physiological levels to 4°C, this enzymatic pump is slowed dramatically, resulting in an intracellular accumulation of Ca^{2+} ions. Upon restoration of the temperature to 37°C, this elevated $[Ca^{2+}]_i$ triggers acrosome reactions in what are then highly susceptible spermatozoa. In addition, as the temperature falls below about 15°–18°C, irreversible phase changes occur in the sperm membrane phospholipids, creating highly fusogenic domains. Combined with the egg yolk phospholipids that intercalate into the sperm membranes, after warming the spermatozoa are obviously in a highly labile state.

Type III protocols apparently provide clinically relevant results (Johnson et al., 1990), but they remain of limited interest outside North America.

Recommended Sperm Preparation Protocol

Sperm preparation for the HEPT falls into two basic steps: (1) preparation of a selected motile sperm population free of seminal plasma, e.g., direct swim-up from semen or discontinuous Percoll gradient methods (see Chapter 12); and (2) the incubation and treatment of this sperm population under conditions that promote capacitation and the acrosome reaction. Although there are numerous alternative methods for the latter process, the one provided here is for the ionophore-enhanced method proposed as an international standard (World Health Organization, 1992). Several patients may be tested in an assay run, along with the obligatory known fertile control donor.

Reagents

Culture medium is any suitable medium, such as HTF, modified Tyrode's, or BWW (see Chapter 12).

A23187 stock is a 5 mM solution in DMSO. It is stored frozen at $-20°C$ in 5- or 10-μl aliquots.

Specimen

Sperm suspension is a selected motile sperm population at 10×10^6 motile cells/ml in culture medium.

Method

1. Two (preferably 3) days before the test, prepare a "ready-to-use" solution of A23187 by diluting 5 μl of stock A23187 in 5.0 ml of sterile culture medium (i.e., 5 μM A23187). This solution is kept at 4°C until use.
2. On the day of the test, the sperm suspension is diluted $1 + 1$ with the ionophore solution (i.e., 5×10^6 motile spermatozoa/ml in 2.5 μM A23187).

N.B. An additional aliquot of the sperm suspension may be treated at 1.25 μM A23187, as some men's spermatozoa respond better to a lower ionophore concentration.

3. Transfer aliquots of ≤ 2.0 ml of the sperm suspension with ionophore into sterile tubes (e.g., Falcon 2096 or 2097), gas with 5% CO_2 in air, and cap tightly.
4. Incubate at 37°C for 3 hours.
5. After incubation, pool up to three tubes from the same sperm suspension and make up to a final volume of 10.1 ml with fresh medium.
6. Put 100 μl of each sperm suspension to one side and centrifuge the remaining 10 ml at 600 g for 6 minutes.
7. While the sample is spinning, determine the concentration and motility of the sperm suspension in the 100-μl aliquot. Calculate the total number of motile

spermatozoa contained in the 10 ml being centrifuged and hence the final resuspension volume to obtain 5×10^6 motile spermatozoa/ml after washing.
8. Discard the supernatant, and resuspend the sperm pellet into the appropriate total volume, as calculated in step 7, using fresh culture medium. This sperm suspension is then used to prepare the gamete coincubation dishes (see below).

Preparation of Fresh Zona-Free Hamster Eggs

Reagents

Pregnant mare's serum gonadotropin (PMSG) is purchased commercially (e.g., Folligon: Intervet, Cambridge, UK).

Human chorionic gonadotropin (hCG) is purchased commercially (e.g., Sigma CG-2).

Saline is either isotonic saline (0.9% w/v NaCl in tissue culture grade water) or, alternatively, additional culture medium.

Culture medium is any suitable medium for use in the HEPT (e.g., HTF, BWW, or modified Tyrode's) (see Chapter 12).

Hyaluronidase solution is 0.1% (w/v) hyaluronidase (type I-S from bovine testes, Sigma H3506) in culture medium. Preweighed 5-mg aliquots of the hyaluronidase may be stored at $-20°C$ in small plastic screw-top vials in a desiccated jar until required. Add 5 ml of medium, mix gently by inversion, and then warm to 37°C for use.

Trypsin solution is 0.1% (w/v) trypsin (type I from bovine pancreas, Sigma T8003, 10,000 BAEE units/mg) in culture medium. Preweighed 5-mg aliquots of the trypsin may be prepared, stored, and used as described for the hyaluronidase solution (above).

Specimen

Mature female golden hamsters are either bred locally or purchased commercially. Although many workers originally started the superovulation injections on day 1 of the estrus cycle, it is now common practice to pay little or no attention to the hamsters' estrus cycle before giving the first injection. It apparently has little influence on the quality or quantity of the eggs obtained and certainly reduces by 75% the number of female hamsters available on any particular day that superovulation is commenced.

Method

1. Hamsters are induced to superovulate by intraperitoneal injections of 40 IU PMSG and 30 IU hCG at 70 and 16 hours before killing, respectively.
2. Hamsters are killed by CO_2 asphyxiation and cervical dislocation. Ether narcotization is not recommended because of the explosion risk associated with its use.

3. The first dissection involves a midline incision from the sternum to the pubic region, with lateral extensions on each side at the anterior end. The fat body containing the ovary, oviduct, and proximal uterine horn is located on each side, excised, and placed in warm saline in a small petri dish (e.g., Falcon 3001). Repeat for each hamster.

4. The second dissection involves first carefully cutting the uterotubal junction and then cutting the oviduct free from the surface of the ovary. The isolated oviducts are transferred into fresh warm saline in another small petri dish. Use small, curved iris scissors and blunt-ended watchmaker's forceps. Repeat for each excised oviduct.

5. Each isolated oviduct is then examined in fresh culture medium under a dissecting microscope. The distended ampullary region is visualized and torn open to release the cumulus masses. Use two pairs of fine, sharp-pointed watchmaker's forceps. Repeat for each isolated oviduct.

N.B. It is strongly recommended that mouth-controlled pipettes be avoided (see Chapter 15), although some authorities still accept the use of mouth control for fine control of extremely small volume transfers (e.g., when handling eggs)—provided a 0.22-μm filter is placed in the line and that there is no risk of aerosol formation or aspiration of a volume large enough to contaminate the filter directly.

6. Transfer the cumulus masses into a small petri dish containing 5 ml of warm hyaluronidase solution (dish should be labeled HYAL). Use either a Pasteur pipette or a pair of watchmaker's forceps for the large pieces of cumulus followed by a pipette for the small cumulus fragments.

7. Incubate on a warming plate at about 35°–37°C until the cumulus masses have dispersed (usually < 20 minutes). Cover with a small box to protect the eggs from light during incubation.

8. Under a dissecting microscope, and using a finely drawn glass pipette, transfer the isolated zona-intact eggs from the hyaluronidase dish into another small dish labeled WASH H1, containing fresh medium.

9. Transfer the zona-intact eggs into a second small dish of fresh medium (WASH H2).

10. Transfer the zona-intact eggs in small groups (25–50 eggs per group) into a small dish containing the trypsin solution (label the dish TRYP). Lay the eggs out in rows and examine under higher power to observe dissolution of the zonae pellucidae. Many eggs acquire a D-shape just before the zona is lost. As soon as the zona has dissolved, remove the eggs immediately and transfer into another small dish (labeled WASH T1) containing fresh medium. It is advisable to have the aspirating pipette prefilled with fresh medium to dilute the trypsin solution as quickly as possible.

11. Transfer the zona-free eggs into a second dish of fresh medium (WASH T2).

12. Repeat steps 10 and 11 until all the eggs recovered from the dispersed cumulus masses have been trypsinized.

13. Transfer all the zona-free eggs into a third dish of fresh culture medium

(WASH T3). These eggs are then ready for setting up the gamete coincubations (see below).

Preparation of Cryopreserved Zona-Free Hamster Eggs

Cryopreserved, zona-intact hamster eggs are available commercially (Cryotech Hamster Ova: Charles River Professional Services, Wilmington, MA, USA) or can be prepared in the laboratory as described for fresh hamster eggs (see above) and cryopreserved after the second posthyaluronidase wash (see Cryopreservation of Zona-Intact Hamster Eggs, below).

Reagents

Culture medium and *trypsin solution* are required as per the method for fresh hamster eggs (see above).

Method

1. Quickly transfer the required number of canes holding the straws of frozen hamster eggs from the liquid nitrogen storage tank to a small wide-neck dewar full of liquid nitrogen.
2. Remove the required number of straws containing frozen hamster eggs from the canes and lay them horizontally on a rack at ambient temperature. Leave to stand for 2 minutes.

N.B. The region of the straw where the eggs are located should not be touched, nor should it come into direct contact with anything (Fig. 10-3).

3. After 2 minutes, slip off the handle portion of the straw (if used) and lightly wipe off the moisture from the outside of the straw. Grasp the straw at the end opposite the label and mix the contents by vigorously "snapping" the straw three or four times (rather like resetting a mercury clinical thermometer) to create a single column of fluid in the straw with one air bubble at the end. This step mixes the column of cryoprotectant containing the oocytes with the large upper column of sucrose-containing diluent that acts as an osmotic buffer during dilution of the cryoprotectant from the oocytes.
4. Place the straws, label end down, in a test tube in a 37°C waterbath for 3 minutes. Make sure the straws are completely submerged.
5. Transfer the straws, label end up, in a test tube containing water at ambient temperature for 2 minutes.
6. Remove the straws from the water and gently dry the outside of the straws. Using scissors, remove the lower heat seal (end opposite the label) by cutting through the middle of the air bubble. Remove the upper heat seal by cutting through the middle of the cotton plug.
7. Using a plastic rod (red plastic stylets are provided with Cryotech straws), push

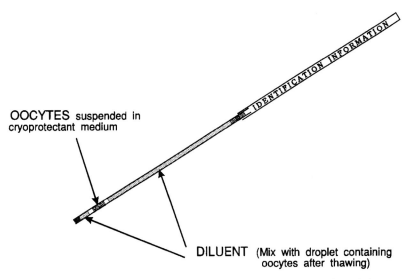

OOCYTES suspended in
cryoprotectant medium

DILUENT (Mix with droplet containing
oocytes after thawing)

Figure 10-3 Cryotech straw containing frozen hamster oocytes. (Adapted from promotional material supplied by Charles River Professional Services, Wilmington, MA, USA.)

the cotton plug to the very bottom end of the straw, expelling its contents into a sterile, small petri dish (e.g., Falcon 3001), labeled CRYO.

8. Using a finely drawn pipette, transfer the eggs into another small dish containing fresh culture medium (labeled WASH C1) and allow them to equilibrate for 10 minutes at ambient temperature.

9. Transfer the eggs into another dish of fresh medium (labeled WASH C2) and incubate at 37°C for 15 minutes under an atmosphere of 5% CO_2 in air.

10. The eggs are now ready for zona dissolution by trypsin as per steps 10–13 described for fresh hamster eggs (see above). After the final wash, the zona-free eggs are ready for setting up the gamete coincubations (see below).

Gamete Coincubation Conditions

Workers use a variety of gamete coincubation conditions for the HEPT, e.g., different volumes of sperm suspension and different concentrations of motile spermatozoa. This method, described below, requires a minimum quantity of spermatozoa and should therefore be applicable to as wide a range of patients as possible.

Reagents

Paraffin oil is a light paraffin oil such as that obtained from BDH Chemicals (B29434). Although the paraffin oil should be equilibrated with culture medium if it is to be used for long-term incubations, this step has not been found necessary for the short-duration incubations used in the HEPT.

Specimens

Sperm suspensions and *zona-free hamster eggs* are prepared as described above.

Method

1. Mark off large petri dishes (e.g., Falcon 3002) into quarters or thirds using a marker pen on the *outside* of the bottom of the dish. Prepare sufficient dishes so that each sperm suspension has sufficient sperm droplets for there to be no more than 15 zona-free eggs per drop. Mark each dish with the patient or donor reference number, and number the section of dish to contain each sperm drop.
2. Dispense the required number of 20-μl droplets of each sperm suspension into the appropriately labeled small petri dishes.
3. Carefully pour warm paraffin oil over the sperm suspension droplets, taking care not to dislodge them. The droplets flatten slightly.
4. Transfer 10–15 zona-free eggs into each sperm droplet using minimal volumes of medium. Take great care not to transfer any spermatozoa between droplets belonging to different men.
5. Cover the dishes and incubate them under an atmosphere of 5% CO_2 in air for 3 hours at 37°C.

Reading the HEPT

After the 3-hour gamete contact coincubation, the degree of sperm penetration into the zona-free hamster eggs is assessed by examining each egg under a compound microscope. Although some workers fix and stain the eggs before scoring, it greatly increases the time required to complete the assay and does not improve the accuracy or ease of scoring. The following protocol is based on the immediate examination of the eggs using phase-contrast microscopy.

Reagents

Culture medium is required for washing the eggs. It should be the same medium as was used for the gamete coincubation.

Silicone grease is used to support the coverslip when making the "squash mounts" of the eggs. Various workers have described Vaseline-paraffin wax mixtures for this mountant, but commercially available high vacuum silicone grease has been found ideal.

Method

1. Remove the gamete coincubation dishes from the incubator, taking great care not to jog them and dislodge a sperm droplet from the bottom of the dish.
2. Under a dissecting microscope and using a finely drawn glass pipette, transfer the zona-free eggs from one sperm droplet into a small petri dish containing

fresh medium. The dish should be labeled with the patient or donor reference number.

3. By carefully drawing the eggs into the pipette and expelling them (being *very* careful not to create bubbles), dislodge loosely adherent spermatozoa from the surface of the eggs.

4. Prepare a clean microscope slide with four small spots of silicone grease in the form of a square, with sides about 15 mm, equidistant about the center of the slide. The optimal size of these grease spots must be learned by trial and error. Transfer the eggs from the wash dish onto the center of the slide in a suitable volume of medium (again learned by experience) and place a No. 1½ coverslip onto the four supporting pillars of silicone grease.

N.B.   Unfortunately, experience has shown that some brands of coverslips (not necessarily the most expensive) are more planar than others. High planarity is essential for uniform squashing of the eggs throughout the preparation.

5. Using two toothpicks, *very* carefully push down on the coverslip over the supporting grease pillars to squash the eggs. Do not allow the meniscus of the medium to flow across the eggs, as it would destroy them. Again, this step must be perfected through experience.

6. Locate each egg in turn under the microscope and examine it at 400× to 500× using phase-contrast optics, looking for the presence of swollen sperm heads or male pronuclei within the ooplasm. If desired, numbers of spermatozoa bound to the oolemma can also be estimated or even counted.

7. Repeat steps 2–6 until all the eggs have been scored. If multiple drops were prepared for each man being tested, score one drop from each sample and then repeat the sequence until all the drops have been examined. This method minimizes the variations in incubation period among men.

Results

Results of the HEPT have been expressed several ways by various authors. All are based on the presence of swollen sperm heads, male pronuclei, or both (Fig. 10-4). A swollen sperm head is a clear space associated with a sperm tail either directly, or close by. A male pronucleus is slightly larger and contains small dark nucleoli; however, it too must be associated with a sperm tail, usually located nearby, to eliminate possible confusion with a fragmented female pronucleus. As a precaution, there must be a sperm tail present for each and every swollen sperm head or male pronucleus counted. The following definitions are reasonably standard and accepted.

Penetration rate is the percentage of eggs that contain one or more swollen sperm heads or male pronuclei (or both). In consideration of the number of eggs usually scored per test (25–50), this result should be expressed only as an integer value.

Polyspermy rate is the average number of penetrated spermatozoa (i.e., swollen sperm heads plus male pronuclei) per penetrated egg. It is usually expressed to one or two decimal places with values beginning at 1.0.

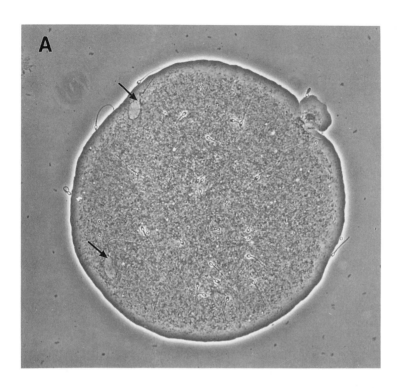

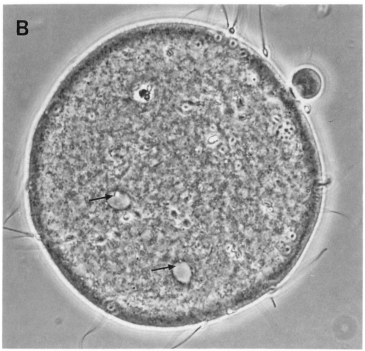

Figure 10-4 Micrographs of fresh (A) and cryopreserved (B) hamster oocytes penetrated by human spermatozoa. *Arrows* denote swollen sperm heads; note the associated sperm tails.

Table 10–1   Rational approach to presenting results of the
zona-free hamster egg penetration test

HEPT Result	Penetration Rate (% Oocytes Penetrated)
Negative	No penetration (i.e., 0%)
Positive	Any penetration (i.e., $\geq 1\%$)
Abnormal	Below some predetermined cutoff, including 0%
Low	Below some predetermined cutoff, excluding 0%
Normal	Above some predetermined cutoff

Penetration index is the average number of penetrated spermatozoa per egg scored, including those showing no penetration. Therefore, unlike the polyspermy rate, it can have a value of < 1.0.

Penetration capacity has been used to facilitate interpretation of simultaneous (e.g., treatment-induced) increases in penetration and polyspermy rates. It is calculated as the product of the penetration rate and the polyspermy rate and is expressed as an integer value; for example, 50% penetration with 1.50 average polyspermy would give a penetration capacity of 75.

To date there has been little interest in relative penetration characteristics directly comparing a patient to a donor (c.f., Expression of Zona Binding Test Results, above). Although heterospermic HEPT methods have been described (e.g., Blazak et al., 1982), no major prospective clinical studies have been reported. The HEPT results are variously described as normal or abnormal, or negative or positive. For general purposes the terminological conventions described in Table 10-1 should be used.

Cryopreservation of Zona-Intact Hamster Eggs

The 3-day period required for hamster superovulation is often a significant inconvenience when scheduling the HEPT for both diagnostic and research purposes. Consequently, there has been considerable interest in using cryopreserved oocytes to the extent that they are available commercially (Cryotech: Charles River Laboratories, Wilmington, MA, USA). Although cryopreserved hamster oocytes are generally considered to show reduced levels of penetration by human sperm populations compared to freshly prepared oocytes, they are acceptable substitutes if cryopreserved appropriately (Hyatt Sachs et al. 1989; Jouannet and Rodrigues, 1990; Leibo et al., 1990). Overall, propanediol seems to be a better cryoprotectant for this application than DMSO.

Principle
The methods provided below are based on the work of Jouannet and Rodrigues (1990). The slow freezing technique was modified after Quinn et al. (1982), and the rapid method was based on the work of Renard et al. (1984). A single step method described by Leibo et al. (1990) and used to prepare the Cryotech commercially available frozen hamster eggs is also provided.

Morphologically abnormal oocytes are discarded before cryopreservation.

Reagents

Phosphate-buffered saline (PBS) is prepared as described for the direct Immunobead test (see Chapter 5).
PBS+BSA is a 1.5% (w/v) solution of Cohn fraction V bovine serum albumin in
   PBS.
PBS+FCS is a 20% (v/v) solution of fetal calf serum in PBS pH 7.4 and 280
   mOsm.
Cryoprotectant solutions (see Methods sections, below) comprise volumetric solutions of propanediol (PROH) in PBS+FCS. Some solutions are supplemented
   with sucrose to increase the osmolarity.
Post-thaw washing solutions (see Methods sections, below) are variants of the culture medium to be used for the HEPT, supplemented with Cohn fraction V human
   serum albumin (HSA) and sucrose.
Hyaluronidase is used to dissociate the cumulus masses (see Preparation of Fresh
   Zona-Free Hamster Eggs, above). It is prepared as a 0.1% (w/v) solution in PBS
   and used at 37°C.

Rapid Freezing Method

1. After hyaluronidase treatment to dissociate the cumulus masses, the zona-intact
   oocytes are transferred to PBS+FCS.
2. Transfer the eggs to a small petri dish (e.g., Falcon 3001) containing 1.5 M
   PROH in PBS at ambient temperature. Leave for 15 minutes.
3. Transfer to another dish containing 2.2 M PROH in PBS supplemented with 0.5
   M sucrose. Leave for 5 minutes at ambient temperature.
4. Package the eggs in groups of 30 in 0.25-ml straws (BICEF, L'Aigle, France).
5. Load the straws into a programable freezing machine and cool according to the
   following protocol.
   Segment 1: −12°C/minute from ambient temperature to −30°C.
   Segment 2: Hold at −30°C for 30 minutes.
   Segment 3: −35°C/minute to −150°C.
   Segment 4: Plunge into liquid nitrogen (−196°C).

Thawing Procedure

6. Transfer the straw(s) from liquid nitrogen to a 37°C waterbath for 2 minutes.
7. Remove the eggs from the straw(s) into a large petri dish (e.g., Falcon 3002)
   containing a large drop (1 ml) of medium with 0.8% HSA and 0.5 M sucrose.
8. Incubate at 37°C for 5 minutes.
9. Slowly add 10 ml medium supplemented with 0.8% HSA and 0.05 M sucrose
   over 5 minutes at 37°C.
10. Wash the eggs by transfer through three changes of medium + 0.8% HSA at
    37°C.
11. Incubate under an atmosphere of 5% CO_2 in air at 37°C for 60 minutes.

12. The eggs are then treated with trypsin to remove their zonae pellucidae (see Preparation of Fresh Zona-Free Hamster Eggs, above).

Slow Freezing Method

1. After hyaluronidase treatment to dissociate the cumulus masses, the zona-intact oocytes are transferred to a small petri dish (e.g., Falcon 3001) containing PBS+BSA.
2. Transfer the eggs to another dish containing 2 M PROH in PBS. Leave for 5 minutes at ambient temperature.
3. Package the eggs in groups of 30 in 0.25-ml straws.
4. Load the straws into a programable freezing machine and cool according to the following protocol:
   Segment 1: $-2°C$/min from ambient temperature to $7°C$.
   Segment 2: Hold at $7°C$. Induce seeding (2 seconds) and hold for another 2 minutes.
   Segment 3: $-3°C$/min to $-40°C$.
   Segment 4: $-35°C$/min to $-150°C$.
   Segment 5: Plunge into liquid nitrogen ($-196°C$).

Thawing Procedure

5. Transfer the straw(s) from liquid nitrogen to a $37°C$ waterbath for 2 minutes.
6. Remove the eggs from the straw(s) into a large petri dish containing a large drop (1 ml) of medium with 0.8% HSA and 0.5 M sucrose.
7. Incubate at $37°C$ for 5 minutes.
8. Wash the eggs by transfer through three changes of medium + 0.8% HSA at $37°C$.
9. Incubate under an atmosphere of 5% CO_2 in air at $37°C$ for 60 minutes.
10. The eggs are then treated with trypsin to remove their zonae pellucidae (see Preparation of Fresh Zona-Free Hamster Eggs, above).

Leibo's Single-Step Freezing Method

The single-step freezing method, described by Leibo et al. (1990), is used to prepare the commercially available Cryotech hamster eggs (see Preparation of Cryopreserved Zona-Free Hamster Eggs, above). These authors emphasized the importance of controlling the age of the oocytes and their exposure to cryoprotectant before freezing: Female hamsters are killed 15 hours post-hCG, and oocyte freezing commences a standard 60 minutes later. A maximum 5-minute exposure to hyaluronidase (1 mg/ml) is used to disperse the cumulus masses, and the entire exposure of oocytes to propanediol ($\equiv$ propylene glycol) at $20°C$ is kept constant at 20 minutes. The post-thaw $37°C$ exposure of oocytes to sucrose is also kept constant at 3 minutes.

1. Zona-intact oocytes recovered from dispersed cumulus masses are rinsed in M2 medium containing BSA 3 mg/ml. *M2 medium* (Quinn et al., 1982) comprises 94.7 mM NaCl, 4.78 mM KCl, 1.19 mM $MgSO_4 \cdot 7H_2O$, 1.19 mM KH_2PO_4, 1.71

mM CaCl$_2$·2H$_2$O, 4.0 mM NaHCO$_3$, 21.0 mM Hepes, 23.3 mM Na lactate, 0.33 mM Na pyruvate, 5.56 mM glucose, and 0.001% (w/v) phenol red.

2. Oocytes are then transferred into M2 medium containing 1.5 M propanediol at ambient temperature for 3–5 minutes.

3. Straws (0.25 ml capacity) are prepared by first aspirating a 66-mm column of M2 medium containing 1.08 M sucrose and 3.0% BSA followed by a 10-mm column of air, a 10-mm column of medium containing propanediol, and a 5-mm column of air.

4. Once the oocytes have reached osmotic equilibrium in the propanediol solution, groups of 15–17 are transferred directly into the 10-mm column of propanediol solution in the straw using a finely drawn glass pipette.

5. Another 10-mm column of propanediol solution is then aspirated into the straw, causing the sucrose solution column to seal the plug at the upper end of the straw.

6. The lower (unplugged) open end of the straw is then heat-sealed.

7. Straws are then transferred directly to −7°C in an alcohol freezing bath (model BC802: FTS Systems Inc., Stone Ridge, NY, USA).

8. Seeding is induced manually at −7°C, and the straws held there for 20 minutes.

9. The straws are then cooled at 0.5°C/minute to below −75°C.

10. At between −75°C and −80°C the straws are transferred directly from the alcohol bath and plunged into liquid nitrogen.

11. For thawing, see Preparation of Cryopreserved Zona-Free Hamster Eggs, above.

Quality Control

The cryopreservation methods described above are reported to give 80–86% cryosurvival and produce highly comparable penetration and polyspermy rates in diagnostic HEPT assays (Jouannet and Rodrigues, 1990). The single-step method (Leibo et al., 1990) is reported to give survival rates of 90–95% and not to affect the clinical results of HEPT assays.

COMPREHENSIVE SPERM FUNCTION TESTING PROTOCOL

Because of the complex series of processes that spermatozoa must accomplish to reach the site of fertilization, successfully penetrate the oocyte–cumulus complex, and achieve syngamy, it is not surprising that the results of single sperm function tests performed in isolation are insensitive and nonspecific in their identification of fertile and infertile/sterile men. However, the idea that there must be one ultimate test of sperm function has still not yet been eradicated. Nevertheless, as comprehensive testing of sperm functional ability in couples undergoing infertility investigations becomes more common, more specific causes of male factor infertility are being defined, and our definition of idiopathic infertility may soon require drastic modification.

Evaluation of a proposed sperm function test by comparison with another, already accepted procedure is inappropriate, although many tests of sperm function do, on a population basis, correlate with each other because they all evaluate various aspects of the same physiological system. Any test of sperm function must be validated by consideration of the following criteria.

1. It must measure a physiologically relevant process.
2. The procedure must be practical and amenable to *routine* clinical use.
3. It must be correlated with an appropriate biological endpoint (e.g., in vivo fertility or IVF success). Another test is not an endpoint of interest.

Consequently, comprehensive sperm function testing protocols should be devised that are constructed to assess as many of the component processes leading to conception as possible. Although some aspects may be covered by more than one test system, such redundancy would not be problematical, as it may allow more reliable conclusions to be reached—or perhaps the future establishment of one test system as preferable to another.

Certainly there is a case for a comprehensive assessment protocol incorporating the following tests.

1. Sperm movement characteristics in semen in relation to sperm–mucus interaction. It may be achieved using either direct CASA analysis (see Chapter 7) or the hyaluronate migration test.
2. Sperm capacitation evaluation, at least using a hyperactivation assay.
3. Acrosome reaction assessments, probably using the ARIC or ARmax approaches rather than some measure(s) of spontaneous acrosome reaction dynamics.
4. A sperm-zona binding test, using, for greatest ease, a competitive format assay.
5. Zona-free hamster egg penetration test using an ionophore-enhanced (type II) method for optimum sensitivity and specificity.

Final assessment of the clinical relevance and value of this approach awaits the publication of large, prospective studies in well-defined patient populations using appropriate clinical endpoints.

References and Recommended Reading

Ahuja, K. K. (1985). Carbohydrate determinants involved in mammalian fertilization. *Am. J. Anat.* **174,** 207.

Aitken, R. J., Best, F., Richardson, D. W., Schats, R., and Simm, G. (1983a). Influence of caffeine on movement characteristics, fertilizing capacity and ability to penetrate cervical mucus of human spermatozoa. *J. Reprod. Fertil.* **67,** 19.

Aitken, R. J., Best, F.S.M., Templeton, A. A., Richardson, D. W., Schats, R., Djahanbakhch, O., and Lees, M. M. (1983b). Fertilizing capacity of human spermatozoa: a study of oligozoospermia and unexplained infertility. In D'Agata, R., Lipsett, M. B., Polosa, P., and van der Molen, H. J. (eds): *Recent Advances in Male Reproduction: Molecular Basis and Clinical Implications.* Raven Press, New York.

Aitken, R. J., Bowie, H., Buckingham, D., Harkiss, D., Richardson, D. W., and West, K. M. (1992). Sperm penetration into a hyaluronic acid polymer as a means of monitoring functional competence. **13,** 44.

Aitken, R. J., Irvine, D. S., and Wu, F.C.W. (1991). Prospective analysis of sperm-oocyte fusion and reactive oxygen species generation as criteria for the diagnosis of infertility. *Am. J. Obstet. Gynecol.* **164,** 542.

Aitken, R. J., Ross, A., Hargreave, T., Richardson, D., and Best, F. (1984). Analysis of human sperm function following exposure to the ionophore A23817: comparison of normospermic and oligozoospermic men. *J. Androl.* **5**, 321.

Aitken, R. J., Thatcher, S., Glasier, A. F., Clarkson, J. S., Wu, F.C.W., and Baird, D. T. (1987). Relative ability of modified versions of the hamster oocyte penetration test, incorporating hyperosmotic medium or the ionophore A23187, to predict IVF outcome. *Hum. Reprod.* **2**, 227.

Aitken, R. J., Wang, Y.-F., Liu, J., Best, F., and Richardson, D. W. (1983c). The influence of medium composition, osmolarity and albumin content on the acrosome reaction and fertilizing capacity of human spermatozoa: development of an improved zona-free hamster egg penetration test. *Int. J. Androl.* **6**, 180.

Bissett, D. L. (1980). Development of a model of human cervical mucus. *Fertil. Steril.* **33**, 211.

Blazak, W. F., Overstreet, J. W., Katz, D. F., and Hanson, F. W. (1982). A competitive *in vitro* assay of human sperm fertilizing ability utilizing contrasting fluorescent sperm markers. *J. Androl.* **3**, 165.

Bolanos, J. R., Overstreet, J. W., and Katz, D. F. (1983). Human sperm penetration of zona-free hamster eggs after storage of the semen for 48 hours at 2°C to 5°C. *Fertil. Steril.* **39**, 536.

Bronson, R. A., and Rogers, B. J. (1988). Pitfalls of the zona-free hamster egg penetration test: protein source as a major variable. *Fertil. Steril.* **50**, 851.

Burkman, L. J., Coddington, C. C., Franken, D. A., Kruger, T. F., Rosenwaks, Z., and Hodgen, G. D. (1988). The hemizona assay (HZA): development of a diagnostic test for the binding of human spermatozoa to the human hemizona pellucida to predict fertilization potential. *Fertil. Steril.* **49**, 688.

Burkman, L. J., Coddington, C. C., Franken, D. R., Oehninger, S. C., and Hodgen, G. D. (1990). The hemizona assay (HZA): Assessment of fertilizing potential by means of human sperm binding to the human zona pellucida. In Keel, B. A., and Webster, B. W. (eds): *Handbook of the Laboratory Diagnosis and Treatment of Infertility.* CRC Press, Boca Raton, FL.

Collins, J. A. (1987). Diagnostic assessment of the infertile male partner. *Curr. Probl. Obstet. Gynecol. Fertil.* **10**, 173.

Cross, N. L., and Overstreet, J. W. (1987). Glycoconjugates of the human sperm surface: distribution and alterations that accompany capacitation in vitro. *Gamete Res.* **16**, 23.

Cross, N. L., Morales, P., Overstreet, J. W., and Hanson, F. W. (1986). Two simple methods for detecting acrosome-reacted human sperm. *Gamete Res.* **15**, 213.

Cummins, J. M., Pember, S. M., Jequier, A. M., Yovich, J. L., and Hartmann, P. E. (1991). A test of the human sperm acrosome reaction following ionophore challenge: Relationship to fertility and other seminal parameters. *J. Androl.* **12**, 98.

Hargreave, T. B. (1983). Non-specific treatment to improve fertility. In Hargreave, T. B. (ed): *Male Infertility.* Springer-Verlag, Berlin.

Holden, C. A., Hyne, R. V., Sathananthan, A. H., and Trounson, A. O. (1990). Assessment of the human sperm acrosome reaction using concanavalin A lectin. *Mol. Reprod. Devel.* **25**, 247.

Hyatt Sachs, H., Pink, M. J., and Gwatkin, R.B.L. (1989). Hamster oocyte penetration tests with oocytes frozen in propanediol: comparison with non-frozen oocytes. *Gamete Res.* **24**, 31.

Johnson, A., Bassham, B., Lipshultz, L. I., and Lamb, D. J. (1990). Methodology for the optimized sperm penetration assay. In Keel, B. A., and Webster, B. W. (eds): *Handbook of the Laboratory Diagnosis and Treatment of Infertility.* CRC Press, Boca Raton, FL.

Johnson, A. R., Syms, A. J., Lipshultz, L. I., and Smith, R. G. (1984). Conditions influencing human sperm capacitation and penetration of zona-free hamster ova. *Fertil. Steril.* **41,** 603.

Jouannet, P., and Rodrigues, D. (1990). Utilisation d'ovocytes congelés de hamster pour evaluer la fonction fusiogène du spermatozoïde humain. *Contraception Fertil. Sexual.* **18,** 557.

Kanwar, K. C., Yanagimachi, R., and Lopata, A. (1979). Effects of human seminal plasma on fertilizing capacity of human spermatozoa. *Fertil. Steril.* **31,** 321.

Lee, M. A., Trucco, G. S., Bechtol, K. B., Wummer, N., Kopf, G. S., Blasco, L., and Storey, B. T. (1987). Capacitation and acrosome reactions in human spermatozoa monitored by a chlortetracycline fluorescence assay. *Fertil. Steril.* **48,** 649.

Leibo, S. P., Giambernard, T. A., Meyer, T. K., Bastias, M. C., and Rogers, B. J. (1990). The efficacy of cryopreserved hamster ova in the sperm penetration assay. *Fertil. Steril.* **53,** 907.

Liu, D. Y., Lopata, A., Johnston, W.I.H., and Baker, H.W.G. (1988). A human sperm-zona pellucida binding test using oocytes that failed to fertilize in vitro. *Fertil. Steril.* **50,** 782.

Lorton, S. P., Kummerfeld, H. L., and Foote, R. H. (1981). Polyacrylamide as a substitute for cervical mucus in sperm migration tests. *Fertil. Steril.* **35,** 222.

Margalioth, E. J., Bronson, R. A., Cooper, G. W., and Rosenfeld, D. L. (1988). Luteal phase sera and progesterone enhance sperm penetration in the hamster egg assay. *Fertil. Steril.* **50,** 117.

McClure, R. D., Tom, R. A., and Dandekar, P. V. (1990). Optimizing the sperm penetration assay with human follicular fluid. *Fertil. Steril.* **53,** 546.

Mortimer, D. (1991). Sperm preparation techniques and iatrogenic failures of in-vitro fertilization. *Hum. Reprod.* **6,** 173.

Mortimer, D., and Camenzind, A. R. (1989). The role of follicular fluid in inducing the acrosome reaction of human spermatozoa incubated *in vitro. Hum. Reprod.* **4,** 169.

Mortimer, D., Chorney, M. J., Curtis, E. F., and Trounson, A. O. (1988). Calcium dependence of human sperm fertilizing ability. *J. Exp. Zool.* **246,** 194.

Mortimer, D., Curtis, E. F., and Camenzind, A. R. (1990a). Combined use of fluorescent peanut agglutinin lectin and Hoechst 33258 to monitor the acrosomal status and vitality of human spermatozoa. *Hum. Reprod.* **5,** 99.

Mortimer, D., Curtis, E. F., and Dravland, J. E. (1986). The use of strontium-substituted media for capacitating human spermatozoa: an improved sperm preparation method for the zona-free hamster egg penetration test. *Fertil. Steril.* **46,** 97.

Mortimer, D., Curtis, E. F., and Miller, R. G. (1987). Specific labelling by peanut agglutinin of the outer acrosomal membrane of the human spermatozoon. *J. Reprod. Fertil.* **81,** 127.

Mortimer, D., Curtis, E. F., Camenzind, A. R., and Tanaka, S. (1989). The spontaneous acrosome reaction of human spermatozoa incubated *in vitro. Hum. Reprod.* **4,** 57.

Mortimer, D., Mortimer, S. T., Shu, M. A., and Swart, R. (1990b). A simplified approach to sperm-cervical mucus interaction using a hyaluronate migration test. *Hum. Reprod.* **5,** 835.

Muller, C. H., Zarutskie, P. W., Stenchever, M. A., and Soules, M. R. (1990). The sperm penetration assay: One of the best methods we have. *Obstet. Gynecol. Rep.* **2,** 412.

Neuwinger, J., Cooper, T. G., Knuth, U. A., and Nieschlag, E. (1991). Hyaluronic acid as a medium for human sperm migration tests. *Hum. Reprod.* **6,** 396.

Osman, R. A., Andria, M. L., Jones, A. D., and Meizel, S. (1989). Steroid induced exocytosis: the human sperm acrosome reaction. *Biochem. Biophys. Res. Commun.* **160,** 828.

Overstreet, J. W., and Hembree, W. C. (1976). Penetration of the zona pellucida of nonliving human oocytes by human spermatozoa in vitro. *Fertil. Steril.* **27**, 815.

Overstreet, J. W., Yanagimachi, R., Katz, D. F., Hayashi, K., and Hanson, F. W. (1980). Penetration of human spermatozoa into the human zona pellucida and the zona-free hamster egg: a study of fertile donors and infertile patients. *Fertil. Steril.* **33**, 534.

Parrish, J. J., and Foote, R. H. (1985). Fertility differences among male rabbits determined by heterospermic insemination of fluorochrome-labelled spermatozoa. *Biol. Reprod.* **33**, 940.

Perreault, S. D., and Rogers, B. J. (1982). Capacitation pattern of human spermatozoa. *Fertil. Steril.* **38**, 258.

Purvis, K., Rui, H., Schølberg, A., Hesla, S., and Clausen, O.P.F. (1990). Application of flow cytometry to studies on the human acrosome. *J. Androl.* **11**, 361.

Quinn, P., Barros, C., and Whittingham, D. G. (1982). Preservation of hamster oocytes to assay the fertilizing capacity of human spermatozoa. *J. Reprod. Fertil.* **66**, 161.

Renard, J. P., Nguyen, B. X., and Garnier, V. (1984). Two step freezing of two cell rabbit embryos after partial dehydration at room temperature. *J. Reprod. Fertil.* **71**, 573.

Rogers, B. J., Perreault, S. D., Bentwood, B. J., McCarville, C., Hale, R. W., and Soderdahl, D. W. (1983). Variability in the human-hamster in vitro assay for fertility evaluation. *Fertil. Steril.* **39**, 204.

Spira, A. (1986). Epidemiology of human reproduction. *Hum. Reprod.* **1**, 111.

Talbot, P., and Chacon, R. (1980). A new procedure for rapidly scoring acrosome reactions of human sperm. *Gamete Res.* **3**, 211.

Talbot, P., and Chacon, R. S. (1981). A triple-stain technique for evaluating normal acrosome reactions of human sperm. *J. Exp. Zool.* **215**, 201.

Talbot, P., and Dudenhausen, E. (1981). Factors affecting triple staining of human sperm. *Stain Technol.* **56**, 307.

Templeton, A. A., and Penney, G. C. (1982). The incidence, characteristics, and prognosis of patients whose infertility is unexplained. *Fertil. Steril.* **37**, 175.

Wikland, M., Wik, O., Steen, Y., Qvist, K., Söderlund, B., and Janson, P. O. (1987). A self-migration method for preparation of sperm for in-vitro fertilization. *Hum. Reprod.* **2**, 191.

World Health Organization (1990). *Progress* **No. 15.** World Health Organization, Geneva.

World Health Organization (1992). *WHO Laboratory Manual for the Examination of Human Semen and Sperm-Cervical Mucus Interaction, 3rd ed.* Cambridge, Cambridge University Press.

Yanagimachi, R. (1984). Zona-free hamster eggs: their use in assessing fertilizing capacity and examining chromosomes of human spermatozoa. *Gamete Res.* **10**, 187.

Yanagimachi, R., Lopata, A., Odom, C. B., Bronson, R. A., Mahi, C. A., and Nicolson, G. L. (1979). Retention of biologic characteristics of zona pellucida in highly concentrated salt solution: the use of salt-stored eggs for assessing the fertilizing capacity of spermatozoa. *Fertil. Steril.* **31**, 562.

Yanagimachi, R., Yanagimachi, H., and Rogers, B. J. (1976). The use of zona-free animal ova as a test-system for the assessment of the fertilizing capacity of human spermatozoa. *Biol. Reprod.* **15**, 471.

Yee, B., and Cummings, L. M. (1988). Modification of the sperm penetration assay using human follicular fluid to minimize false negative results. *Fertil. Steril.* **50**, 123.

11

Clinical Relevance of Diagnostic Procedures

Numerous instances of fertility despite one or more abnormal semen characteristics and the many occasions where semen analysis and all other factors seem normal yet the couple remains infertile testify to the inadequacy of the traditional "descriptive" approach for predicting an individual's fertility potential. Because the major part of the spermatozoon's functional life is spent in the female reproductive tract, descriptive semen analysis clearly cannot be expected to provide all the answers. Obviously, an assessment of a suspected infertile man's reproductive potential must incorporate some evaluation of the various processes that take place between ejaculation and conception in the relative inaccessibility of the female tract. This chapter discusses the availability, limitations, and relevance of current laboratory procedures for the assessment of human sperm function or functional potential.

SEMEN ANALYSIS

Several general principles relevant to performing and interpreting semen analyses were discussed in Chapter 1. This chapter deals in greater depth with the clinical interpretation of semen analysis characteristics and discusses their clinical relevance in terms of infertility diagnosis and fertility prognosis.

Extrinsic Effects

Abstinence
A significant influence of sexual (or, more correctly, ejaculatory) abstinence on semen characteristics is well established. The production of spermatozoa and the accessory gland secretions that comprise the seminal plasma are continuous processes. Therefore for the purpose of standardization, a fixed period of abstinence is necessary, 3 days being the most commonly used interval. A large component of sample variation, on a population basis, can be attributed to variations in prior abstinence, so although it is not vital that all samples for analysis be produced after 3 days of ejaculatory abstinence, correct interpretation of results does require that the actual duration of abstinence be known. In some cases in which samples have been produced after longer periods of abstinence and the results cannot be interpreted with reasonable accuracy, repeat analyses are needed with a more appropriate period of abstinence.

Continuous sperm production means that each additional day of abstinence results in the availability of many more spermatozoa for ejaculation. The daily sperm production rate is the combined number of spermatozoa produced per 24 hours by both testes. Although this number is difficult to determine, values have been reported using various methods. As would be expected, there is an appreciable variation among men, but a "normal" range of 80×10^6 to 100×10^6 spermatozoa per day has been suggested, although there is evidence that it may be as high as 140×10^6 to 190×10^6/day (Johnson, 1982). Many male partners of infertile couples obviously have lower values.

Production of the accessory glands secretions is also continuous, but their reserve capacities seems to be reached within 3–4 days, so marked regular increases are not usually seen after this time. Obviously the situation varies among individual men as the relationships between the variations in the production of spermatozoa and the seminal plasma constituents are not constant. Abstinence in terms of the duration of storage of spermatozoa in the caudae epididymides also influences the qualitative aspects of the spermatozoa with a range of 2–5 days' abstinence being optimal for analysis.

Illness

Various illnesses may affect semen characteristics. For example, a semen sample produced for analysis 10–12 weeks after a bout of influenza or some other febrile illness (this being the time interval between spermatogonial division and the appearance of the resulting spermatozoa in the ejaculate) would be expected to have a low sperm concentration and the spermatozoa present to be of poor quality. A sample produced 2 weeks or so later may be more typical for the individual.

Drugs

Drug use or abuse may also affect semen characteristics. Excessive alcohol consumption and smoking have been reported to be detrimental, although the true significance, and extent, of these effects remain disputed. Sulfasalazine, which was introduced as a treatment for ulcerative colitis some 40 years ago, is now known to have direct side effects causing infertility. Although the induced oligozoospermia can improve quickly when sulfasalazine is withdrawn, it does seem that either the drug itself or a metabolite is toxic to spermatogenesis.

Aspects of Sperm Quality

The relationship between sperm concentration and fertility is rather poor, although there is a definite positive correlation (Smith et al., 1977; Bostofte et al., 1982). With regard to sperm quality, assessments of these characteristics (i.e., sperm motility, morphology and vitality) are intrinsic to a complete semen analysis. Whereas motility is assessed on the fresh material in a wet preparation, both morphology and vitality are evaluated from stained smears prepared from the fresh liquefied semen at the time of the initial examination (see Chapter 3).

Sperm Motility

The motility of ejaculated spermatozoa has long been recognized as an important functional characteristic that must be evaluated as an integral part of semen analysis. The likelihood of achieving a pregnancy increases with decreasing proportions of immotile spermatozoa (Bostofte et al., 1984a) and with increasing quality of sperm progression (Bostofte et al., 1983).

It is not just the proportion of spermatozoa that are motile or even their concentration that is of greatest importance. The objective and quantitative measurement of sperm movement characteristics derived from observations on individual cells has been found to be more predictive of functional ability (see Sperm Movement Analysis and CASA, below) and hence a man's potential fertility. Clearly, motility is a vitally important characteristic of spermatozoa that we need to measure objectively and accurately. Furthermore, it is apparent that we need to concentrate on those approaches that provide reliable measurements of specific aspects of sperm movement, not just simple motility (reviews: Aitken, 1990; Mortimer, 1990).

Sperm Morphology

Although the pleomorphism of the human spermatozoon is legendary and the assessment of sperm morphology subject to great observer bias, careful technician training and internal standardization do allow reliable morphological assessments. Immature spermatozoa showing a droplet of residual cytoplasm may be found in large numbers associated with frequent ejaculation (i.e., repeated, short periods of abstinence). The presence of many spermatozoa with coiled tails may indicate that the spermatozoa have been exposed to hypotonic stress, although coiling of the tail is also associated with sperm senescence. Large numbers of spermatozoa with tapered heads have been associated with "testicular stress" such as may be experienced in cases of severe varicocele, although it has been denied by other workers. Scrotal heating (possibly associated with prolonged periods spent seated) may result in high proportions of morphologically abnormal spermatozoa, although not necessarily associated with any specific type of structural defect.

Sperm morphology in terms of the proportion of normal forms has been shown to be significantly related to in vivo conception (Bostofte et al., 1984b), in vitro fertilization (Kruger et al., 1986, 1988), and in vitro tests of sperm function (Aitken et al., 1982b; Rogers et al., 1983; Mortimer et al., 1986a). In addition, assessment of acrosomal normality is predictive of IVF success (Jeulin et al., 1986; Liu and Baker, 1988). These correlations seem to be best if strict criteria for morphological normality are employed.

Finally, the extent of morphological abnormality, usually derived from multiparametric scoring and expressed as the average number of defects per abnormal spermatozoon, has been found to be predictive not only of sperm function in vitro (Mortimer et al., 1990) but also of spontaneous in vivo fertility (Jouannet et al., 1988).

Sperm Vitality

Vital staining makes it possible to differentiate between spermatozoa that are immotile from those that are dead. In all semen samples it is to be expected that the percentage of vital cells slightly exceeds that of motile cells; not all the immotile cells are necessarily dead. Such a measurement is of particular value in samples where the motility is low (i.e., below 40%) to distinguish between dead and immotile live cells. A specific example would be Kartagener syndrome, where there is an ultrastructural defect of the axoneme and all the spermatozoa are immotile and yet exclude eosin. Confirmation of the presence of this type of sterilizing sperm defect can be obtained by TEM of thin-sectioned spermatozoa.

Relationships Between Characteristics of Sperm Quality

Because of the complex nature of spermiogenesis it should not be surprising that the qualitative aspects of the process, as reflected in the various characteristics of sperm quality (i.e., morphological normality, cellular integrity, and motile ability) are interrelated not only with each other but also with the quantitative aspect of spermatogenesis (i.e., the number of spermatozoa produced). Statistically significant positive correlations exist between all the various combinations of sperm concentration, motility, vitality, and normal morphology, with higher correlations being found between the three characteristics of sperm quality themselves than between any one of them and the sperm count. An important corollary of these relationships is that in cases of oligozoospermia the quality of those few spermatozoa present in the semen must be expected to be reduced as well. This situation obviously results in a lower proportion of (and therefore even fewer in number) potentially functional spermatozoa in the ejaculates of these men.

Clearly, a valuable seminal characteristic would be the concentration of morphologically normal motile spermatozoa. Unfortunately, this parameter is difficult to measure by any technique amenable to routine use, although methods for its determination do exist (e.g., Katz et al., 1982). As an alternative, the concentration of live normal spermatozoa may be obtained by scoring sperm morphology and vitality simultaneously in eosin-nigrosin preparations. If it were not for the relatively poor staining of spermatozoa in eosin-nigrosin preparations, this type of differential score might be more likely to replace the present separate morphology and vitality counts in the future.

A point of the utmost importance is that those men with oligozoospermia but apparently normal sperm quality (see Tables 1-4 and 1-5) should not be treated clinically the same as those oligozoospermic individuals with poor sperm quality. Immediate referral for mechanically assisted fertilization (e.g., subzonal insemination or partial zona dissection) or donor insemination is presently the most efficient management for the latter group of men; but, if possible, the first group should be allowed more time to try to conceive their own child.

The ideal of needing to develop more efficacious treatments than donor insemination for those men whose only problem is fewer spermatozoa than normally found in fertile men is being realized with the increasing availability of mechanically assisted fertilization techniques in conjunction with clinical IVF programs. Such approaches are also useful for mildly oligozoospermic men, allowing us to bypass the deficiency.

It must be stressed that management decisions are the perogative and responsibility of a patient's physician, but it does not preclude laboratory identification of suitable or possible options according to principles and standard practices established by referring physicians.

Relationships with Fertility

The interpretation of semen characteristics is made in relation to the likelihood of achieving a conception. Studies by Smith et al. (1977) and Bostofte et al. (1981, 1982, 1983, 1984a,b) provide good evidence for positive associations between semen characteristics and the likelihood of achieving a pregnancy. At the same time, however, they illustrate clearly that there are no absolute limits for distinguishing fertile from infertile men. Almost 40% of patients with $< 5 \times 10^6$ motile spermatozoa/ml achieved pregnancies, usually within 12 months (Smith et al., 1977); moreover, almost 50% of men with 60–80% morphologically abnormal spermatozoa and $> 20\%$ of men with only 20% motile spermatozoa had living children at follow-up 20 years later (Bostofte et al., 1984a).

In a prospective study of 739 couples, Dunphy et al. (1989) found that the only significant predictor of pregnancy was the concentration of spermatozoa showing progressive motility with substantial lateral head displacement (ALH) (see Chapter 7). In fact, when this semen characteristic fell below 5×10^6/ml, no conceptions were reported among 35 couples over a 32-month follow-up. Of further interest was the finding that semen characteristics were of no predictive value when there were fewer than 48 months of infertility prior to investigation, nor when the female partner had ovulatory dysfunction or pelvic pathology.

Finally, the presence of multiple defects in the population of morphologically abnormal spermatozoa may be the most significant semen characteristic related to spontaneous in vivo fertility (Jouannet et al., 1988).

In conclusion, future studies should probably focus attention on the concentration of progressively motile spermatozoa with good ALH, the percentage of normal forms using strict morphological criteria, and the multiple anomalies or teratozoospermia index.

ANTISPERM ANTIBODIES

That postmeiotic male germ cells, spermatozoa, or sperm antigens can induce the production of auto- and isoantibodies that may interfere with fertility has been established since the beginning of the century (Behrman, 1968; Rose et al., 1976; Jones, 1980; Bronson et al., 1984; Haas and Beer, 1986; Mortimer, 1991). However, despite the plethora of publications on immunological infertility, no absolute

246 Practical Laboratory Andrology

etiology, or protocols for diagnosis or treatment have emerged. Rather, an ever increasing list of unanswered questions has arisen, which has led to substantial skepticism on the relevance and clinical significance of antisperm antibodies in human infertility.

This section briefly summarizes some of the more important findings in this area and develops a critical overview of the mechanisms whereby antisperm antibodies influence human fertility. Appropriate diagnostic tests for their identification and to determine their prevalence in patient populations are discussed.

Effects of Antisperm Antibodies in Men

In extreme cases, male autoimmunity to postmeiotic germ cell antigens can result in the destruction of all spermatogenic cells in the testicular germinal epithelium, e.g., mumps orchitis. However, clinical infertility is more often confronted with less clear-cut problems caused by the presence of circulating antisperm antibodies or those present in genital tract secretions.

Traditionally these antibodies were termed either spermagglutinating, if they induced the agglutination of motile donor spermatozoa, or spermotoxic, when they induced a complement-dependent loss of vitality. The latter type are also often called spermimmobilizing antibodies because they induce a loss of motility as a consequence of sperm death. However, the discovery of sperm-specific antibodies that cause neither effect but induce a "shaking" pattern of motility when such antibody-coated spermatozoa are exposed to cervical mucus can cause some confusion with regard to the term immobilization; such antibodies are not spermotoxic.

Antibodies present in men may be suspected if the semen analysis shows many motile spermatozoa specifically involved in agglutinates or a low percentage of live cells (assessed by vital staining, not motility). Agglutinates can usually be distinguished microscopically from aggregates (which are not immunologically mediated) by their involvement of mostly immotile spermatozoa in conjunction with other nonspermatozoal cells and debris. To have such effects the antibodies must be present in the seminal plasma either as a result of transudation from the blood or by local secretory activity within the accessory glands of the male genital tract.

Specific assays exist for the titration of these seminal plasma antibodies and are described in Chapter 5. The same or similar antibodies may also be sought in serum, although one source of confusion over the years has been the measurement of circulating antisperm antibodies in men who do not have any detectable activity in their seminal plasma, even though it is generally accepted there is an association (unfortunately not a 1:1 equivalence) between the presence of antisperm antibodies in serum and seminal plasma. Because seminal plasma is so readily available, along with tests for detecting antibody bound to the spermatozoa (see below), perhaps antibodies should not be assayed in male serum.

The classic spermagglutinating and spermotoxic antibodies obviously impair a man's fertility potential by reducing the availability of spermatozoa in his ejaculate that are competent to penetrate the cervical mucus, a process dependent on adequate numbers of progressively motile spermatozoa. Other, sperm-coating antibodies are often not apparent at semen analysis but cause negative or poor mucus penetration when evaluated under in vivo (postcoital test) or in vitro (Kremer test) conditions.

Congenital aplasia of the vasa deferentia can result in autosensitization to sperm antigens and the presence of antibodies even in epididymal fluid. This point not only demonstrates that antisperm antibodies can enter the proximal male genital tract but also provides evidence of local antibody production at this level of the tract. Obstruction of the efferent ducts, as at vasectomy, also results in the presence of antisperm antibodies in the male tract secretions, which may decrease the expected fecundity after vasovasostomy by interfering with sperm function. Indeed, the combination of IgA antibodies on the surface of all motile spermatozoa and a strong humoral immune response ($\geq$ 1:256 titer) has been associated with a zero conception rate after vasovasostomy (Meinertz et al., 1990).

Effects of Antisperm Antibodies in Women

Circulating antibodies may be transuded into the female genital tract secretions and follicular fluid, and local secretion of antibodies can occur at the cervix. Obviously, antibodies in cervical mucus may impair sperm penetration and the initiation of sperm transport, and those present in the higher levels of the female tract can interfere with sperm–egg interaction (see below). The latter mechanism is difficult to establish in vivo, but several studies in conjunction with IVF procedures have demonstrated that female serum containing antisperm antibodies can inhibit, and even prevent, fertilization when used as a culture medium supplement.

Prevalence and Significance of Antisperm Antibodies

Antisperm Antibodies in Serum

The SIT and TAT assays on sera from 698 couples with primary or secondary idiopathic infertility revealed antisperm antibodies in 16.5% of men and 21.6% of women; spermagglutinating activity was present in 14.8% of men and 19.6% of women, and the incidence of sperm-immobilizing activity was 5.6% for men and 6.4% for women (Menge et al., 1982). Overall, 31.1% of the couples had at least one individual with a positive result, and in 7.2% both partners had significant titers (TAT $\geq$ 1:16 and SIT $\geq$ 1:4); and although these prevalences appear high, they are comparable with reports from other centers using similar assay methods. However, it should be remembered that this group was a selected population with apparently idiopathic infertility, not a general referral population.

Furthermore, the incidence of subsequent pregnancy in 376 of these couples was reduced significantly if one or both partners had antisperm antibodies in either their serum or genital tract secretions (including cervical mucus; see below). With the antibodies in the male partners the pregnancy rate fell significantly from 42.7% to 7.1% with TAT titers > 1:16 (28.1% at TAT = 1:16); if the female partners had TAT titers $\geq$ 1:16, the incidence of pregnancy was only 4.0% compared to 46.2% in the TAT-negative group. Both partners had significantly lower pregnancy rates with serum SIT titers ≥ 1:4 (19.2% for men and 12.5% for women).

Such unequivocal data clearly establish the clinical significance of antisperm antibodies in the etiology of infertility. Naturally, the relationship is not absolute: All patients with a positive result do not fail to achieve a pregnancy. This immunological factor cannot be ignored, however, and serum antisperm antibody determinations must be integral to a basic infertility workup.

Antisperm Antibodies in Cervical Mucus

Sperm penetration of cervical mucus is significantly reduced in the presence of serum sperm-immobilizing activity (i.e., shaking) in both partners of 459 couples with otherwise unexplained infertility, as well as with SIT-positive results in cervical mucus (Menge et al., 1982).

The indirect Immunobead test (IBT) evaluation of bromelain-treated cervical mucus from 78 infertile women revealed that seven (8.9%) were positive for IgG or IgA class antibodies, but none tested positive for IgM (Clarke, 1984). Of the positive samples, almost 60% contained both IgG and IgA. In another study, positive IgA IBT reactions were found in 13 of 102 women (12.7%), all of whom had histories of negative or poor postcoital tests and otherwise unexplained infertility (Clarke et al., 1984). IgA-positive mucus samples also showed negative or poor penetration by normal donor spermatozoa in in vitro tests; and in those cases where spermatozoa did penetrate the mucus, they displayed the characteristic shaking phenomenon.

Antisperm Antibodies on the Sperm Surface

Routine screening for sperm-bound antibodies using the isotype-specific IBT in 813 men revealed that 63 (7.8%) had IgG or IgA class antibodies (or both) bound to ≥ 20% of their motile spermatozoa (De Almeida et al., 1986). Results of crossed-inhibition tests with purified human immunoglobulins and comparison of IBT results with serum SIT titers and spermagglutination in semen indicated that the IBT procedure is an immunologically specific test for antisperm antibodies (Clarke et al., 1985a). Using the GAM-IBT screening method, 32 of 300 men (10.7%) showed ≥ 10% IBT-bound motile spermatozoa and were considered positive (Pattinson and Mortimer, 1987). The lower cutoff for positive results in the GAM-IBT procedure is a margin of safety to avoid missing any men who should be retested later using the isotype-specific IBT, because although there is excellent correspondence between the two tests the absolute levels of Immunobead binding are not always identical.

In 94 infertile couples with negative postcoital tests, failure of spermatozoa to penetrate the semen–mucus interface was closely correlated with the presence of antisperm antibodies in the semen, as determined using the MAR and TAT assays, and vice versa with the tests agreeing in 81% of cases (Glazener and Hull, 1987). In another group of infertile men with suspected autoimmunity to spermatozoa, 53 of 120 (44%) showed ≥ 10% of their motile spermatozoa to be antibody-coated using a direct IBT (De Almeida et al., 1986). Both IgG and IgA were present in 88.7% of cases, and in 97.6% of cases there was decreased sperm penetration into cervical mucus.

In eight couples where the male partner had $\geq$ 80% of his motile spermatozoa coated with IgG and IgA class antibodies (assessed by IBT) an overall fertilization rate in IVF of only 27% was obtained in contrast to a normal fertilization rate of 72% seen in a group of nine men with < 80% sperm coating with IgA class antibodies (Clarke, 1988). In three men with $\geq$ 90% IgG but < 70% IgA Immunobead binding, a good IVF fertilization rate of 76% was obtained, indicating that it is IgA class antibodies that interfere with sperm–egg interaction. Further evidence from an indirect IBT on serum used to supplement IVF culture medium demonstrated that in cases where the IgG and IgA IBT titers were both $\geq$ 1:10 the fertilization rate was reduced to 15%. However, when only the IgG titer was $\geq$ 1:10 (IgA < 1:10), the fertilization rate was normal.

Taken in conjunction with the results of a study where passive transfer of antibodies was used to inhibit the fertilization of supernumerary oocytes from a GIFT program (Clarke et al., 1988), these studies demonstrate that serum containing antisperm antibodies must not be used in IVF procedures.

SPERM–CERVICAL MUCUS INTERACTION TESTING

Because cervical mucus receptivity to penetration by spermatozoa is cyclic, and optimal during the periovulatory period, it is clearly essential that any diagnostic test of sperm–mucus interaction must be performed during this window (see Chapter 9). Before final interpretation of a test booked prospectively for the expected day of ovulation its relationship to the ovarian cycle must be established from knowledge of the date of the next menstrual period. Tests performed on days outside the optimum window must be interpreted with caution.

Sperm–cervical mucus interaction assessments may be made either in vivo using the postcoital test or in vitro with the slide or the capillary tube test in conjunction with sperm–cervical mucus contact testing to show the shaking pattern of motility, preferably in a crossed hostility format.

Postcoital Test

There is still much debate as to the true clinical value and significance of the postcoital test (PCT). Even reliable studies have provided conclusions that are at variance with each other. Hull et al. (1982), using strict criteria for determining the time of ovulation and performing their PCTs, along with cumulative conception rates for analysis of their results were able to demonstrate a good prognostic value of the PCT investigation for subsequent conception. However, Collins et al. (1984), also employing meticulous criteria for their PCTs, were unable to find any predictive value of the test for the later occurrence of pregnancy in a large group of infertile couples. In a prospective study comparing both the PCT and Kremer-type in vitro sperm–mucus interaction testing to spontaneous fertility, Eggert-Kruse et al. (1989b) reported that whereas the Kremer test was predictive of fertility, the PCT was not. A clinical review of the PCT concluded that it lacks validity and should be used more selectively and interpreted with greater caution (Griffith and Grimes, 1990).

Furthermore, although the presence of antibodies against spermatozoa in the cervical mucus may be involved in causing poor PCTs (see above; also Kremer and Jager, 1988), technical problems in the assay methodology may also be responsible. Consequently, great care should be taken when attributing poor PCTs to immunologically hostile mucus.

Notwithstanding these problems and limitations of the PCT, many clinicians still consider it a required, if not essential, part of an infertile couple's workup, and consequently diagnostic laboratories are obliged to continue offering the procedure for some time to come.

In Vitro Tests

Because penetration of cervical mucus is the first obstacle that spermatozoa must face if conception is to be achieved in vivo, such assessments are clearly physiologically relevant to infertility diagnosis. This process has also been shown to be dependent on semen analysis assessments of both sperm motility and morphology, as well as the presence of certain types on antisperm antibodies either on the sperm surface or locally secreted by the cervical epithelium. Furthermore, several groups have demonstrated an influence of sperm movement characteristics on the outcome of sperm–cervical mucus interaction (see Sperm Movement Analysis and CASA, below).

In terms of fertility prediction, Eggert-Kruse et al. (1989a) reported that the pregnancy rate at 6 months in couples with good Kremer-SMIT results was higher than that for couples with poor results (2.3% versus 29.0%; $P < 0.001$). In addition, these authors reported that human cervical mucus was superior to bovine cervical mucus as a penetration medium for providing information about sperm function.

In another study comparing the clinical significance of in vitro and in vivo tests of sperm–mucus interaction (PCT and Kremer-SMIT methods), although the PCT result was not predictive of pregnancy (24% with good PCTs versus 20% with poor PCTs), significant differences were found in the pregnancy rate according to homologous SMIT results: 30.5% with good SMITs versus 8.5% with poor SMITs (Eggert-Kruse et al., 1989b).

A study of 56 couples for whom Kremer-SMIT assessments were made on the same ejaculates provided for IVF reported that not only was mucus-penetrating ability independently related to fertilization, but that there were no false-negative results; that is, no fertilization occurred in all five cases where the spermatozoa failed to penetrate cervical mucus (Barratt et al., 1989). Furthermore, only one case with an abnormal Kremer-SMIT result showed successful fertilization.

SPERM MIGRATION TESTS

In vitro tests of sperm migration in media other than cervical mucus have been considered for many years in attempts to assess the quality of sperm motility. Some studies have used simple culture media, whereas others have employed high viscosity media as surrogates for cervical mucus. The basis of such tests is that their outcome must depend on the same sperm characteristics as govern penetration into cervical mucus. Most recently, studies using migration media based on sodium hyaluronate polymers have shown the greatest potential. For example, the outcome of Kremer-SMITs can be predicted with high success and confidence (Mortimer et al., 1990). In addition, the outcome of such a hyaluronate migration test (HMT) accounted for all the variance components due to sperm factors when predicting the outcome of these Kremer tests. In other words, an HMT evaluates mucus-penetrating ability on a "global" scale, including both traditional semen analysis and sperm kinematic characteristics.

The HMT effectively assesses the mucus-penetrating potential of a semen sample without the need for large quantities of midcycle cervical mucus, and it could therefore augment (as an internal control), although not necessarily replace, the homologous Kremer test and thereby reduce the quantity of both patient and donor mucus needed for comprehensive crossed-hostility format testing of sperm–mucus interaction. Furthermore, the HMT could also be used as an independent test of sperm function, as it is a standardized test system that would provide a stable, objective assay over long time frames.

ZONA-FREE HAMSTER EGG PENETRATION TEST

Most published studies have applied the hamster egg penetration test (HEPT) to groups of patients preselected on the basis of ill-defined seminological criteria (e.g., oligozoospermia or asthenozoospermia versus normozoospermia) or clinical categories such as infertile men (i.e., the male partners in infertile couples) and fertile donors (often selected highly fertile individuals used for donor insemination). Very few papers have reported prospective studies using a clinically relevant endpoint.

Appropriate endpoints of clinical interest are the achievement of conception in vivo or in vitro fertilization (IVF). HEPT results are variously described as normal or abnormal, or negative or positive. For the present purposes the terminological conventions listed in Table 10-1 are used.

A low HEPT score indicates probably reduced fecundity, not sterility—a situation similar to that for low sperm counts. There are also men who achieve a good HEPT score yet remain unable to conceive in vivo (i.e., false positives). Consequently, the question is how to distinguish between men with low fecundity and those with significant sperm defects that impair sperm–egg interaction. The HEPT is not the absolute test system because it cannot evaluate sperm–cumulus or, more importantly, sperm–zona interactions.

HEPT and In Vivo Conception

Sperm kinematics and the HEPT allowed a 76.5% correct prediction of spontaneous in vivo fertility, defined as pregnancy, during a 2.3-year follow-up of 68 idiopathic infertile couples (Aitken et al., 1984). Of those men with abnormal HEPT results, 5 of 21 (23.8%) with low (1–10%) HEPT penetration and none of the four men with a negative HEPT achieved a pregnancy.

In another study of 74 infertile men from couples with no identified female factor, 68% of men who had shown normal ($\geq$ 11%) HEPT penetration rates had achieved a spontaneous pregnancy, whereas only 27% of those with abnormal HEPT results had done so (Shy et al., 1988). Only 1 of 14 men with a negative HEPT achieved a pregnancy.

Normal HEPT penetration ($\geq$ 11%) was indicative of a twofold higher likelihood of pregnancy over a 2.5-year period in a mixed population of 227 couples selected primarily because of the presence of abnormal semen characteristics, poor postcoital tests, a history of varicocele, or idiopathic infertility: 40% versus 20% (Corson et al., 1988).

Most recently, in a population of 369 infertile couples with no apparent female factor, a normal ($\geq$ 20% penetration) HEPT result was predictive of a higher pregnancy rate in 192 men with an abnormal semen analysis (41% versus 17%) and in the 177 couples with idiopathic infertility (52% versus 24%) over a 2- to 5-year follow-up period (Margalioth et al., 1989). Overall, 16% of men with a negative HEPT (21 of 131) and 23.3% of men with low (< 10%) penetration (28 of 120) achieved a pregnancy. Of the 118 men with a normal HEPT, 57 (48.3%) achieved a pregnancy.

HEPT and In Vitro Fertilization

With the increasing clinical use of IVF as a treatment for infertility, several groups evaluated the correlation between the HEPT and IVF success or failure. Although some early studies reported that, in general terms, HEPT results correlated well with IVF outcome and that the HEPT should be considered as a selection criterion for patients contemplating IVF treatment, closer inspection revealed the relation to be less useful.

In one study of 24 tubal factor patients, 27.3% of men (6 of 22) with normal HEPT results (> 10%) failed to fertilize the human eggs; and both patients with abnormal HEPT results did achieve successful homologous fertilization in vitro (Wolf et al., 1983). Another study of 20 tubal factor couples undergoing IVF treatment reported that all seven patients with abnormal HEPT penetration (< 20%, including two negative HEPT results) subsequently failed to fertilize in vitro (Margalioth et al., 1983). However, 3 of 13 patients with normal ($\geq$ 20%) HEPT penetration did fail to fertilize at IVF, giving a 23.1% false-positive rate. When the HEPT was performed on 15 men whose spermatozoa had consistently failed to fertilize human oocytes in vitro, 9 showed positive results but at lower penetration rates than seen in men who did achieve IVF success (Foreman et al., 1984).

In a mixed-diagnosis population of patients undergoing IVF treatment, a normal HEPT result ($\geq$ 20% penetration) was generally a good predictor of IVF fertilization, although there was a 15% (16 of 107 couples) false-positive rate (Margalioth et al., 1986). An abnormal HEPT result was subject to a 22.2% (6 of 27 couples) false-negative rate. Considering only the tubal and idiopathic infertility couples, none of the 11 men with an abnormal HEPT achieved fertilization in vitro. Among the 29 couples with male factor infertility, 6 of 16 (37.5%) of the cases with an abnormal HEPT result showed homologous fertilization. This lack of association between HEPT and IVF results in couples with male factor infertility must be taken to indicate that the HEPT should not be relied on to predict male factor IVF outcome.

Another study on 54 IVF couples also showed that an abnormal HEPT result was not always indicative of fertilization failure in that four of five men with < 15% penetration were successful in homologous fertilization in vitro (Ausmanas et al., 1985). Furthermore, 3 of 12 patients who established an IVF pregnancy had shown HEPT penetration rates of < 15%, including one negative result. These authors concluded that a lower limit of HEPT penetration for defining male infertility could not be conclusively established.

Yet another report on 29 IVF couples described the existence of substantial false-positive and false-negative rates—20% (5 of 25) and 75% (3 of 4), respectively—using a 15% cutoff for HEPT penetration rate (Belkien et al., 1985). Although all six cases with abnormal semen characteristics were incorrectly classified by the HEPT result (four falsely positive and two falsely negative), there was only one case each of false-positive or false-negative results among the 23 couples with normal semen characteristics, with one of the two cases of IVF failure being correctly identified. These results again led to the conclusion that the HEPT was of limited value for predicting IVF outcome in men with abnormal semen characteristics.

Finally, HEPT results on 19 couples who failed to fertilize any eggs in 31 IVF attempts were 31 ± 4% (range 0–70%), compared to HEPT results of 38 ± 5% (range 3–100%) in IVF couples with tubal factor infertility, again indicating that the HEPT is not predictive of IVF failure (Vazquez-Levin et al., 1990). When nine of these couples went on to 12 repeat IVF cycles incorporating zona drilling, all were able to achieve fertilization, including two with abnormal HEPT results (0% and 8% penetration). The authors suggested that although patients should not be unduly optimistic after a positive HEPT result, they should also not be eliminated from consideration for IVF in conjunction with zona drilling on the basis of negative HEPT results.

Influence of HEPT Methodology

It must be recognized that all the studies described above employed HEPT protocols relying on spontaneous capacitation and acrosome reactions. When the relative ability of such protocols to predict IVF outcome was compared to one employing A23187, stimulation of the acrosome reaction was far superior (Aitken et al., 1987). When the HEPT was performed on semen samples different from those used for the IVF attempts, a false-negative rate of 14.3% was observed for negative HEPT results (1 of 7 cases) and a false-positive rate of 15.5% (9 of 58 cases) was seen for positive HEPT results. These results were even better when the HEPT was performed on the semen sample used for the IVF attempt: 0% false negatives and 5.3% false positives.

From a prospective study using an ionophore-enhanced HEPT, Aitken et al.

(1991) demonstrated that, over a 4-year follow-up, abnormal penetration rates (0–10%) resulted in a cumulative pregnancy rate of about 8% (plateau reached at 30 months) compared to a cumulative pregnancy rate of about 30% for those patients with normal (11–100%) HEPT penetration rates (plateau reached by 42 months).

When evaluating a follicular fluid-optimized HEPT, 19 men were studied using both conventional and human follicular fluid (hFF) protocols in conjunction with the outcome of IVF (McClure et al., 1990). In terms of predicting IVF outcome, although the false-positive rate was approximately the same by the two methods (10% and 6.7%), the false-negative rate was reduced from 66.7% to 25.0% by the incorporation of hFF into the HEPT assay.

Future Use of HEPT

It is clear that to improve the diagnostic sensitivity and specificity of the HEPT, as well its predictive value in terms of either in vivo conception or IVF outcome, we must abandon protocols relying on spontaneous capacitation and acrosome reactions. The problems caused by interindividual variation in the optimum capacitation preincubation period, low levels of spontaneous acrosome reactions in many men, the likely induction of the physiological acrosome reaction by one or more component(s) of the products of ovulation (probably as a consequence of sperm–zona binding) (see Chapter 2), and the other sources of methodological variation such as protein source, make such assays inherently technically crude and insensitive. Furthermore, any reliance on a biological product such as serum or follicular fluid as a medium supplement makes interassay standardization difficult and certainly precludes any real attempts at major interlaboratory standardization.

For such reasons, the WHO has decided to recommend an ionophore-based protocol for the future (World Health Organization, 1992). Because the WHO is the only international organization involved in infertility diagnosis and treatment at this level, all laboratories should give serious consideration to accepting the WHO's recommendations and thereby facilitate not only standardization of sperm function testing in andrology but also establishment of the clinical relevance and significance of such diagnostic tests.

SPERM–ZONA PELUCIDA BINDING TESTS

A major criticism frequently leveled against the HEPT is its inability to test the species-specific binding of spermatozoa to the zona pellucida. It has long been established that sperm dysfunction causing impaired fertilizing ability may be expressed at one or more steps in the fertilization process.

1. Failure to bind to the zona pellucida
2. Successful sperm–zona binding but with impaired ability to penetrate the zona matrix
3. Successful sperm binding to, and penetration of, the zona but with reduced ability to fuse with the oolemma

4. Successful fusion with the oolemma but with impaired sperm incorporation into the oocyte or male pronucleus formation

Although an assessment of sperm–zona pellucida binding using a homologous zona-binding test (ZBT) (see Chapter 10) is probably a valuable adjunct to the HEPT, few studies on the clinical relevance of ZBT results have been published to date. Those available do support its significance for predicting IVF outcome.

Using the hemizona assay (HZA) method, 5 of 6 cases (83.3%) with ≤ 36% HZA index showed poor IVF fertilization rates (i.e., ≥ 65% of oocytes fertilized), whereas 21 of 22 cases (95.5%) with > 36% HZA index showed good (≥ 65%) IVF fertilization (Oehninger et al., 1989).

Results of a heterospermic, competitive ZBT were found to be the most significant factor related to IVF success by logistic regression analysis (Liu et al., 1989) and ranged from about 0.2 (≈ 20%) in patients showing failure to fertilize human eggs in vitro to 0.75 (75%) or higher in patients with > 50% IVF fertilization rates. There were a few patients with low sperm–zona pellucida binding ratios who had high IVF fertilization rates; conversely, a few with high zona binding (> 0.8, or > 80%) had low IVF fertilization rates. Indeed, in one case spermatozoa with a very high zona binding ratio (> 1.0, or > 100%) failed to fertilize any of six morphologically normal human oocytes.

The latter study also considered ZBT results in a subgroup of 33 patients with poor sperm morphology (< 30% normal forms) where there was a highly significant relation between ZBT results and IVF fertilization rate. Applying the HZA index 36% cutoff in these men gave a false-positive rate of only 12.5% for predicting an IVF success rate of > 65%, and only 2 of 17 men (11.8%) with ZBT results > 36% fertilized < 50% of human oocytes at IVF.

SPERM ACROSOME REACTION ASSESSMENTS

The essential role of the acrosome in fertilization has led numerous authors to propose acrosome status and acrosome reaction assessments as potential sperm function tests. Acrosomal morphology is known to be related to impaired sperm function (Jeulin et al., 1986), and extensive studies on acrosomal biochemistry and acrosome reactions have tried to define associations between these structure-function relationships of the organelle and sperm fertilizing ability (e.g., Schill et al., 1988). The percentage of acrosome-reacted spermatozoa was not found to be correlated with sperm fertilizing ability assessed using either spontaneous capacitation or follicular fluid-enhanced HEPTs (Fukuda et al., 1989).

With regard to IVF outcome, although spontaneous acrosome reactions apparently have no relation to fertilizing ability (Plachot et al., 1984; Cummins et al., 1991), induced acrosome reactions (using the ARIC protocol described in Chapter 10) were significantly reduced or absent in subfertile men, indicating acrosomal dysfunction as a likely cause of fertilization failure (Cummins et al., 1991).

During the next few years, the establishment of standardized protocols for acrosome reaction induction and assessment as a diagnostic procedure should facilitate the establishment of this aspect of sperm physiology as a clinically relevant test of sperm function.

SPERM MOVEMENT ANALYSIS AND CASA

Semen Analysis

The commonest application of CASA systems is to provide values for sperm concentration and sperm motility more rapidly and (supposedly) more accurately than those obtained using traditional semen analysis methods. For many small or nonspecialized laboratories where specially trained andrology technicians are not available, this task is not difficult. However, in a center providing tertiary level infertility services and following WHO-recommended methods with appropriate standardization and quality control, CASA systems may not yet be sufficiently accurate for them to replace traditional methods (review: Mortimer, 1990; see also Chapter 7).

The total sperm concentration is well known to have little diagnostic value; it is the progressively motile spermatozoa in a semen sample (and their movement characteristics) that are of biological, and hence clinical, significance. Therefore these semen characteristics are the ones that ought to be measured (along with sperm morphology, vitality, and so on). It seems pointless expending great effort trying to use modern technology to make unreliable and inaccurate measurements of semen characteristics with little diagnostic value.

What we should use CASA systems for is determining the concentration of progressively motile spermatozoa in semen along with their movement characteristics. We should take the opportunity to apply modern technology to the assessment of sperm functional potential, thereby making a significant advance in clinical andrology. Because penetration of cervical mucus is the first obstacle that spermatozoa must face if conception is to be achieved in vivo, movement analysis of seminal spermatozoa is of greatest significance in studies evaluating sperm functional potential when in vivo fertility prediction is the biological endpoint. Unfortunately, at the time of writing, no studies have yet been published on the predictive value of sperm kinematics in relation to in vivo fertility.

Sperm Kinematics and SMIT Results

Several groups have demonstrated an influence of sperm movement characteristics on the outcome of sperm–cervical mucus interaction (Aitken et al., 1985, 1986; Feneux et al., 1985; Mortimer et al., 1986b). Good progression (e.g., mean VSL $\geq$ 25 μm/second) with large mean ALH (e.g., $\geq$ 7.5 μm using TEP) are important discriminators in predicting in vitro sperm–mucus interaction test (SMIT) outcome. Using these values in conjunction with a minimum concentration of progressively motile spermatozoa ($\geq$ 25 $\times$ 10^6 spermatozoa/ml with mean VSL $\geq$ 10 μm/second) we were able to show that 25 of 30 "good" semen samples produced normal SMIT results, whereas all 13 samples that failed to meet these three criteria produced abnormal SMIT results (Mortimer et al., 1986b). In addition, a small number of men have been identified whose motile spermatozoa are incapable of penetrating cervical mucus or migrating through it, a defect caused by extremely small ALH (Feneux et al., 1985).

Sperm Kinematics and HEPT

Aitken and his colleagues have provided substantial evidence of a relationship between sperm movement characteristics and sperm fertilizing ability as evaluated by the HEPT (Aitken et al., 1982a,b, 1983, 1984, 1985). The best discrimination between normal or abnormal HEPT results was obtained using movement characteristics of the washed, preincubated sperm suspension. Such sperm populations show higher VSL and larger ALH values than do seminal spermatozoa (Mortimer et al., 1984), and the apparent relationship between smaller mean ALH values and normal HEPT results cannot be explained physiologically, although its discriminant power is unquestioned.

Sperm Hyperactivation

No studies on sperm hyperactivation in relation to the HEPT have yet been performed. Because there is no biological requirement for hyperactivated motility in the case of sperm interaction with zona-free oocytes, as there are no egg vestments to penetrate, a clearly definable relationship may not be apparent. The HEPT is an indirect bioassay of human sperm functional potential, so one should expect relationships between it and other sperm function tests (e.g., laparoscopic sperm recovery) (Templeton et al., 1982) or movement analysis. However, these correlations do not necessarily reflect a direct biological involvement, as the parameters being assessed may themselves be secondary events.

Increased intracellular calcium causes increased flagellar curvature, and it is flagellar curvature that determines ALH. Calcium influx is associated with the later stage(s) of capacitation and induction of the acrosome reaction; therefore one would expect to see (1) larger ALH values and (2) increased proportions of hyperactivated cells in capacitating and capacitated sperm populations. Perhaps it is the cells with the largest ALH values that develop hyperactivated motility and thereby reduce the mean ALH of the progressive sperm population. Certainly the identification of hyperactivated cells is not easy using TEP.

Objective descriptions now exist for hyperactivated human spermatozoa and allow their automated detection using CASA technology (Burkman, 1984, 1990; Robertson et al., 1988; Mortimer and Mortimer, 1990; Mortimer et al., 1991). Several groups are trying to establish a clinical relationship between sperm hyperactivation and IVF outcome.

Sperm Kinematics and IVF

Sperm motility is clearly essential for fertilization *in vivo* and *in vitro*. In the in vivo situation motility is also necessary for successful sperm transport, a step that is bypassed with IVF. Little has been published to date on any relation between clinical IVF and sperm movement analysis, although Jeulin et al. (1986) reported that preincubated post-swim-up spermatozoa from men who fertilized ≤ 33% of human oocytes in vitro showed lower mean ALH values (analyzed using TEP) and more morphologically abnormal acrosomes.

Obviously, this area is one in which we shall see a proliferation of literature over the next few years, hopefully leading to the establishment of clearly defined relationships between sperm movement characteristics and their dynamic changes associated with capacitation, which can be used in clinical management.

LAPAROSCOPIC SPERM RECOVERY

With the increasing use of laparoscopy in the primary investigation of female infertility, aspiration of peritoneal fluid represents an ideal approach for investigating sperm transport. In couples with idiopathic infertility, a positive laparoscopic sperm recovery (LSR) had a good prognosis for subsequent spontaneous pregnancy of 50% within a year or so, and a negative LSR result had a poor prognosis of only about 10% within 2 years (Templeton and Mortimer, 1982). However, only 50% of appropriately scheduled LSRs in couples with completely normal semen characteristics were positive. Consequently, although LSR false negatives cannot be excluded, sperm transport failure appears to be implicated as a cause of infertility. Whether it is due to a sperm defect or female tract abnormality remains unknown, but such a dysfunction may underlie the successful treatment of idiopathic infertility by GIFT.

EVALUATION OF A SPERM FUNCTION TEST

Although during its development a sperm function test may be evaluated by comparison to other, more established tests, its final validation must consider a relevant clinical endpoint (see Comprehensive Sperm Function Testing Protocol in Chapter 10). In statistical terms, several analytical techniques may be used depending on the purpose and needs of the analysis. Such techniques include discriminant function (DF) analysis, Cox regression, multiple regression, receiver operating characteristics (ROC), and simple sensitivity and specificity calculations.

The complex procedures of DF, Cox, and multiple regression analysis should be used to analyze one data set (the "learning" set) and the results of the analysis subsequently validated by prospective application to a second, independent data set (the "validation" set). They are also powerful tools for investigating the complex relationships between numerous independent predictor variables and a particular dependent variable (i.e., the endpoint of choice). For such purposes, although it is statistically impure, such analyses remain very useful. Indeed, the purpose of their application under such conditions is not to try to establish an absolute relationship between the predictor and dependent variables but, rather, to understand the relationships within a particular data set.

Appropriate methods should be used depending on the nature of the dependent variable. If it is a continuous variable (e.g., time to conception, expected cryosurvival rate), a method such as multiple regression should be used; DF analysis cannot be used because it requires a binary dependent variable (e.g., pregnant versus not pregnant, survival versus death).

The ROC analysis is a method for establishing the best cutoff value of a variable to discriminate between two outcomes such as normal versus abnormal test results or pregnant versus not pregnant. Once the best delimiting value has been established, optimum sensitivity and specificity calculations can be performed.

If such calculations are used to evaluate the performance of, for example, a new kit for measuring something for which there is already an established but perhaps more expensive or more complicated method, the situations considered are as follows.

A = **true positive** = kit and other method both positive
B = **false positive** = kit positive but other method negative
C = **false negative** = kit negative but other method positive
D = **true negative** = kit and other method both negative

Using these situations, the following characteristics of the new kit are established:

Sensitivity $= A \div (A + C) \times 100$
Specificity $= D \div (B + D) \times 100$
Positive predictive value $= A \div (A + B) \times 100$
Negative predictive value $= D \div (C + D) \times 100$
Accuracy $= (A + D) \div (A + B + C + D) \times 100$

References and Recommended Reading

Aitken, R. J. (1990). Motility parameters and fertility. In Gagnon, C. (ed): *Controls of Sperm Motility: Biological and Clinical Aspects.* CRC Press, Boca Raton, FL.

Aitken, R. J.Best, F.S.M., Richardson, D. W., Djahanbakhch, O., and Lees, M. M. (1982a). The correlates of fertilizing capacity in normal fertile men. *Fertil. Steril.* **38**, 68.

Aitken, R. J., Best, F.S.M., Richardson, D. W., Djahanbakhch, O., Mortimer, D., Templeton, A. A., and Lees, M. M. (1982b). An analysis of sperm function in cases of unexplained infertility: conventional criteria, movement characteristics and fertilizing capacity. *Fertil. Steril.* **38**, 212.

Aitken, R. J., Best, F.S.M., Warner, P., and Templeton, A. (1984). A prospective study of the relationship between semen quality and fertility in cases of unexplained infertility. *J. Androl.* **5**, 297.

Aitken, R. J., Irvine, D. S., and Wu, F.C.W. (1991). Prospective analysis of sperm-oocyte fusion and reactive oxygen species generation as criteria for the diagnosis of infertility. *Am. J. Obstet. Gynecol.* **164**, 542.

Aitken, R. J., Sutton, M., Warner, P., and Richardson, D. W. (1985). Relationship between the movement characteristics of human spermatozoa and their ability to penetrate cervical mucus and zona-free hamster oocytes. *J. Reprod. Fertil.* **73**, 441.

Aitken, R. J., Thatcher, S., Glasier, A. F., Clarkson, J. S., Wu, F.C.W., and Baird, D. T.

(1987). Relative ability of modified versions of the hamster oocyte penetration test, incorporating hyperosmotic medium or the ionophore A23187, to predict IVF outcome. *Hum. Reprod.* **2,** 227.

Aitken, R. J., Warner, P., Best, F.S.M., Templeton, A. A., Djahanbakhch, O., Mortimer, D., and Lees, M. M. (1983). The predictability of subnormal penetrating capacity of sperm in cases of unexplained infertility. *Int. J. Androl.* **6,** 212.

Aitken, R. J., Warner, P. E., and Reid, C. (1986). Factors influencing the success of sperm-cervical mucus interaction in patients exhibiting unexplained infertility. *J. Androl.* **7,** 3.

Ausmanas, M., Tureck, R. W., Blasco, L., Kopf, G. S., Ribas, J., and Mastroianni, L., Jr. (1985). The zona-free hamster egg penetration assay as a prognostic indicator in a human in vitro fertilization program. *Fertil. Steril.* **43,** 433.

Barratt, C.L.R., Osborn, J. C., Harrison, P. E., Monks, N., Dunphy, B. C., Lenton, E. A., and Cooke, I. D. (1989). The hypo-osmotic swelling test and the sperm mucus penetration test in determining fertilization of the human oocyte. *Hum. Reprod.* **4,** 430.

Behrman, S. J. (1968). The immune response and infertility. In Behrman, S. J. and Kistner, R. W. (eds): *Progress in Infertility, 2nd ed.* Little, Brown, Boston.

Belkien, L., Bordt, J., Freischem, C. W., Hano, R., Knuth, U. A., and Nieschlag, E. (1985). Prognostic value of the heterologous ovum penetration test for human in vitro fertilization. *Int. J. Androl.* **8,** 275.

Bostofte, E., Serup, J., and Rebbe, H. (1981). Hammen semen quality classification and pregnancies obtained during a twenty-year follow-up period. *Fertil. Steril.* **36,** 84.

Bostofte, E., Serup, J., and Rebbe, H. (1982). Relation between sperm count and semen volume, and pregnancies obtained during a twenty-year follow-up period. *Int. J. Androl.* **5,** 267.

Bostofte, E., Serup, J., and Rebbe, H. (1983). Relation between spermatozoa motility and pregnancies obtained during a twenty-year follow-up period: spermatozoa motility and fertility. *Andrologia* **15,** 682.

Bostofte, E., Serup, J., and Rebbe, H. (1984a). Relation between number of immotile spermatozoa and pregnancies obtained during a twenty-year follow-up period: immotile spermatozoa and fertility. *Andrologia* **16,** 136.

Bostofte, E., Serup, J., and Rebbe, H. (1984b). Interrelations among the characteristics of human semen, and a new system for classification of male infertility. *Fertil. Steril.* **41,** 95.

Bronson, R., Cooper, G., and Rosenfeld, D. (1984). Sperm antibodies: their role in infertility. *Fertil. Steril.* **42,** 171.

Burkman, L. J. (1984). Characterization of hyperactivated motility by human spermatozoa during capacitation: comparison of fertile and oligozoospermic sperm populations. *Arch. Androl.* **13,** 153.

Burkman, L. J. (1990). Human sperm hyperactivation. In Gagnon, C. (ed): *Controls of Sperm Motility: Biological and Clinical Aspects.* CRC Press, Boca Raton, FL.

Clarke, G. N. (1984). Detection of antispermatozoal antibodies of IgG, IgA, and IgM immunoglobulin classes in cervical mucus. *Am. J. Reprod. Immunol.* **6,** 1985.

Clarke, G. N. (1988). Immunoglobulin class and regional specificity of antispermatozoal autoantibodies blocking cervical mucus penetration by human spermatozoa. *Am. J. Reprod. Immunol. Microbiol.* **16,** 135.

Clarke, G. N. (1988). Sperm antibodies and human fertilization. *Am. J. Reprod. Immunol. Microbiol.* **17,** 65.

Clarke, G. N., Elliott, P. J., and Smaila, C. (1985a). Detection of sperm antibodies in semen using the Immunobead test: A survey of 813 consecutive patients. *Am. J. Reprod. Immunol. Microbiol.* **7,** 118.

Clarke, G. N., Hyne, R. V., du Plessis, Y., and Johnston, W.I.H. (1988). Sperm antibodies and human in vitro fertilization. *Fertil. Steril.* **49,** 1018.

Clarke, G. N., McBain, J. C., Lopata, A., and Johnston, W.I.H. (1985b). In vitro fertilization results for women with antibodies in plasma and follicular fluid. *Am. J. Reprod. Immunol. Microbiol.* **8,** 130.

Clarke, G. N., Stojanoff, A., Cauchi, M. N., and Johnston, W. I. H. (1985c). The immunoglobulin class of antispermatozoal antibodies in serum. *Am. J. Reprod. Immunol. Microbiol.* **7,** 143.

Clarke, G. N., Stojanoff, A., Cauchi, M. N., McBain, J. C., Speirs, A. L., and Johnston, W. I. H. (1984). Detection of antispermatozoal antibodies of IgA class in cervical mucus. *Am. J. Reprod. Immunol.* **5,** 61.

Collins, J. A., So, Y., Wilson, E. H., Wrixon, W., and Casper, R. F. (1984). The postcoital test as a predictor of pregnancy among 355 infertile couples. *Fertil. Steril.* **41,** 703.

Corson, S. L., Batzer, F. R., Marmar, J., and Maislin, G. (1988). The human sperm-hamster egg penetration assay: prognostic value. *Fertil. Steril.* **49,** 328.

Cummins, J. M., Pember, S. M., Jequier, A. M., Yovich, J. L., and Hartmann, P. E. (1991). A test of human sperm acrosome reaction following ionophore challenge: Relationship to fertility and other seminal parameters. *J. Androl.* **12,** 98.

De Almeida, M., Soumah, A., and Jouannet, P. (1986). Incidence of sperm-associated immunoglobulins in infertile men with suspected autoimmunity to sperm. *Int. J. Androl.* **9,** 321.

Dunphy, B. C., Neal, L. M., and Cooke, I. D. (1989). The clinical value of conventional semen analysis. *Fertil. Steril.* **51,** 324.

Eggert-Kruse, W., Gerhard, I., Tilgen, W., and Runnebaum, B. (1989a). Clinical significance of crossed in vitro sperm-cervical mucus penetration test in infertility investigation. *Fertil. Steril.* **52,** 1032.

Eggert-Kruse, W., Leinhos, G., Gerhard, I., Tilgen, W., and Runnebaum, B. (1989b). Prognostic value of in vitro sperm penetration into hormonally standardized human cervical mucus. *Fertil. Steril.* **51,** 317.

Feneux, D., Serres, C., and Jouannet, P. (1985). Sliding spermatozoa: a dyskinesia responsible for human infertility? *Fertil. Steril.* **44,** 508.

Foreman, R., Cohen, J., Fehilly, C. B., Fishel, S. B., and Edwards, R. G. (1984). The application of the zona-free hamster egg test for the prognosis of human in vitro fertilization. *J. In Vitro Fert. Embryo Transf.* **1,** 166.

Fukuda, M., Cross, N. L., Cummings-Paulson, L., and Yee, B. (1989). Correlation of acrosomal status and sperm performance in the sperm penetration assay. *Fertil. Steril.* **52,** 836.

Glazener, C.M.A., and Hull, M.G.R. (1987). The sperm-mucus interface: patterns of disorder in the diagnosis of specific causes of penetration failure causing infertility. *Hum. Reprod.* **2,** 673.

Griffith, C. S., and Grimes, D. A. (1990). The validity of the postcoital test. *Am. J. Obstet. Gynecol.* **162,** 615.

Haas, G. G., Jr., and Beer, A. E. (1986). Immunologic influences on reproductive biology: sperm gametogenesis and maturation in the male and female genital tracts. *Fertil. Steril.* **46,** 753.

Hull, M.G.R., Savage, P. E., and Bromham, D. R. (1982). Prognostic value of the postcoital test: prospective study based on time-specific conception rates. *Br. J. Obstet. Gynaecol.* **89**, 299.

Jeulin, C., Feneux, D., Serres, C., Jouannet, P., Guillet-Rosso, F., Belaisch-Allart, J., Frydman, R., and Testart, J. (1986). Sperm factors related to failure of human in-vitro fertilization. *J. Reprod. Fertil.* **76**, 735.

Johnson, L. (1982). A reevaluation of daily sperm output of men. *Fertil. Steril.* **37**, 811.

Jones, W. R. (1980). Immunologic infertility—fact or fiction? *Fertil. Steril.* **33**, 577.

Jouannet, P., Ducot, B., Feneux, D., and Spira, A. (1988). Male factors and the likelihood of pregnancy in infertile couples. I. Study of sperm characteristics. *Int. J. Androl.* **11**, 379.

Katz, D. F., Diel, L., and Overstreet, J. W. (1982). Differences in the movement of morphologically normal and abnormal human seminal spermatozoa. *Biol. Reprod.* **26**, 566.

Kremer, J., and Jager S. (1988). Sperm-cervical mucus interaction, in particular in the presence of antispermatozoal antibodies. *Hum. Reprod.* **3**, 69.

Kruger, T. F., Acosta, A. A., Simmons, K. F., Swanson, R. J., Matta, J. F., and Oehninger, S. (1988). Predictive value of abnormal sperm morphology in in vitro fertilization. *Fertil. Steril.* **49**, 112.

Kruger, T. F., Menkveld, R., Stander, F.S.H., Lombard, C. J., Van der Merwe, J. P., van Zyl, J. A., and Smith, K. (1986). Sperm morphologic features as a prognostic factor in in vitro fertilization. *Fertil. Steril.* **46**, 1118.

Liu, D. Y., and Baker, H.W.G. (1988). The proportion of human sperm with poor morphology but normal intact acrosomes detected with pisum sativum agglutinin correlates with fertilization in vitro. *Fertil. Steril.* **50**, 288.

Liu, D. Y., Clarke, G. N., Lopata, A., Johnston, W.I.H., and Baker, H. W. G. (1989). A sperm-zona pellucida binding test and in vitro fertilization. *Fertil. Steril.* **52**, 281.

Liu, D. Y., Lopata, A., and Baker, H.W.G. (1990). Use of oocytes that failed to be fertilized *in vitro* to study human sperm-oocyte interactions: comparison of sperm-oolemma and sperm-zona pellucida binding, and relationship with results of IVF. *Reprod. Fertil. Dev.* **2**, 641.

Margalioth, E. J., Feinmesser, M., Navot, D., Mordel, N., and Bronson, R. A. (1989). The long-term predictive value of the zona-free hamster ova sperm penetration assay. *Fertil. Steril.* **52**, 490.

Margalioth, E. J., Navot, D., Laufer, N., Lewin, A., Rabinowitz, R., and Schenker, J. G. (1986). Correlation between the zona-free hamster egg sperm penetration assay and human in vitro fertilization. *Fertil. Steril.* **45**, 665.

Margalioth, E. J., Navot, D., Laufer, N., Yosef, S. M., Rabinowitz, R., Yarkoni, S., and Schenker, J. G. (1983). Zona-free hamster ovum penetration assay as a screening procedure for in vitro fertilization. *Fertil. Steril.* **40**, 386.

McClure, R. D., Tom, R. A., and Dandekar, P. V. (1990). Optimizing the sperm penetration assay with human follicular fluid. *Fertil. Steril.* **53**, 546.

Meinertz, H., Linnet, L., Fogh-Anderson, P., and Hjort, T. (1990). Antisperm antibodies and fertility after vasovasostomy: a follow-up study of 216 men. *Fertil. Steril.* **54**, 315.

Menge, A. C., Medley, N. E., Mangione, C. M., and Dietrich, J. W. (1982). The incidence and influence of antisperm antibodies in infertile human couples on sperm-cervical mucus interactions and subsequent fertility. *Fertil. Steril.* **38**, 439.

Mortimer, D. (1990). Objective analysis of sperm motility and kinematics. In Keel, B. A., and Webster, B. W. (eds): *Handbook of the Laboratory Diagnosis and Treatment of Infertility.* CRC Press, Boca Raton, FL.

Mortimer, D. (1991). Clinical significance of antisperm antibodies. *J. Soc. Obstet. Gynaecol. Can.* **13,** 69.

Mortimer, D., Courtot, A. M., Giovangrandi, Y., Jeulin, C., and David, G. (1984). Human sperm motility after migration into, and incubation in, synthetic media. *Gamete Res.* **9,** 131.

Mortimer, D., Mortimer, S. T., Shu, M. A., and Swart, R. (1990). A simplified approach to sperm-cervical mucus interaction testing using a hyaluronate migration test. *Hum. Reprod.* **5,** 835.

Mortimer, D., Mortimer, S. T., Anderson, S. J., and Robertson, L. (1991) Hyperactivated motility of human spermatozoa. In Baccetti, B. (ed): *Comparative Spermatology 20 Years After.* Raven Press, New York.

Mortimer, D., Pandya, I. J., and Sawers, R. S. (1986a). Human sperm morphology and the outcome of modified Kremer tests. *Andrologia* **18,** 376.

Mortimer, D., Pandya, I. J., and Sawers, R. S. (1986b). Relationship between human sperm motility characteristics and sperm penetration into human cervical mucus in vitro. *J. Reprod. Fertil.* **78,** 93.

Mortimer, S. T., and Mortimer, D. (1990). Kinematics of human spermatozoa incubated under capacitating conditions. *J. Androl.* **11,** 195.

Oehninger, S., Coddington, C. C., Scott, R., Franken, D. A., Burkman, L. J., Acosta, A. A., and Hodgen, G. D. (1989). Hemizona assay: assessment of sperm dysfunction and prediction of in vitro fertilization outcome. *Fertil. Steril.* **51,** 665.

Pattinson, H. A., and Mortimer, D. (1987). Prevalence of sperm surface antibodies in the male partners of infertile couples as determined by Immunobead screening. *Fertil. Steril.* **48,** 466.

Plachot, M., Mandelbaum, J., and Junca, A.-M. (1984). Acrosome reaction of human sperm used for in vitro fertilization. *Fertil. Steril.* **42,** 418.

Robertson, L., Wolf, D. P., and Tash, J. S. (1988). Temporal changes in motility parameters related to acrosomal status: identification and characterization of populations of hyperactivated human sperm. *Biol. Reprod.* **39,** 805.

Rogers, B. J., Bentwood, B. J., Van Campen, H., Helmbrecht, G., Soderdahl, D., and Hale, R. W. (1983). Sperm morphology assessment as an indicator of human fertilizing capacity. *J. Androl.* **4,** 119.

Rose, N. R., Hjort, T., Rumke, P., Harper, M.J.K., and Vyazov, O. (1976). Techniques for detection of iso- and auto-antibodies to human spermatozoa. *Clin. Exp. Immunol.* **23,** 175.

Schill, W.-B., Töpfer-Petersen, E., and Heissler, E. (1988). The sperm acrosome: functional and clinical aspects. *Hum. Reprod.* **3,** 139.

Shy, K. K., Stenchever, M. A., and Muller, C. H. (1988). Sperm penetration assay and subsequent pregnancy: A prospective study of 74 infertile men. *Obstet. Gynecol.* **71,** 685.

Smith, K. D., Rodriguez-Rigau, L. J., and Steinberger, E. (1977). Relation between indices of semen analysis and pregnancy rate in infertile couples. *Fertil. Steril.* **28,** 1314.

Templeton, A. A., and Mortimer, D. (1982). The development of a clinical test of sperm migration to the site of fertilization. *Fertil. Steril.* **37,** 410.

Templeton, A. A., Aitken, J., Mortimer, D., and Best, F.S.M. (1982). Sperm function in patients with unexplained infertility. *Br. J. Obstet. Gynaecol.* **89,** 550.

Tsukui, S., Noda, Y., Yano, J., Fukuda, A., and Mori, T. (1986). Inhibition of sperm penetration through human zona pellucida by antisperm antibodies. *Fertil. Steril.* **46,** 92.

Vazquez-Levin, M., Kaplan, P., Sandler, B., Garrisi, G. J., Gordon, J., and Navot, D. (1990). The predictive values of zona-free hamster egg sperm penetration assay for failure of human in vitro fertilization and subsequent successful zona drilling. *Fertil. Steril.* **53,** 1055.

Wolf, D. P., Sokoloski, J. E., and Quigley, M. M. (1983). Correlation of human in vitro fertilization with the hamster egg bioassay. *Fertil. Steril.* **40,** 53.

World Health Organization (1992). *WHO Laboratory Manual for the Examination of Human Semen and Sperm-Cervical Mucus Interaction, 3rd ed.* Cambridge University Press, Cambridge.

III

Therapeutic Procedures

12

Sperm Washing

To be potentially functional ejaculate spermatozoa must be separated from seminal plasma quickly and efficiently. Prolonged exposure to seminal plasma results in marked declines in both sperm motility and vitality, which is not the case if spermatozoa are incubated for comparable periods in synthetic culture medium free of seminal plasma contamination. By virtue of constituents that inhibit or reverse capacitation, the presence of seminal plasma in in vitro fertilization systems inhibits the occurrence of acrosome reactions and hence the fertilizing ability of the spermatozoa.

Prolonged exposure to seminal plasma after ejaculation for periods of more than 30 minutes can permanently diminish the fertilizing capacity of human spermatozoa in vitro (Rogers et al., 1983). Furthermore, contamination of prepared sperm populations with only small concentrations of seminal plasma can diminish, or even totally inhibit, their fertilizing capacity (Kanwar et al., 1979). It is clearly essential, therefore, that spermatozoa for clinical procedures such as IVF, GIFT, or IUI and for laboratory tests of sperm fertilizing ability, must be separated from the seminal environment as soon as possible after ejaculation.

In general terms, four basic approaches exist for separating spermatozoa from semen: (1) simple dilution and washing; (2) sperm migration; (3) selective washing procedures; and (4) adherence methods for the elimination of debris and dead spermatozoa. The success of such methods is often assessed by their yield of motile spermatozoa (see below). Other relevant considerations include the cost of a procedure in terms of the time taken, materials used, and necessary apparatus, as well as the likely level of contamination with seminal components and the possible exposure of the spermatozoa to deleterious influences during the process. Obviously, the fertilizing capacity of a sperm population after processing is another significant factor that may be particularly important with compromised sperm populations such as those recovered from postretrograde ejaculation urine or cryopreserved spermatozoa.

YIELD CALCULATIONS

The success or applicability of a sperm-washing method can be considered in terms of either the absolute or relative yield of motile spermatozoa one obtains at the end of the technique. Usually, progressive motility is used, as nonprogressive spermatozoa are unlikely to be potentially functional. Although hyperactivation starts to

267

appear soon after the separation of human spermatozoa in a suitable culture medium, it affects only a small proportion of the cells at this time; and they are switching between progressive patterns of motility and true hyperactivation anyway.

Relative Yield

Relative yield is the proportion of progressively motile spermatozoa one submits to a preparative procedure that are present in the final preparation. It is calculated as:

$$\text{Yield (\%)} = \frac{v \times c \times \text{pm\%}}{V \times C \times \text{PM\%}} \times 100$$

where:
v = volume of sperm preparation (ml)
V = volume of semen used for the procedure (ml)
c = sperm concentration in the prepared population (10^6/ml)
C = sperm concentration in the semen sample (10^6/ml)
pm% = progressive motility of the prepared sperm population (decimal)
PM% = progressive motility in the semen sample (decimal)

Asbolute Yield

Absolute yield is simply the total number of progressively motile spermatozoa one can obtain from a whole ejaculate submitted to the preparative procedure. One usually makes some allowance for the aliquots needed to perform a standard semen analysis (see Chapter 3) and then extrapolates from a relative yield derived from a preparation trial to the remainder of the ejaculate.

Yield Quality

If the product is not a clean preparation of motile spermatozoa, the quality of the product may also be important. This point may be considered in terms of the proportions of progressively motile or morphologically normal spermatozoa. The useful sperm preparative techniques recommended below give a high proportion of motile spermatozoa.

The ultimate selection criterion clearly is the established functional capacity of the prepared sperm populations (see above).

CULTURE MEDIA FOR HUMAN SPERMATOZOA

Many culture media are used experimentally and clinically for human spermatozoa, and it is impossible to provide detailed recipes for them all. However, a selection of more commonly used media is provided in Table 12-1. Instructions for the preparation of a medium commonly used in andrology laboratories to prepare spermatozoa for such clinical uses as IVF, GIFT, or IUI (human tubal fluid, or HTF medium) (Quinn et al., 1985) are provided below.

Table 12–1 Commonly used culture media for human spermatozoa

Medium	Acronym	Refs.
Biggers, Whitten, & Whittingham	BWW	1
Earle's balanced salts	EBS	2
Ham's F10	F10	2–4
Human tubal fluid	HTF	5
Lopata's medium		6
Ménézo's B_2	B_2	7,8
Ménézo's B_3	B_3	8
Modified Krebs-Ringer-bicarbonate	KRB	9
Synthetic tubal fluid	STF	10
Whittingham's T6 (modified Tyrode's)	T6	11,12

1. Biggers, J. D., Whitten, W. K., and Whittingham, D. G. (1971). The culture of mouse embryos *in vitro*. In Daniel, J. C., Jr. (ed): *Methods in Mammalian Embryology*. W. H. Freeman, San Francisco.

2. Purdy, J. M. (1982). Methods for fertilization and embryo culture *in vitro*. In Edwards, R. G., and Purdy, J. M. (eds): *Human Conception* in Vitro. Academic Press, London.

3. Lopata, A., Johnston, I. W. H., Hoult, I. J., and Speirs, A. I. (1980). Pregnancy following intrauterine implantation of an embryo obtained by in vitro fertilization of a preovulatory egg. *Fertil. Steril.* **33,** 117.

4. Dandekar, P. V., and Quigley, M. M. (1984). Laboratory setup for human in vitro fertilization. *Fertil. Steril.* **42,** 1.

5. Quinn, P. J., Kerin, J. F., and Warnes, G. M. (1985). Improved pregnancy rate in human in vitro fertilization with the use of a medium based on the composition of human tubal fluid. *Fertil. Steril.* **44,** 493.

6. Lopata, A., Patullo, M. J., Chang, A., and James, B. (1976). A method for collecting motile spermatozoa from human semen. *Fertil. Steril.* **27,** 677.

7. Ménézo, Y. (1976). Milieu synethétique pour la survie et la maturation des gamètes et pour la culture de l'oeuf fécondé. *C. R. Acad. Sci. [D]* **272,** 1967.

8. Menezo, Y., Testart, J., and Perrone, D. (1984). Serum is not necessary in human in vitro fertilization, early embryo culture, and transfer. *Fertil. Steril.* **42,** 750.

9. Nishimoto, T., Yamada, I., Niwa, K., Mori, T., Nishimura, T., and Iritani, A. (1982). Sperm penetration *in vitro* of human oocytes matured in a chemically defined medium. *J. Reprod. Fertil.* **64,** 115.

10. Mortimer, D. (1986). Elaboration of a new culture medium for physiological studies on human sperm motility and capacitation. *Hum. Reprod.* **1,** 247.

11. Quinn, P., Warnes, G. M., Kerin, J. F., and Kirby, C. (1984). Culture factors in relation to the success of human in vitro fertilization and embryo transfer. *Fertil. Steril.* **41,** 202.

12. Caro, C. M., and Trounson, A. (1986). Successful fertilization, embryo development, and pregnancy in human in vitro fertilization (IVF) using a chemically defined culture medium containing no protein. *J. In Vitro Fert. Embryo Transf.* **3,** 215.

Preparation of HTF Culture Medium

Principle

Various laboratory and clinical applications require preparations of washed, selected motile spermatozoa in a culture medium capable of sustaining their metabolism in vitro. This simple culture medium was developed from the composition of human oviduct fluid (Quinn et al., 1985) and has proved useful for in vitro studies and clinical applications including IVF, GIFT, and IUI. A Hepes-buffered variant is best for sperm-washing applications (see below).

Reagents

Water must be of tissue culture grade prepared using a combination of activated carbon filtration, reverse osmosis, deionization, organic substances and pyrogen extraction, and ultrafiltration.

Chemicals should all be of at least analytical grade, and preferably tissue culture tested (see Chapter 1).

Method

1. Dissolve the following chemicals in about 600 ml tissue culture grade water in a 1000-ml volumetric flask:

    5.938 g NaCl
    0.350 g KCl
    0.049 g $MgSO_4·7H_2O$
    0.050 g KH_2PO_4
    0.420 g $NaHCO_3$
    0.036 g Na pyruvate
    0.501 g Glucose
    0.003 g Phenol red
    4.766 g Hepes free acid
    3.136 ml Na lactate (60% syrup)
    2.400 ml NaOH 5 N

2. Mix until dissolved.
3. Separately, dissolve 0.300g $CaCl_2·2H_2O$ in about 100 ml tissue culture grade water. Add slowly, with thorough mixing, to the stock HTF solution.
4. Make up to 1000 ml with additional tissue culture grade water and mix thoroughly by inversion.
5. Add 10.0 g HSA (see Quality Control, point 1, below) and mix thoroughly but carefully by inversion. Beware of frothing.
6. Adjust to pH 7.5–7.6 using 1 N HCl or 1 N NaOH. These solutions must also be prepared in tissue culture grade water.
7. Check that the osmolarity is 280–290 mOsm.
8. Filter-sterilize into sterile plastic containers (e.g., Falcon 3013 or 3024 flasks) under positive pressure through either:
    a. Autoclaved Millipore Swinnex 25 units containing a Durapore (GVWP) 0.22-μm membrane and AP-25 depth type prefilter; or
    b. 60 mm Millipak-20 filter unit.
9. Label HTF+HSA and store at 4°C for a maximum of 6 months (probably less if it is to be used for IVF, e.g., 35 days, but see item 1 under Quality Control, below). Discard if there are any signs of contamination or sedimentation.
10. Warm to 37°C before use. Discard any unused portions of opened containers.

N.B. For sperm capacitation the Hepes and NaOH 5N should be omitted and the $NaHCO_3$ increased to 2.100 g.

Quality Control

1. Clinical applications of sperm washing where the sperm suspension is to be inseminated into the female reproductive tract require that albumin from hepatitis- and HIV-screened donors be used in the culture medium. Although the commonly used HSA fraction V preparations (e.g., Sigma A-1653) are acceptable for experimental applications and are probably suitable for this purpose, they are *not* licensed for any such in vivo use. Other products should be used for clinical procedures involving transfer of any culture medium into the body, e.g., Cat. No. 5020 fraction V HSA preparation from Irvine Scientific (Santa Ana, CA, USA), which has been shown, by Food and Drug Administration (FDA)-approved methods, to be free of hepatitis B and HIV-I. It should also be noted that the high-concentration HSA solutions (e.g., 25% w/v) available from some suppliers contain chemicals to stabilize the protein from flocculating. A common substance used for this purpose is sodium caprilate, a detergent that is certainly harmful to mouse embryos and must be considered potentially dangerous to human gametes and embryos (see also Chapter 13).
2. The osmometer and balance should be calibrated against appropriate standards before use.
3. For some clinical applications each batch of medium should be tested in a suitable bioassay to verify its acceptability. Although the two-cell mouse embryo to blastocyst culture system is commonly used, it is probably insufficiently sensitive; and a zygote to blastocyst culture system should be considered (Fleetham et al., 1993).

DILUTION AND WASHING TECHNIQUES

Simple dilution of the semen with a relatively large volume of culture medium, typically 5–10 times volume, and separation of the spermatozoa by centrifugation is the simplest method for washing spermatozoa. Repeat centrifugation of the spermatozoa resuspended from the pellet (usually two or three times) is commonly used to ensure adequate removal of contaminating seminal plasma. During these centrifugation steps it is essential that forces greater than 800 *g* are not used (Jeulin et al., 1982).

This procedure has the great disadvantage that all the spermatozoa, including the dead, moribund, and abnormal ones present in the original semen remain in the final sperm population. The presence of these nonfunctional gametes may be detrimental by inhibiting capacitation and increasing the risk of developing antisperm antibodies if inseminated into the uterine cavity at IUI.

Furthermore, it has been demonstrated that if semen is centrifuged prior to the isolation of motile spermatozoa, resulting in the good spermatozoa being pelleted along with the dead and moribund spermatozoa and other cellular elements of semen, the functional potential of the motile cells, even when isolated later, is impaired (Aitken and Clarkson, 1988). These authors demonstrated that centrifugal pelleting of unselected sperm populations from human ejaculates caused the production of reactive oxygen species (superoxide and hydroxyl radicals) within the pellet that induced irreversible damage to the spermatozoa and impairment of their fertilizing ability in the HEPT. Superoxide radicals cause peroxidation of sperm plasma membrane phospholipids, and elevated superoxide production has been implicated in defective sperm function at the cellular level (Aitken and Clarkson, 1987).

Within the pellet there are "good" spermatozoa, senescent and dead spermatozoa, numerous types of leukocytes, germinal line cells, some epithelial cells, anucleate cytoplasmic bodies [presumably residual cytoplasmic masses (RCMs) from round spermatids released from the seminiferous epithelium at spermiation] and particulate debris. The reactive oxygen species generated in these pellets come not only from the spermatozoa themselves but also from neutrophils and macrophages present in the original semen sample. In particular, it is a population of low-density spermatozoa (as isolated on Percoll gradients) (Aitken and Clarkson, 1988) that produce superoxide radicals, i.e., spermatozoa with a relatively high cytoplasmic volume. This defective subpopulation therefore includes immature spermatozoa, which typically have cytoplasmic droplets, and some morphologically abnormal spermatozoa with excess residual cytoplasm.

This evidence clearly indicates that any sperm preparation method involving the centrifugal pelleting of unselected seminal sperm populations should be abandoned (review: Mortimer, 1991). Whether the same problem occurs with techniques whereby spermatozoa are spun onto a soft, fluid cushion (which is considered to minimize mechanical damage) before being allowed to resuspend themselves by virtue of their own motility (e.g., Makler et al., 1984) remains to be determined.

MIGRATION TECHNIQUES

In vivo the potentially functional sperm population is separated from liquefied semen by virtue of their migration into cervical mucus (see Chapter 2). Consequently, sperm preparation techniques involving a self-migration step are widely used. Variations on this theme are numerous, including the classic "swim-up" from liquefied semen into an overlay of culture medium (which may or may not contain other substances such as Ficoll to help stabilize the interface); "swim-down" into one or more layers of culture medium containing bovine serum albumin; swimming through porous membranes or meshes; or the "jump-over," or migration-sedimentation, approach, which uses a combination of migration and gravitational sedimentation.

Swim-Up from Semen

For the swim-up procedure aliquots of semen are taken from a sample as soon as it is liquefied and placed in tubes underneath a layer of culture medium. A series of tubes is prepared with each tube containing the required volume of culture medium. Round-bottom tubes (e.g., Falcon No. 2001 or 2037) should be used to optimize the surface area of the interface between the semen layer and the culture medium; and although the tubes may be prepared by gently layering culture medium over the liquefied semen, the reverse procedure provides a much cleaner interface zone.

The semen to be used for underlayering is gently aspirated into a sterile plastic syringe of a brand known not to have any deleterious effects on spermatozoa (de Ziegler et al., 1987). A 19-gauge needle is attached, the syringe plunger depressed to expel the air deadspace, and the needle tip passed through the culture medium layer to the bottom of the tube. After careful expulsion of the required volume of semen, the needle is withdrawn from the tube and the process repeated along the series of tubes. A sterile Pasteur pipette and volumetric controller may also be used.

With viscous semen samples, culture medium may be mixed with the semen prior to loading into the syringe; "needling" of viscous semen (i.e., its forceful expulsion one or more times through a 19- or 22-gauge needle) should be avoided except in extreme cases due to deleterious effects of the high shear forces on the spermatozoa (see Viscous Semen Samples, below).

To maximize the yield of this method, multiple tubes with relatively small volumes of semen per tube are used to increase the total interface area between semen and culture medium. We typically use 200-250 µl of semen under 500–800 µl of culture medium per tube. Tubes are usually incubated at an angle (typically 20–45 degrees to the horizontal), which again serves to increase the interface. After an appropriate period of incubation at 37°C—the longer the incubation the greater the yield, although it should not exceed 60 minutes—most of the upper culture medium layer is removed. This step is done carefully, working from the upper miniscus downward using a sterile Pasteur pipette or an automatic pipette. Typically, 75–80% of the culture medium layer is removed, taking great care not to aspirate directly from the interface region.

Each migration tube is harvested separately and the individual preparations combined only after ascertaining that they contain high proportions of motile spermatozoa (typically > 90% or even 95% motile) and are not contaminated with debris or other cellular elements from the semen fraction.

This combined preparation is then usually centrifuged at 600 g for 6–10 minutes and resuspended into fresh culture medium at the desired concentration of motile spermatozoa. If a small aliquot of the preparation is kept back while the rest is being centrifuged, Makler chamber or Microcell sperm concentration and motility counts may be completed during the centrifugation period.

Swim-Up from a Washed Pellet

The swim-up procedure using a washed pellet typically involves two or three dilution and centrifugation steps to produce a pellet of spermatozoa on the bottom of a centrifuge tube that is then overlayered with a volume of culture medium; the tube, or tubes, are then incubated at 37°C to allow the spermatozoa to "rise" from the pellet. Although the pellet was originally gently resuspended into a small residual volume of supernatant before being overlayered with medium, this small, yet important point has apparently been omitted by many workers (review: Mortimer, 1991).

Although this "sperm rise" method, by virtue of the initial washing steps, is considered to give a "cleaner" sperm preparation after migration, it must now be considered suspect because of the possible deleterious effects of reactive oxygen produced in these pelletings of unselected spermatozoa (Aitken and Clarkson, 1988). The technique also suffers from a low yield, as many of the spermatozoa in the lower levels of the pellet never reach the interface with the culture medium layer, especially if conical-bottom centrifuge tubes are used.

This method has clearly been used successfully in many clinical IVF programs, demonstrating that the initial washing steps are insufficiently deleterious to completely destroy the fertilizing ability of many men's spermatozoa. Although the level of impairment that may have been induced in borderline cases is unknown, it is certainly well known that the level of IVF success achieved by male factor infertility patients is low using this procedure. Overall, although many men's spermatozoa may not be impaired to the extent of inhibiting fertilization, some couples' chances of successful IVF are certainly compromised. Clearly, one cannot justify continuing to use a technique that incorporates steps known to be prejudicial to sperm function in a significant subpopulation of patients (review: Mortimer, 1991).

Swim-Up from a Washed Sperm Preparation

The swim-up method using a washed sperm preparation also uses one or two initial washing steps to separate the unselected spermatozoa from seminal plasma and resuspend them in culture medium, from which they migrate into an overlayer of fresh medium (Russell and Rogers, 1987). Often the lower sperm suspension layer is made more viscous, to stabilize the interface, by addition of a higher concentration of albumin or a substance such as Ficoll (Cummins and Breen, 1984). Although it may produce a cleaner sperm preparation (less contamination by seminal plasma components) than swim-up from a washed pellet, like the washed pellet method this technique should also now be considered suspect (review: Mortimer, 1991).

Swim-Down Migration

The swim-down migration procedure is based on the original description of Ericsson whereby spermatozoa were prepared by layering on top of one or more layers of medium containing bovine serum albumin (Ericsson et al., 1973). During a 1-hour incubation at 37°C the most motile spermatozoa migrate down into the albumin gradient. Sperm migration down through Percoll gradients has also been proposed as a preparative technique for human spermatozoa (Pousette et al., 1986).

The albumin gradient method was originally proposed as a means for separating Y-chromosome-bearing spermatozoa, although many subsequent workers have not been able to achieve this separation, and great skepticism remains regarding its value as a method of preconceptional gender selection (Gledhill, 1988). Albumin columns have also been used in clinical IVF, where it was found to give a higher yield than the swim-up from a washed pellet method (Perrone and Testart, 1985).

Sperm Select

The commercial product Sperm Select (Select Medical Systems, Williston, VT, USA), uses a highly purified preparation of sodium hyaluronate (average 3000 kDa) at a final concentration of 1 mg/ml in culture medium. In a clinical IVF program, swim-up from semen into Sperm Select gave a significantly higher percentage of motile spermatozoa compared to swim-up from a washed pellet and, ultimately, a higher pregnancy rate (Wikland et al., 1987). Although this initial study did not establish whether these improved results were due specifically to the use of the hyaluronate rather than a method that did not involve the initial pelleting of unselected spermatozoa, a follow-up study has shown that Sperm Select is equivalent to direct swim-up from semen and confirmed that the latter method is superior to swim-up from a washed pellet (Sjöblom and Wikland, 1991).

Combined Migration-Sedimentation

The approach that combines swim-up from semen with gravitional settling of spermatozoa from the upper medium layer is referred to as combined migration-sedimentation (Tea et al., 1984). Basically, spermatozoa migrate from semen contained in a ring-shaped well that is completely overlaid with a layer of culture medium (Fig. 12-1). The central hole of the ring constitutes the collection well into which motile spermatozoa settle. This approach remains interesting and may represent a useful method for dealing with male factor semen samples. The method should be used only for samples with sluggish motility; a direct swim-up from semen is the preferred method for samples with average or better progression. Tea-Jondet tubes for this method are available commercially (BICEF/IMV, L'Aigle, France).

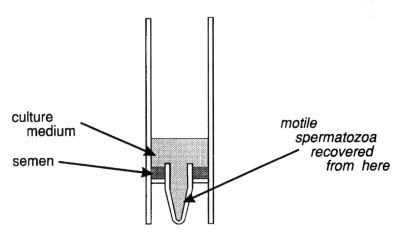

Figure 12-1 Tea-Jondet tube for the combined migration-sedimentation method for preparing spermatozoa.

Transmembrane Migration

Transmembrane migration uses an apparatus in which a motile sperm population is separated from culture medium by a Nuclepore membrane filter (Nuclepore, Pleasanton, CA, USA). These filters are unusual in that their pores are cylindrical and at right angles to the plane of the membrane. The spermatozoa therefore have straight channels in which to swim through the membrane. Unfortunately, these membranes have a low transparency (transparency = ratio of the combined cross-sectional area of the pores to the total membrane area), and as a consequence the yield is low. Primarily, this method has been used for testing the motility of sperm populations treated with various pharmacological agents, not as a preparative method (Raoof et al., 1987).

Migration Across Meshes

A study on the morphological selection of human spermatozoa resulting from self-migration utilized a double-chamber system in which the lower (semen) chamber was separated from the upper (culture medium) chamber by a nickel mesh (Mortimer et al., 1982). These meshes had relatively large pore sizes (11 μm) and high transparency. Although good yields of spermatozoa with high motility were obtained, the complicated assembly of the chambers and the fragility of the nickel mesh make it unsuitable for routine clinical use.

SELECTIVE WASHING TECHNIQUES

Selective washing techniques are based on the use of density gradient centrifugation to fractionate subpopulations of spermatozoa. During centrifugation the spermatozoa reach a position of the density gradient that matches their own density or specific gravity (their isopycnic point).

Gradient materials such as sucrose or cesium chloride are far too osmotically active to be used with live cells such as spermatozoa. Sodium metrizoate (metrizamide: Nyegaard, Oslo, Norway) was initially evaluated as a material for separating human spermatozoa but has not seen wide use. Ficoll (Pharmacia, Uppsala, Sweden) has been used as a gradient material for preparing spermatozoa (Harrison, 1976), but by far the most widely used has been Percoll (Kabi-Pharmacia; see below). Finally, Nycodenz (Nyegaard) is the latest substance to be used as a density gradient material for preparing human spermatozoa (see below).

For any of these methods the gradients may be continuous or discontinuous. With continuous gradients there is a gradual increase in density from the top of the gradient to its bottom; they are usually prepared with expensive gradient mixing machines (which cannot be kept sterile and are therefore not amenable to clinical use for sperm preparation purposes) or sometimes by "self-generation," whereby the layers of a discontinuous gradient are allowed to diffuse into each other to a limited degree, or a single solution of the gradient material is subjected to very high centrifugal forces and the gradient is generated by gravitational separation of the gradient substance particles. A discontinuous gradient is composed of several layers with more or less discrete boundaries between them. These layers can lead to the problem of "rafting" of cells at the interface(s), although passage through such interfaces may be advantageous when selecting the best spermatozoa.

Percoll

Numerous Percoll-based gradients have been described of both the continuous and discontinuous types (review: Mortimer, 1990). Some authors have reported deleterious effects of Percoll gradient centrifugation on the ultrastructural integrity of human spermatozoa and on their longevity as measured by motility maintenance. However, normal sperm function as assessed in the zona pellucida-free hamster egg penetration test, as well as in human IVF, GIFT, and SUZI procedures, clearly indicate differences between Percoll gradient methods.

Sperm populations prepared by Percoll gradients, although having the advantage of being essentially free of any bacteria that were present in the original semen, may contain small quantities of Percoll particles. There has been great concern over the possible dangers of using such preparations for IUI, as Percoll consists of polyvinylpyrrolidone-coated silica particles, and silica is an established tissue irritant. This preparation method has been used for some time by several IUI programs with no untoward effects.

Another concern is the finding that some batches of Percoll contain high levels of endotoxin contamination, which although they may not affect sperm fertilizing ability may be deleterious to zygotes and early cleavage stages, as well as perhaps having some possible untoward effect in vivo. It is strongly advised that each new batch of Percoll be tested for endotoxins using the *Limulus polyphemus* amebocyte lysate (LAL) assay (e.g., Sigma Kit 210 E-TOXATE assay) and used only if shown to be endotoxin-free.

These concerns, in conjunction with the low yields usually seen with Percoll gradients for abnormal semen samples (especially those with low sperm motility), has led to the investigation of alternative gradient materials.

Although highly specialized Percoll gradients have been reported to separate human X- and Y-bearing spermatozoa (Mohri et al., 1987), recent studies have refuted this claim (van Kooij and van Oost, 1992). Furthermore, it must be remembered that such gradients are much more complex than the simple ones used to prepare washed motile spermatozoa. There are no indications that these simple gradients have any influence on the sex ratio of the prepared sperm populations. The most practical Percoll gradient procedures use small, discontinuous gradients with only two, occasionally three, layers. A detailed method for a simple two-step discontinuous Percoll gradient with optimized quantitative and sperm motility yields compared to other Percoll gradients (c.f., Dravland and Mortimer, 1985: 0.5 ml layers of 95.0% and 47.5% v/v Percoll; or World Health Organization, 1992: 3.0-ml layers of 72% and 36% v/v Percoll) is provided below.

A reduced-volume, discontinuous mini-Percoll gradient has also been described for particular use with severe oligoasthenozoospermic male factor cases (total motile count $< 5 \times 10^6$/ejaculate) (Ord et al., 1990). This gradient uses three 0.3-ml layers of 50%, 70%, and 95% isotonic Percoll (i.e., 45%, 63%, and 85.5% v/v Percoll), respectively. The requirement for an initial washing step in this method must cause some concern, and it is interesting to note that the inclusion of pentoxifylline (a potent scavenger of reactive oxygen radicals; see below) in this initial wash produced a substantial improvement in fertilization rates at IVF (Ord et al., 1991). Mini-Percoll gradients, prepared in conical centrifuge tubes and loaded with the washed sperm pellet resuspended in 0.3 ml of culture medium, are centrifuged at 300 g for 30–45 minutes. After centrifugation the lower Percoll layer is removed and the spermatozoa washed twice using fresh medium.

One study has reported improved yields using a high osmolarity Percoll gradient; that is, one whose osmolarity is closer to that of semen than serum: 360 mOsm versus 290 mOsm (Velez de la Calle, 1991). This approach warrants further investigation.

Reagents

Percoll is purchased from Kabi-Pharmacia (Uppsala, Sweden).

Culture medium is whatever is to be used for the final resuspension of the prepared sperm population: for the present purpose it is assumed that HTF medium, supplemented with HSA 10 mg/ml (1.0% w/v) is used.

10× Buffer is a 10× concentrated version of the standard HTF recipe, including 10.0% HSA. Adjust the pH to 7.4 and filter-sterilize (see Preparation of HTF Culture Medium, above).

Method

1. Prepare the isotonic (90% v/v) Percoll solution by mixing 9 volumes of stock Percoll with 1 volume of 10× buffer.
2. Take two sterile conical-bottom centrifuge tubes (e.g., Falcon 2095, 2096, or 2097) and mark one B (bottom layer) and the other T (top layer). Measure the required materials using *sterile* pipettes and mix thoroughly by inversion after tightly recapping the tubes.
   a. *Top layer:* Mix 4.5 ml isotonic 90% Percoll and 5.5 ml HTF medium.
   b. *Bottom layer:* Mix 9.0 ml isotonic 90% Percoll with 1.0 ml HTF medium.
3. Place 1.5 ml of layer B into the bottom of each of two sterile Falcon *conical* bottom centrifuge tubes. Carefully layer 1.5 ml of layer T on top of these bottom layers. Use an automatic (e.g., Gilson) pipettor and sterile tips.
4. Layer up to 1.5 ml liquefied semen onto each gradient using sterile pipette tips. Additional pairs of gradients are required to process more than 3.0 ml of semen.

5. Centrifuge the gradients at 300 g for 20 minutes.
6. Remove the seminal plasma and upper interface material and discard.
7. Using a clean sterile 9-inch Pasteur pipette, remove the soft pellets from the bottom of the gradients and combine in a clean centrifuge tube. Measure the combined volume and bring to 6.1 ml total volume using culture medium.
8. Remove 100 µl and determine the sperm concentration and motility using a Makler chamber or Microcell. While doing this procedure the remaining 6.0 ml is centrifuged at 600 g for 6–10 minutes in a conical-bottom tube.
9. Remove the supernatant, leaving about 0.2 ml to resuspend the pellet. Make up to an appropriate total volume with fresh medium to give a sperm suspension of the required concentration of motile spermatozoa.

Nycodenz

Concern over the possible inflammatory responses that could be induced by the insemination of sperm populations contaminated with Percoll (Percoll being approved for in vitro use only) and the poor yields obtained from male factor semen samples on Percoll gradients prompted the evaluation of possible alternative gradient materials. Nycodenz (Nyegaard, Oslo, Norway) is the same molecule, iohexol, as used in the x-ray contrast medium Omnipaque commonly employed for angiography. Continuous and discontinuous Nycodenz gradients have been evaluated, and a five-layer discontinuous gradient was found to produce populations of highly motile spermatozoa with better yields and survival than either swim-up or Percoll gradients from oligozoospermic and asthenozoospermic semen samples (Gellert-Mortimer et al., 1988).

A study comparing Nycodenz and Percoll gradient prepared spermatozoa for use in the HEPT reported comparable results for the two methods, with both being significantly better than swim-up from a washed pellet (Serafini et al., 1990). This technique clearly has great potential in the preparation of motile spermatozoa from poor quality semen for IVF use and warrants further investigation.

ADHERENCE METHODS

Adherence methods are based on the "sticking-to-glass" phenomenon. It is well known that dead and moribund spermatozoa are "sticky" and attach to glass surfaces even in the presence of relatively high concentrations of protein.

Glass Wool Column Filtration

The use of a glass wool column, prepared by filling Pasteur pipettes with glass wool fibers, has been reported to remove most of the debris as well as agglutinated and dead spermatozoa from semen samples (Paulson and Polakoski, 1977; Rhemrev et al., 1989). In addition, the total viscosity of semen samples is usually reduced.

Although this simple procedure was considered to have potential clinical significance, a subsequent report indicated that filtration by glass wool induces damage to the sperm plasma membrane and acrosome in some spermatozoa (Sherman et al., 1981). Furthermore, the real danger of glass wool fragments in the final sperm population urges caution when using such preparations for artificial insemination.

It has been shown that glass wool column filtration yields a higher recovery of viable spermatozoa than the swim-up procedure and that the sperm preparations retain their ability to fertilize human oocytes in vitro (Van der Ven et al., 1988). This technique therefore has clear application for clinical IVF, perhaps especially for men with poor quality semen because of its high yield. Application of this technique to GIFT procedures must, however, be viewed with concern.

Glass Beads

The glass beads method, which is used widely for the preparation of hamster spermatozoa for in vitro capacitation, has been shown to select motile human spermatozoa from semen efficiently and with high yields (Daya et al., 1987). The relatively large size of the glass beads also alleviates concerns regarding their possible carry-over into an inseminate preparation.

It should be noted that, as with glass wool column filtration, this method prepares motile spermatozoa from diluted semen. Consequently, the initial preparation should be subjected to at least one cycle of subsequent washing before using for IVF, GIFT, IUI, or in vitro capacitation.

Sephadex Columns

Another selective filtration method uses Sephadex columns (SpermPrep: ZBL Inc., Lexington, KY, USA) and has been reported to achieve qualitative improvements in sperm motility and morphology, coupled with decreased debris contamination, similar to those with a washed pellet swim-up. In addition to providing a significantly higher yield, processing time is substantially reduced.

Unfortunately, the need to wash the specimen prior to loading it onto the column made the original version of this method of suspect application for any but normal men due to the problems of free radical generation (see above). However, the development of an improved column (SpermPrep II), which allows filtration of semen that has simply been diluted 1:1 with culture medium (Zavos, 1991), could well make this approach of great future interest.

CLINICAL APPLICATIONS

Sperm Washing and Microbiology

It is important that sperm preparations for clinical use (IVF, GIFT, or IUI) or for long-term incubation in vitro should be free of microbiological contaminants that may be present in semen (see Chapter 6). Several studies have examined the carryover of bacterial contaminants during sperm washing and have concluded that both sperm migration and Percoll gradient procedures yield sperm preparations essentially free of bacteria (review: Mortimer, 1990). The use of culture medium supplemented with antibiotics is certainly advantageous in this respect, although problems may be encountered when preparing spermatozoa for IUI in patients allergic to, for example, penicillin.

Choice of Sperm-Washing Method

The swim-up from semen procedure remains the simplest means of obtaining populations of highly motile human spermatozoa, and it has been recommended for sperm fertilizing ability tests by the WHO (World Health Organization, 1987, 1992). Depending on the absolute yield required, it can also be a rapid procedure when working with normal semen samples that contain large concentrations of highly motile spermatozoa. Abnormal semen samples, especially those with increased viscosity, may benefit from prior filtration on a glass bead column. The initial motile sperm preparation should be washed centrifugally once (perhaps twice) to ensure minimum seminal plasma contamination of the final preparation.

For normal semen samples there are several two-layer discontinuous Percoll gradients described in the literature that are both rapid and simple procedures giving excellent yields. However, for asthenozoospermic samples the results are often disappointing, and a Nycodenz gradient may be the method of choice for such samples.

Because of the risks of potentially severe detrimental effects on the spermatozoa, methods involving initial centrifugal washing steps resulting in the pelleting of unselected spermatozoa (e.g., swim-up from a washed pellet or a washed sperm suspension) should clearly be discontinued forthwith (review: Mortimer, 1991).

The acceptable yield from a preparative method requires consideration of the ultimate use of the sperm population. For example, IUI requires some 5 million motile spermatozoa in a 100-μl volume for insemination, whereas IVF or GIFT require only 50,000–100,000 motile spermatozoa per oocyte or per oviduct, although one may need larger numbers in male factor cases to improve the likelihood of successful fertilization. Finally, experimental studies on human sperm physiology often require large numbers of spermatozoa, and the ultimate clinical applicability of such studies depends on being able to obtain sufficient numbers of spermatozoa not only from donor samples but also from the ejaculates of patients undergoing infertility investigations.

Choosing an appropriate sperm preparation method should take into account not only the relative simplicity and rapidity of a method, for reasons of laboratory efficiency but also the quality of the semen samples that are likely to be encountered and the absolute yield required. One must also remember that an individual man's response to a given preparation method, in terms of the motile sperm yield, is not necessarily constant with time. Furthermore, there may well be substantial interindividual variability in the method providing optimum yield even for samples of apparently comparable semen quality.

Viscous Semen Samples

Obtaining satisfactory sperm yields from highly viscous semen samples remains a major problem for laboratories providing services to assisted conception programs. Because the practice of needling viscous semen (forcibly passing it through a 19- or 22-gauge syringe needle one or more times) to reduce its viscosity is now eschewed (Knuth et al., 1989), other, less drastic, approaches must be employed.

The simplest alternative is to mix culture medium with the viscous semen and then use the less viscous mixture for loading onto Percoll gradients or underlayering for direct swim-up migration. Mixing is achieved by swirling the sample container, nonvigorous agitation, or gentle pipetting through a wide-bore serological or Pasteur pipette.

Alternatively, enzymatic liquefaction can be attempted. Early studies used trypsin, although chymotrypsin is now used more routinely (Cohen and Aafjes, 1982; Tucker et al., 1990). The semen coagulum is mixed with an approximately equal volume of protein-free culture medium containing 5 mg α-chymotrypsin (type IV-S from bovine pancreas: Sigma CHY-5S). Upon liquefaction (typically 1–5 minutes at 37°C), the sample can be processed by the chosen preparative procedure.

Stimulation of Sperm Motility

The idea of using phosphodiesterase inhibitors, principally caffeine, to stimulate sperm motility, especially that of cryopreserved spermatozoa, has been around for some time (e.g., Barkay et al., 1977). Various reports have considered theophylline, dibutyryl-cAMP, pentoxifylline, and isobutylmethylxanthine (IBMX). Unfortunately, the few clinical trials published do not support this approach (Vandeweghe et al., 1982; Barkay et al., 1984), with the exception of pentoxifylline (Yovich et al., 1990; see also below). Indeed, although caffeine may stimulate the motility of poorly motile spermatozoa, it has been shown to have detrimental effects on the most motile spermatozoa in a sample (Serres et al., 1982). Another problem for in vivo clinical use is that once spermatozoa penetrate cervical mucus or are diluted within the uterine cavity the effect of the stimulant is lost (Aitken et al., 1983). In vitro use, in conjunction with IVF, has not found great application, although again with the exception of pentoxifylline (see below).

There is some evidence to support using dibutyryl-cGMP to influence processes regulated by G proteins, although such treatments seem to act through induction of the acrosome reaction rather than via mediating motility changes. This approach may well be beneficial for clinical procedures involving mechanically assisted fertilization, where high levels of acrosome-reacted spermatozoa are required.

Treatment of human spermatozoa with pentoxifylline has been shown to stimulate fertilization in vitro and, by some (although by no means all) workers, to stimulate sperm motility (e.g., Yovich et al., 1990). Evidence has indicated, however, that the beneficial effect of pentoxifylline on human sperm function is probably not mediated through phosphodiesterase inhibition but, rather, via its powerful scavenging capacity for reactive oxygen radicals (Gavella et al., 1991). Nevertheless, its use at concentrations of the order of 3–5 mM seem to be clinically useful in male factor situations for IVF or mechanically assisted fertilization. Pentoxifylline-treated spermatozoa must, however, be used for in vitro insemination of human oocytes within 60 minutes of exposure to the drug (J. Yovich, personal communication). Although this rider does not relate to the use of such spermatozoa for SUZI, it may be prejudicial if used in conjunction with IUI.

References and Recommended Reading

Aitken, R. J., Best, F., Richardson, D. W., Schats, R., and Simm, G. (1983). Influence of caffeine on movement characteristics, fertilizing capacity and ability to penetrate cervical mucus of human spermatozoa. *J. Reprod. Fertil.* **67**, 19.

Aitken, R. J., and Clarkson, J. S. (1987). Cellular basis of defective sperm function and its association with the genesis of reactive oxygen species by human spermatozoa. *J. Reprod. Fertil.* **81**, 459.

Aitken, R. J., and Clarkson, J. S. (1988). Significance of reactive oxygen species and antioxidants in defining the efficacy of sperm preparation techniques. *J. Androl.* **9**, 367.

Barkay, J., Bartoov, B., Ben-Ezra, S., Langsam, J., Feldman, E., Gordon, S., and Zuckerman, H. (1984). The influence of in vitro caffeine treatment on human sperm morphology and fertilizing capacity. *Fertil. Steril.* **41**, 913.

Barkey, J., Zuckerman, H., Sklan, D., and Gordon, S. (1977). Effect of caffeine on increasing the motility of frozen human sperm. *Fertil. Steril.* **28**, 175.

Biggers, J. D., Whitten, W. K., and Whittingham, D. G. (1971). The culture of mouse embryos *in vitro.* In Daniel, J. C., Jr. (ed): *Methods in Mammalian Embryology.* W. H. Freeman, San Francisco.

Caro, C. M., and Trounson, A. (1986). Successful fertilization, embryo development, and pregnancy in human in vitro fertilization (IVF) using a chemically defined culture medium containing no protein. *J. In Vitro Fert. Embryo Transf.* **3**, 215.

Cohen, J., and Aafjes, J. H. (1982). Proteolytic enzymes stimulate human spermatozoal motility and in vitro hamster egg penetration. *Life Sci.* **30**, 899.

Cummins, J. M., and Breen, T. M. (1984). Separation of progressively motile spermatozoa from human semen by "sperm-rise" through a density gradient. *Aust. J. Med. Lab. Sci.* **5**, 15.

Daya, S., Gwatkin, R. B. L., and Bissessar, H. (1987). Separation of motile human spermatozoa by means of a glass bead column. *Gamete Res.* **17**, 375.

De Ziegler, D., Cedars, M. I., Hamilton, F., Moreno, T., and Meldrum, D. R. (1987). Factors influencing maintenance of sperm motility during in vitro processing. *Fertil. Steril.* **48**, 816.

Dravland, J. E., and Mortimer, D. (1985). A simple discontinuous Percoll gradient procedure for washing human spermatozoa. *IRCS Med. Sci.* **13**, 16.

Ericsson, R. J., Langevin, C. N., and Nishino, M. (1973). Isolation of fractions rich in human Y sperm. *Nature.* **246**, 421.

Fleetham, J. A., Pattinson, H. A., and Mortimer, D. (1993). The mouse embryo culture system: improving the sensitivity for use as a quality control assay for human in vitro fertilization. *Fertil Steril.* **59**, 192.

Gavella, M., Lipovac, V., and Marotti, T. (1991). Effect of pentoxifylline on superoxide anion production by human sperm. *Int. J. Androl.* **14,** 320.

Gellert-Mortimer, S. T., Clarke, G. N., Baker, H. W. G., Hyne, R. V., and Johnston, W. I. H. (1988). Evaluation of Nycodenz and Percoll density gradients for the selection of motile human spermatozoa. *Fertil. Steril.* **49,** 335.

Gledhill, B. L. (1988). Selection and separation of X- and Y-chromosome-bearing mammalian spermatozoa. *Gamete Res.* **20,** 377.

Harrison, R. A. P. (1976). A highly efficient method for washing mammalian spermatozoa. *J. Reprod. Fertil.* **48,** 347.

Jeulin, C., Serres, C., and Jouannet, P. (1982). The effects of centrifugation, various synthetic media and temperature on the motility and vitality of human spermatozoa. *Reprod. Nutr. Dev.* **22,** 81.

Kanwar, K. C., Yanagimachi, R., and Lopata, A. (1979). Effects of human seminal plasma on fertilizing capacity of human spermatozoa. *Fertil. Steril.* **31,** 321.

Knuth, U. A., Neuwinger, J., and Nieschlag, E. (1989). Bias to routine semen analysis by uncontrolled changes in laboratory environment—detection by long-term sampling of monthly means for quality control. *Int. J. Androl.* **12,** 375.

Lopata, A., Johnston, I. W. H., Hoult, I. J., and Speirs, A. I. (1980). Pregnancy following intrauterine implantation of an embryo obtained by in vitro fertilization of a preovulatory egg. *Fertil. Steril.* **33,** 117.

Lopata, A., Patullo, M. J., Chang, A., and James, B. (1976). A method for collecting motile spermatozoa from human semen. *Fertil. Steril.* **27,** 677.

Makler, A., Murillo, O., Huszar, G., Tarlatzis, B., DeCherney, A., and Naftolin, F. (1984). Improved techniques for separating motile spermatozoa from human semen. II. An atraumatic centrifugation method. *Int. J. Androl.* **7,** 71.

Ménézo, Y. (1976). Milieu synthétique pour la survie et la maturation des gamètes et pour la culture de l'oeuf fécondé. *C. R. Acad. Sci. [D]* **272,** 967.

Menezo, Y., Testart, J., and Perrone, D. (1984). Serum is not necessary in human in vitro fertilization, early embryo culture, and transfer. *Fertil. Steril.* **42,** 750.

Mohri, H., Oshio, S., Kaneko, S., Kobayashi, T., and Iizuka, R. (1987). Separation and characterization of mammalian X- and Y-bearing sperm In Mohri, H. (ed): *New Horizons in Sperm Cell Research.* Gordon & Breach, New York.

Mortimer, D. (1986). Elaboration of a new culture medium for physiological studies on human sperm motility and capacitation. *Hum. Reprod.* **1,** 247.

Mortimer, D. (1990). Semen analysis and sperm washing techniques. In Gagnon, C. (ed): *Controls of Sperm Motility: Biological and Clinical Aspects,* CRC Press, Boca Raton, FL.

Mortimer, D. (1991). Sperm preparation techniques and iatrogenic failures of in-vitro fertilization. *Hum. Reprod.* **6,** 173.

Mortimer, D., Leslie, E. E., Kelly, R. W., and Templeton, A. A. (1982). Morphological selection of human spermatozoa *in vivo* and *in vitro. J. Reprod. Fertil.* **64,** 391.

Nishimoto, T., Yamada, I., Niwa, K., Mori, T., Nishimura, T., and Iritani, A. (1982). Sperm penetration *in vitro* of human oocytes matured in a chemically defined medium. *J. Reprod. Fertil.* **64,** 115.

Ord, T., Patrizio, P., Marello, E., Balmaceda, J. P., and Asch, R. H. (1990). Mini-Percoll: a new method of semen preparation for IVF in severe male factor infertility. *Hum. Reprod.* **5,** 987.

Ord, T., Patrizio, P., Silber, S. J., Jones, G., Marello, E., and Asch, R. H. (1991). A new technique for sperm preparation in cases of epididymal aspiration. *Fertil. Steril. Suppl.* S29, (abstract O-067).

Paulson, J. D., and Polakoski, K. L. (1977). A glass wool column procedure for removing extraneous material from the human ejaculate. *Fertil. Steril.* **28**, 178.

Perrone, D., and Testart, J. (1985). Use of bovine serum albumin column to improve sperm selection for human in vitro fertilization. *Fertil. Steril.* **44**, 839.

Pousette, A., Akerlof, E., Rosenborg, L., and Fredricsson, B. (1986). Increase in progressive motility and improved morphology of human spermatozoa following their migration through Percoll gradients. *Int. J. Androl.* **9**, 1.

Purdy, J. M. (1982). Methods for fertilization and embryo culture *in vitro*. In Edwards, R. G., and Purdy, J. M. (eds): *Human Conception In Vitro*. Academic Press, London.

Quinn, P., Warnes, G. M., Kerin, J. F., and Kirby, C. (1984). Culture factors in relation to the success of human in vitro fertilization and embryo transfer. *Fertil. Steril.* **41**, 202.

Quinn, P. J., Kerin, J. F., and Warnes, G. M. (1985). Improved pregnancy rate in human in vitro fertilization with the use of a medium based on the composition of human tubal fluid. *Fertil. Steril.* **44**, 493.

Raoof, N. T., Pearson, R. M., and Turner, P. (1987). A modified trans-membrane migration method for measuring the effect of drugs on sperm motility. *Br. J. Clin. Pharmacol.* **24**, 319.

Rhemrev, J., Jeyendran, R. S., Vermeiden, J. P. W., and Zaneveld, L. J. D. (1989). Human sperm selection by glass wool filtration and two-layer, discontinuous Percoll gradient centrifugation. *Fertil. Steril.* **51**, 685.

Rogers, B. J., Perreault, S. D., Bentwood, B. J., McCarville, C., Hale, R. W., and Soderdahl, D. W. (1983). Variability in the human-hamster in vitro assay for fertility evaluation. *Fertil. Steril.* **39**, 204.

Russell, L. D., and Rogers, B. J. (1987). Improvement in the quality and fertilization potential of a human sperm population using the rise technique. *J. Androl.* **8**, 25.

Serafini, P, Blank, W., Tran, C., Mansourian, M., Tan, T., and Batzofin, J. (1990). Enhanced penetration of zona-free hamster ova by sperm prepared by Nycodenz and Percoll gradient centrifugation. *Fertil. Steril.* **53**, 551.

Serres, C., Feneux, D., and David, G. (1982). Microcinematographic analysis of the motility of human spermatozoa incubated with caffeine. *Andrologia* **14**, 454.

Sherman, J. K., Paulson, J. D., and Liu, K. C. (1981). Effect of glass wool filtration on ultra-structure of human spermatozoa. *Fertil. Steril.* **36**, 643.

Sjöblom, P., and Wikland, M. (1991). A follow-up study of sperm preparation for IVF by swim-up in a solution of hyaluronate. *Hum. Reprod.* **6**, 722.

Tea, N. T., Jondet, M., and Scholler, R. (1984). A 'migration-gravity sedimentation' method for collecting motile spermatozoa from human semen. In Harrison, R. F., Bonnar, J., and Thompson, W. (eds): *In Vitro Fertilization, Embryo Transfer and Early Pregnancy*. MTP Press, Lancaster.

Tucker, M., Wright, G., Bishop, F., Wiker, S., Cohen, J., Chan, Y. M., and Sharma, R. (1990). Chymotrypsin in semen preparation for ARTA. *Mol. Androl.* **2**, 179.

Van der Ven, H. H., Jeyendran, R. S., Al-Hasani, S., Tunnerhoff, A., Hoebbel, K., Diedrich, K., Krebs, D., and Perez-Pelaez, M. (1988). Glass wool column filtration of human semen: relation to swim-up procedure and outcome of IVF. *Hum. Reprod.* **3**, 85.

Vandeweghe, M., Vermeulen, L., and Comhaire, F. (1982). Adverse effect of caffeine on fertilizing capacity of cryopreserved human sperm. In Spira, A., and Jouannet, P. (eds): *Human Fertility Factors*, Vol. 103. INSERM, Paris.

van Kooij, R. J., and van Oost, B. A. (1992). Determination of sex ratio of spermatozoa with a deoxyribonucleic acid-probe and quinacrine staining: a comparison. *Fertil. Steril.* **58,** 384.

Velez de la Calle, J. F. (1991). Human spermatozoa selection in improved discontinuous Percoll gradients. *Fertil. Steril.* **56,** 737.

Wikland, M., Wik, O., Steen, Y., Qvist, K., Söderlund, B., and Janson, P. O. (1987). A self-migration method for preparation of sperm for in-vitro fertilization. *Hum. Reprod.* **2,** 191.

World Health Organization (1987). *WHO Laboratory Manual for the Examination of Human Semen and Semen-Cervical Mucus Interaction, 2nd ed.* Cambridge University Press, Cambridge.

World Health Organization (1992). *WHO Laboratory Manual for the Examination of Human Semen and Sperm-Cervical Mucus Interaction,* 3rd ed. Cambridge University Press, Cambridge.

Yovich, J. M., Edirisinghe, W. R., Cummins, J. M., and Yovich, J. L. (1990). Influence of pentoxifylline in severe male factor infertility. *Fertil. Steril.* **53,** 715.

Zavos, P. M. (1991). A new simple method for preparing spermatozoa for insemination using the new SpermPrep™ filtration method. *J. Androl. Suppl.* P-58 (abstract 133).

13

Therapeutic Insemination Procedures

Increasingly andrology laboratories are becoming involved in the preparation of spermatozoa for therapeutic procedures. In almost all situations these procedures require spermatozoa free of seminal plasma and usually a selected motile sperm population. These requirements are based on a number of fundamental physiological principles.

1. Prolonged exposure of spermatozoa to seminal plasma causes irreversible decreases in sperm motility, vitality, and functional potential.
2. Seminal plasma, acellular debris, and the other cellular elements commonly seen in human ejaculates do not ascend beyond the semen–mucus interface at the external cervical os. Of particular significance are the high levels of prostaglandins found in human semen, which, if instilled into the uterine cavity, will probably cause severe cramping.
3. Seminal plasma contains factors that inhibit sperm capacitation; therefore its presence as a contaminant in prepared sperm populations diminishes sperm-fertilizing ability.
4. In situations involving insemination into the female reproductive tract beyond the cervix, only small volumes of sperm suspension may be used, e.g., 100–200 μl for IUI, up to 50 μl for GIFT, and 5 or 10 μl for ITI. Insemination of a large volume into the uterine cavity can cause severe cramping, and deposition of excess volumes into the fallopian tubes results in spillage of the inseminate.
5. The presence of excessive numbers of spermatozoa, especially of moribund or dead spermatozoa, beyond the cervix may induce the production of antibodies against sperm antigens, resulting in isoimmunization and possible immunological infertility.

SPERM PREPARATION FOR THERAPEUTIC INSEMINATION PROCEDURES

As a consequence of the requirements described above, specific procedural differences exist among the various clinical scenarios that are discussed in more detail in the following sections. A number of aspects, however, are fundamental to all sperm preparation procedures when the spermatozoa are to be used for therapeutic purposes.

Sterile Technique

Although semen is not a sterile fluid, great care should be exercised to ensure that the bacterial and viral contamination of sperm populations being prepared for insemination beyond the cervix is minimized. It requires that semen specimens that are to be used for any form of artificial insemination procedure must be collected under optimally sterile conditions (see Chapter 6) and that all subsequent analyses and processing be performed under sterile conditions in a laminar flow hood.

Although many culture media used for making sperm preparations include antibiotics (commonly penicillin and streptomycin) in their formulation, it is not an excuse for sloppy laboratory technique. More importantly, it is probably best that antibiotics *not* be used in such media owing to the relatively high incidence of allergies to common antibiotics such as penicillin.

Protein Supplementation of Culture Media

Human spermatozoa require the presence of a suitable macromolecule in culture media for optimum survival. The most commonly used medium supplement is human serum albumin (HSA), typically the Cohn fraction V crystalline or powdered preparation for diagnostic purposes, and as a constituent of serum for therapeutic purposes. Both supplements raise concerns regarding infection control.

Most crystalline or powdered HSA preparations are not licensed for internal use and should not be used for such procedures. Indeed, many suppliers no longer sell such products to laboratories, even research laboratories in clinical departments. Even though these HSA preparations are made from blood obtained from hepatitis- and HIV-screened donors, suppliers are now taking every precaution to avoid any possible misuse of their products, which may occur even when they are clearly labeled "For In Vitro Diagnostic Use Only." Interestingly, in the case of HIV the ethanol precipitation step when making fraction V albumin certainly kills the virus so there is no measurable risk of infection, although an infinitesimally small risk of seroconversion in response to dead virus is present in the miniscule quantities of albumin included in the inseminate does exist.

Although for IVF programs and many IUI programs obtaining and processing patient serum for medium supplementation is a matter of routine, it is far less practical for a service andrology laboratory, especially one performing a variety of sperm preparation procedures for diagnostic and therapeutic purposes. Nevertheless, unless an acceptable alternative source of albumin can be established, it may be necessary to use the recipient's (or her partner's) serum for all procedures that result in transfer of any culture medium to the female tract.

Laboratories should identify a local supplier that can provide an HSA product licensed for clinical use if they wish to use this form of protein supplementation in their media (e.g., Cat. No. 5020: Irvine Scientific, Santa Ana, CA, USA). Great caution should be exercised when selecting an albumin preparation. The high-concentration HSA solutions (e.g., 25% w/v) available from some suppliers, intended for intravenous administration to patients with severe burn injuries, contain chemicals to stabilize the protein from flocculating. A commonly used substance for this purpose is sodium caprilate, a detergent that is certainly harmful to mouse embryos and must therefore be considered potentially dangerous to human gametes and embryos.

Sperm Preparation Techniques

Clearly, spermatozoa to be used for therapeutic purposes must be prepared using techniques that are neither suspected nor known to be detrimental to sperm function (see Chapter 12). There is now more than adequate information available in the literature to support the opinion that any method involving the centrifugal pelleting of unselected sperm populations (e.g., simple washing or variations of the sperm-rise method) must be discontinued (review: Mortimer, 1991a). Chapter 12 discusses the various sperm preparation methods currently considered suitable for clinical use and provides some guidance for selecting a sperm preparation technique appropriate for a particular application.

RETROGRADE EJACULATION

Retrograde ejaculation is a clinical condition in which spermatozoa are not ejaculated in the antegrade direction along the ureter and expelled to the exterior but, because of an incompetent bladder neck, reflux in the retrograde direction into the bladder. It occurs despite all the apparent sensations of normal ejaculation. The origin of this problem can be due to a variety of reasons, e.g., diabetes, iatrogenic surgical damage to the bladder neck innervation, or pharmacological side effects of hypertensive therapy such as α-adrenergic blockers. Exposure to urine is highly deleterious to spermatozoa due to the combined effects of osmotic stress, low pH, and urea toxicity (Crich and Jequier, 1978).

Two therapeutic approaches exist: various sperm washing methods and achieving antegrade ejaculation. The latter approach involves the patient ejaculating with a (painfully) full bladder. Initially it is done by masturbation, but eventually he may be able to use the technique in combination with intercourse. This noninvasive full-bladder technique has been particularly useful in diabetics (Crich and Jequier, 1978) and should perhaps be the first approach attempted because, if successful, it minimizes clinical interference.

Sperm-washing techniques are used in conjunction with alkalinization of the urine and recovery of the spermatozoa either by catheterization and washing of the bladder or by urination immediately after ejaculation. The former approach is a clinical procedure and therefore outside the scope of this book. Examination of postejaculatory urine is the usual diagnostic method for confirming retrograde ejaculation. Alkalinization of the urine is commonly achieved by administering oral sodium bicarbonate (see Retrograde Ejaculation Evaluation, below). When spermatozoa are to be prepared from the urine for subsequent artificial insemination either pericervically or by IUI, monitoring the urine osmolarity and pH can be advantageous for modifying the sodium bicarbonate dosage to optimize the recovery of motile spermatozoa. Recommended ranges are 300–500 mOsm and pH $\geq$ 7.0; human spermatozoa are highly sensitive to acidic pH and exposure to hypotonic stress (see Sperm Osmotic Fragility: Hypoosmotic Swelling Test in Chapter 3).

Retrograde Ejaculation Evaluation

Principle

In some men the semen passes back into the bladder at ejaculation, resulting in aspermia or no apparent ejaculate. Confirmation of this situation is obtained by examining a sample of postejaculatory urine for the presence of spermatozoa.

Urine has a number of deleterious actions on spermatozoa: osmotic shock, urea toxicity, and acidic pH. Consequently, the exposure of spermatozoa to the urinary environment should be minimized in terms of duration and by prior alkalinization of the urine.

Reagents

HTF +HSA is human tubal fluid culture medium with human serum albumin. It is prepared by dissolving HSA at 10 mg/ml in HTF medium (see Preparation of HTF Culture Medium in Chapter 12). Store at 4°C until needed. Discard if there are any signs of contamination or sedimentation. Warm to 37°C before use. Discard any opened containers.

Specimen

1. Three days of ejaculatory abstinence are recommended before the examination of postejaculatory urine.
2. The patient should take sodium bicarbonate on the day prior to the appointment at the laboratory: one tablespoon dissolved in tap water morning and evening.
3. On the morning of sample collection, upon rising the patient should:
   a. Take a tablespoon of bicarbonate dissolved in tap water.
   b. Pass urine.
   c. Have breakfast, preferably including several cups of coffee.
4. Upon arrival at the laboratory the patient should pass urine and then wait until he feels there is some urine in his bladder before masturbating. Additional fluid intake may be necessary.
5. As soon after ejaculation as possible the patient should collect a urine sample in the container provided and hand it to the laboratory staff.

Method

1. Measure the volume of the urine using a 10-ml pipette and aliquot the specimen into 50- or 15-ml disposable conical centrifuge tubes (e.g., Falcon 2070 or

2098, or 2096 or 2097, respectively). Divide the urine equally between an even number of tubes, using as few as possible.

2. Measure the pH of the urine using ColorpHast test strips.
3. Centrifuge at 600 g for 10 minutes.
4. Discard all the supernatants and resuspend the pellets in small (≤ 5 ml) volumes of HTF+HSA.
5. Combine the resuspended pellets and make up to a total volume of 20 ml with more HTF+HSA. Transfer 10 ml to each of two 15-ml disposable conical centrifuge tubes.
6. Centrifuge at 600 g for 10 minutes.
7. Discard the supernatants and resuspend each pellet in < 0.5 ml of HTF+HSA.
8. Combine the suspensions in one tube and make up to a total volume of 1.0 ml with more HTF+HSA. Use this "extra" medium to rinse out the now empty 15-ml tube.
9. Perform a standard semen analysis on this suspension (see Chapter 3).

Sperm Preparation for Insemination
If the spermatozoa are being recovered from the urine for insemination, the following steps should be inserted *between* steps 6 and 7.

6a. Discard the supernatants and resuspend each pellet in 2–3 ml of HTF+HSA.
6b. Combine the two suspensions in one 15-ml tube and make up to a total volume of 10 ml with more HTF+HSA. Use this "extra" medium to rinse out the now empty tube.
6c. Centrifuge at 600 g for 10 minutes.

N.B. Obviously the instruction in step 8 to "combine the suspensions. . . ." should now be ignored.

The resulting sperm suspension can be used for pericervical insemination without further processing (see below). Additional steps should be included at the end of the procedure if the spermatozoa are to be prepared for insemination beyond the cervix:

10. Prepare a motile sperm population using either a direct swim-up or discontinuous Percoll gradient method as described in Chapter 12.
11. Determine the yield of motile spermatozoa that can be obtained (see Chapter 12).

Results

For the diagnostic procedure, results are expressed as for a semen analysis but with the specimen being clearly identified as a postejaculation urine specimen. For pretherapy evaluations the total number of motile spermatozoa that could be recovered from a whole specimen should be noted on the report. For samples processed for therapeutic use, the number of motile spermatozoa recovered should be noted.

Quality Control

There are no quality control aspects to this procedure beyond those required for semen analysis.

PERICERVICAL INSEMINATION

Pericervical insemination is the simplest approach used for homologous artificial insemination, often termed AIH. It can be performed with either fresh semen, cryopreserved semen, or spermatozoa prepared from postejaculatory urine specimens (see above). It is also the commonest method for insemination using cryopreserved donor semen.

For small-volume inseminates (e.g., 0.25- or 0.50-ml straws of cryopreserved semen, many physicians simply deposit the material directly into the lower cervical canal after having taken a sample of cervical mucus for assessment of its quality (see Cervical Mucus Sampling and Assessment in Chapter 9). Special insemination instruments are available for use with straws (Fig. 13-1). For larger-volume inseminates a cervical cup may be employed, although with fresh semen the inseminate is often merely deposited into the lower cervical canal and around the external cervical os, leaving a pool in the posterior fornix of the vagina.

INTRAUTERINE INSEMINATION

For patients in whom cervical hostility to spermatozoa has been demonstrated it may be appropriate to bypass the cervix and inseminate the spermatozoa directly into the uterus. However, because only motile spermatozoa normally reach the uterine cavity under in vivo conditions and seminal plasma (which contains high concentrations of prostaglandins) does not pass beyond the external cervical os, sperm preparation for intrauterine insemination (IUI) must involve preparation of a subpopulation of motile spermatozoa free of seminal plasma. Because the uterine cavity is more a virtual space than a true lumen, especially in nulliparous women, inseminates to be deposited here must not be of large volume in order to minimize the risk of cramping. Typically, volumes of 100–200 µl should be used for clinical IUI procedures.

An ejaculate semen specimen produced by masturbation must be provided at the laboratory so the sperm preparation procedure can be started as soon as possible after liquefaction. Ideally, a special room should be set aside for the purpose of producing samples. A prior 2- to 5-day period of ejaculatory abstinence is required.

Selected populations of motile spermatozoa to be used for clinical IUI must be prepared using an appropriate technique (see above). Because motile sperm yields are often unpredictable from semen quality assessments, the proposed preparative procedure(s) should be evaluated before commencing clinical treatment. Only if one can expect to obtain a yield of the order of 5×10^6 motile spermatozoa from a whole ejaculate should IUI be contemplated, although an absolute lower limit may be more like 2×10^6 motile spermatozoa.

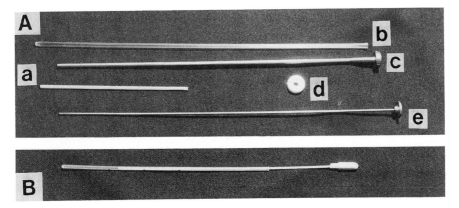

Figure 13-1   Artificial insemination devices for use with straws of cryopreserved semen. (**A**) Insemination gun from BICEF/IMV for 0.5-ml straws. This unit comprises a stainless steel cylindrical "gun" (c) into the distal end of which (the end without the hub and tapered section) and straw (a) is inserted after cutting off the plugged end at the air bubble. The straw is held in place by the sterile disposable plastic sheath (b), which slides over the gun cylinder and is held in place by the plastic retaining ring (d), which slides over the proximal end of the sheath, trapping it on the tapered section of the gun cylinder adjacent to its hub. The stainless steel plunger (e) is then inserted into the gun cylinder and expels the contents of the straw by pushing the sealant plug along the straw. (**B**) "Baby-Stick" disposable plastic device from Laboratoire CCD (Paris) for 0.25-ml straws. This device consist of an outer cylinder into which the straw (after cutting off the plugged end at the air bubble) is loaded proximally and the plunger rod then inserted. Again the contents of the straw are expelled by pushing the sealant plug along the straw.

Because inseminating large numbers of spermatozoa into the uterine cavity may induce isoimmunity to sperm antigens (Friedman et al., 1991), it is recommended that the maximum number of motile spermatozoa inseminated not exceed 10 million, a figure that already exceeds the numbers typically recoverable from the uterine cavity postcoitum. This recommendation is reasonable, as the selection processes used to prepare spermatozoa for IUI are intended to produce populations of quality comparable to those that would reach the uterine cavity in vivo after migration through the cervix (see Chapters 2 and 12). A reasonable inseminate might be 100 µl of a prepared sperm population at 50×10^6 motile spermatozoa per milliliter.

INTRATUBAL INSEMINATION

In patients with cervical hostility, a more extreme approach may be to inseminate the spermatozoa directly into the fallopian tube. This technique also has the advantage that even fewer spermatozoa are required, typically no more than 50,000 motile spermatozoa per oviduct. As a consequence, this approach may be considered in couples with severe male factor infertility, although evidence of sperm fertilizing ability from in vitro function tests would be a recommended prerequisite.

The actual insemination has been achieved by a number of methods: (1) into the tubal ampulla under laparoscopic guidance; (2) into the tubal isthmus under hysteroscopic guidance; and (3) into the tubal isthmus under ultrasound guidance. In any of these scenarios the volume of the inseminate should be as small as can be managed technically, ideally 5 or 10 µl for isthmic inseminations and 50 µl for ampullary inseminations. Handling such small volumes is relatively easy using Hamilton syringes and fine catheters filled with culture medium: The sperm suspension is aspirated into the tip of the catheter after a small air bubble, which separates it from the medium column.

Only limited clinical series using this approach have been published to date. Interested readers are therefore recommended to seek up-to-date information by searching bibliographic databases.

GAMETE INTRAFALLOPIAN TRANSFER

Originally developed by Ricardo Asch as a treatment for couples with idiopathic infertility, GIFT is a modification of IVF in that both oocytes and spermatozoa are transferred into the tubal ampulla, originally at laparotomy but now usually under laparoscopic guidance, so fertilization occurs at the normal site. Ultrasound-guided GIFT is also practiced in some centers using a transvaginal approach. The small volumes of culture medium containing the oocytes and spermatozoa are sometimes separated by a small bubble of air so that contact between male and female gametes does not occur until after their deposition in the female tract.

Although in the early days two oocytes and 50,000 (sometimes as many as 100,000) motile spermatozoa were transferred to each patent oviduct, increasing numbers of programs are transferring a maximum of two or three oocytes (often nowadays into only one oviduct) to reduce the incidence of multiple pregnancies. Ideally, the total volume transferred into the oviductal ampulla should not exceed 50 µl. Motile spermatozoa are prepared as for IUI or IVF.

In couples with a concurrent male factor, increased sperm numbers (100,000 or more) of motile spermatozoa per oviduct may be used. However, GIFT is not recommended for male factor cases where definitive evidence of sperm fertilizing ability is unavailable without a parallel IVF attempt on surplus oocytes.

INTRAPERITONEAL INSEMINATION

Direct intraperitoneal insemination (DIPI) has been used in some centers as an indirect method of ampullary insemination, bypassing sperm transport. Often large numbers of unselected spermatozoa are used, causing some anxiety about the risk of inducing isoimmunity to sperm antigens. This risk must be a major concern as intraperitoneal injection of spermatozoa is the usual means of inducing mice to produce antibodies to sperm surface antigens.

Both transabdominal and (reverse) culdocentesis routes have been reported. The transabdominal route requires ultrasound guidance; passing a needle through the posterior vaginal fornix into the pouch of Douglas can be achieved with less risk. A special device has been described to facilitate the latter approach (Cupido system: Medical Development and Technology bv, Tilburg, The Netherlands). The advantages of DIPI over other tubal insemination techniques, other than its crude simplicity, are unclear; and many centers are unwilling to risk the possibility of inducing sperm isoimmunity.

INSEMINATION OF HUMAN OOCYTES IN VITRO

With simple in vitro fertilization (IVF), oocytes are exposed individually to a prepared motile sperm population at a concentration of 50,000 motile spermatozoa per milliliter, usually in a volume of 0.8–1.0 ml. In cases of male factor infertility high sperm concentrations (100,000 motile spermatozoa/ml and sometimes higher) are used to achieve better fertilization rates, as sperm populations from such men are known to have impaired fertilizing capacity.

An ejaculate semen specimen, produced by masturbation, must be provided at the laboratory so the sperm preparation procedure can be started as soon as possible after liquefaction. Ideally, a special room should be set aside for the purpose of producing samples. A prior 2- to 5-day period of ejaculatory abstinence is required.

Selected populations of motile spermatozoa to be used for IVF inseminations must be prepared free of seminal plasma contamination using an appropriate technique (see above). Because motile sperm yields are often unpredictable from semen quality assessments, the proposed preparative procedure(s) should be evaluated before commencing clinical treatment. Only if one can expect to obtain a minimum yield of the order of 10^6 motile spermatozoa from a whole ejaculate should IVF be contemplated, although in extreme cases oocytes may be exposed to the sperm suspension in groups of two or three, or even all together.

MECHANICALLY ASSISTED FERTILIZATION

There are now many variations to basic IVF for extreme male factor cases in which the spermatozoa bypass the zona pellucida. Whether the reduced or absent fertilizing ability of spermatozoa from these men is due to their impaired ability to undergo acrosome reactions or hyperactivation is not clear. However, spermatozoa from men with Kartagener (immotile cilia) syndrome, which are immotile but capable of undergoing an acrosome reaction, can penetrate zona-free hamster eggs in the HEPT (Aitken et al., 1983) and even fuse with human oocytes after subzonal insemination (Bongso et al., 1989).

These mechanically assisted fertilization (MAF) techniques all involve micromanipulation and can be divided into two major groups: zona opening and microinjection. Zona opening procedures include techniques such as partial zona dissection (PZD) or zona drilling, cracking, and tearing. Sperm microinjection into the perivitelline space (SMI) is also often referred to as subzonal or sperm-under-zona insemination (SZI or SUZI) or microinsemination by sperm transfer (MIST).

Although microinjection of spermatozoa directly into the ooplasm (intracytoplasmic sperm injection or ICSI) is now entering clinical use, it has only been used successfully in one center in Brussels and is not considered further.

For all these MAF procedures spermatozoa should be acrosome-reacted (see Chapter 2). Consequently, after sperm preparation as for traditional IVF, additional treatment is required to induce high levels of acrosome reactions (review: Mortimer, 1993). Because this area of assisted reproductive technology is so new and there are no established methods, any attempt to even suggest methods for routine application would be inappropriate.

TREATMENT OF ANTIBODY-COATED SPERMATOZOA

Methods for the detection, characterization, and quantitation of antisperm antibodies (ASABs) are described in Chapter 5. Although there is evidence that some ASABs may be present in the epididymis and therefore become bound to the spermatozoa before ejaculation, it is a general assumption that most male ASABs bind to spermatozoa at or immediately after ejaculation. Consequently, various attempts have been made to either reduce the opportunity for seminal ASABs to bind to spermatozoa or remove them from the sperm surface afterward.

Attempts to Reduce ASAB Binding to Spermatozoa

Probably the earliest approach required that the patient ejaculate into a specimen container containing a relatively large volume of culture medium in an attempt to "dilute out" the antibody titers. In general, this method has met with little success, which is probably not surprising in view of the high affinity of antibody-antigen binding. More recently, a variation of this approach has been to include ultrasonically disrupted spermatozoa in the collection medium in an attempt to bind (and so neutralize) much of the antibody. Clinical results with this method are sparse.

Attempts to Separate Antibody-Free Spermatozoa

More elegant—but to date no more successful in terms widespread use with clinical results—techniques have employed affinity immunochromatography and immunomagnetic methods (Kiser et al., 1987). Readers wishing to use such a technique employing Sephadex G-200, the antisperm antibody processing (ASAP) technique, are referred to the review by Fulgham and Alexander (1990).

Attempts to Remove ASABs from the Sperm Surface

Because reduction in the quantity (or even perhaps the molecular size) of sperm surface antibodies may improve sperm functional potential, approaches based on attempting to remove ASABs from the sperm surface also bear investigation. IgA1 protease has been shown to improve the mucus-penetrating capacity of spermatozoa in vitro (Bronson et al., 1987), but in vivo application with pregnancy as the endpoint has not yet been reported. Trypsin (500 IU/ml) has also been used to disagglutinate spermatozoa that had been exposed to sera containing high titers of sperm agglutinins (Pattinson et al., 1990). Although sperm–mucus interaction was not improved after trypsin treatment, fertilizing ability as assessed using the zona-free hamster egg penetration test was. These findings suggest that protease treatment may be clinically useful in conjunction with IUI or IVF, provided the residual immunoglobulin fragments do not interfere with sperm–zona or sperm–oolemma interaction. Further research is still needed in this area before routine clinical application should be considered.

Influence of Sperm-Surface Antibodies on Sperm Function

A decrease in the extent of sperm agglutination is often used as the endpoint when considering sperm preparation techniques for antibody-coated spermatozoa. Several workers have reported that high proportions of the spermatozoa still show Immunobead binding after treatment, indicating that the resultant sperm population is certainly not free of sperm-coating antibodies. Certainly for in vitro insemination applications, antibody-coated spermatozoa may be able to fertilize so long as agglutination is minimized and the ASABs neither impair capacitation nor impede sperm–zona or sperm–oolemma interaction. For in vivo insemination, ASABs may hamper sperm transport or expose spermatozoa to increased detection by macrophages or other components of cell-mediated immunity.

Antisperm antibodies bound to the sperm head probably hinder capacitation or fertilization in vivo and in vitro, whereas antibodies bound to the sperm tail are more likely to interfere only with sperm transport at the cervical level. ASABs directed against the tail tip do not seem to impair sperm function. It is unclear how head-directed ASABs interfere with fertilization, but mechanisms based on membrane glycoprotein stabilization and steric hindrance seem probable.

Clinical Treatment of ASABs

Although treatment for ASABs is clearly a clinical matter, laboratory staff are often asked about the possibilities of such treatment. It is therefore appropriate that at least some background be presented here.

ASABs in Men

Several corticosteroid preparations have been used in various regimens in trials attempting to treat sperm-mediated autoimmune infertility, including methylprednisolone, betamethasone, dexamethasone, and prednisolone. Probably the most successful and best tolerated protocol is intermittent prednisolone administered during the early follicular and midfollicular phases of the female partner's cycle (Hendry et al., 1986; review: Mortimer, 1991b). Over a 9-month period one-third of the patients conceived—more than twice the expected pregnancy rate for an unselected group of infertile patients. However, the ever-present risk of severe side effects (e.g., necrosis of the hip joint requiring its replacement) has made this approach unacceptable to many physicians.

ASABs in Women

Attempts to reduce the titers of circulating antibodies in women using condom therapy to prevent recurrent exposure to sperm antigens (i.e., reduce the immunological challenge) have not been successful (e.g., Kremer et al., 1978). Other workers, however, have reported high success rates for condom therapy in reducing sperm agglutinin titers, although not for sperm-immobilizing antibodies (Windt et al., 1989).

References and Recommended Reading

Aitken, R. J., Ross, A., and Lees, M. M. (1983). Analysis of sperm function in Kartagener's syndrome. *Fertil. Steril.* **40,** 696.

Bongso, T. A., Sathananthan, A. H., Wong, P. C., Ratnam, S. S., Ng, S. C., Anandakumar, C., and Ganatra, S. (1989). Human fertilization by micro-injection of immotile spermatozoa. *Hum. Reprod.* **4,** 175.

Bronson, R. A., Cooper, G. W., Rosenfeld, D. L., Gilbert, J. V., and Plaut, A. G. (1987). The effect of an IgA$_1$ protease on immunoglobulins bound to the sperm surface and sperm cervical mucus penetrating ability. *Fertil. Steril.* **47,** 985.

Crich, J. P., and Jequier, A. M. (1978). Infertility in men with retrograde ejaculation: the action of urine on sperm motility, and a simple method for achieving antegrade ejaculation. *Fertil. Steril.* **30,** 572.

Friedman, A. J., Juneau-Norcross, M., and Sedensky, B. (1991). Antisperm antibody production following intrauterine insemination. *Hum. Reprod.* **6,** 1125.

Fulgham, D. L., and Alexander, N. J. (1990). Spermatozoa washing and concentration techniques. In Keel, B. A., and Webster, B. W. (eds): *CRC Handbook of the Laboratory Diagnosis and Treatment of Infertility.* CRC Press, Boca Raton, FL.

Hendry, W. F., Hughes, L., Scammell, G., Pryor, J. P., and Hargreave, T. B. (1990). Comparison of prednisolone and placebo in subfertile men with antibodies to spermatozoa. *Lancet* **335,** 85.

Hendry, W. F., Treehuba, K., Hughes, L., Stedronska, J., Parslow, J. M., Wass, J.A.H., and Besser, G. M. (1986). Cyclic prednisolone therapy for male infertility associated with autoantibodies to spermatozoa. *Fertil. Steril.* **45,** 249.

Kiser, G. C., Alexander, N. J., Fuchs, E. F., and Fulgham, D. L. (1987). In vitro absorption of antisperm antibodies with Immunobead-rise, immunomagnetic, and immunocolumn separation techniques. *Fertil. Steril.* **47,** 466.

Kremer, J., Jager, S., and Kuiken, J. (1978). Treatment of infertility caused by antisperm antibodies. *Int. J. Fertil.* **23,** 270.

Mortimer, D. (1991a). Sperm preparation techniques and iatrogenic failures of in-vitro fertilization. *Hum. Reprod.* **6,** 173.

Mortimer, D. (1991b). Clinical significance of antisperm antibodies. *J. Soc. Obstet. Gynaecol. Can.* **13,** 69.

Mortimer, D. (1993). Techniques for the preparation of spermatozoa and the need for capacitation and the acrosome reaction. In Fishel, S. B., and Symonds, E. M. (eds): *Gamete and Embryo Micromanipulation in Human Reproduction.* Edward Arnold, Sevenoaks Kent, U. K. (in press).

Pattinson, H. A., Mortimer, D., and Taylor, P. J. (1990). Treatment of spermagglutination with proteolytic enzymes II. Sperm function after enzymatic disagglutination. *Hum. Reprod.* **5,** 174.

Windt, M.-L., Menkveld, R., Kruger, T. F., Van der Merwe, J. P., and Van Zyl, J. A. (1989). Effect of sperm washing and swim-up on antibodies bound to sperm membrane: Use of Immunobead/sperm cervical mucus contact tests. *Arch. Androl.* **22,** 55.

14

Semen Cryopreservation

Cryopreservation is the branch of cryobiology concerned with the maintenance or, more correctly, suspension of life during (prolonged) storage in the frozen state at ultralow temperatures. The fundamental principle of cryopreservation is that if the water inside a cell is converted to ice at temperatures low enough to effectively arrest molecular movement (freezing), the biochemical processes of cellular metabolism are suspended. Successful cryopreservation also requires that the biological system can be subsequently returned to normal temperatures (thawing) without sustaining biochemical or structural injuries that cause the cell to die. In the frozen state the cell is effectively in suspended animation.

Exhaustive discussions of the many aspects of cryobiology that impinge on human semen cryopreservation are clearly extraneous to the present text. However, some consideration is made of the most salient points contributory to the successful implementation of semen banking for clinical purposes.

HISTORICAL PERSPECTIVES

Certainly the most significant, albeit accidental, discovery pertaining to semen cryopreservation was the effectiveness of glycerol as a cryoprotective agent for bovine spermatozoa by Polge and colleagues in 1949. Even though at that time the emphasis in semen cryopreservation was focused on farm animals (principally bulls), shortly afterward Sherman reported the successful cryopreservation and storage of human spermatozoa on dry ice ($-78°C$) with the production of normal offspring. The use of liquid nitrogen vapor freezing was described, also by Sherman, during the early 1960s along with the first normal births from this method. The still commonly used glycerol-egg yolk-citrate (GEYC) cryoprotectant medium for human spermatozoa was originally described by Ackerman during the late 1960s. Detailed historical reviews of this period have been published by Sherman (1973, 1977, 1986, 1990).

Greater appreciation of the potential and applications of human semen cryobanking developed with wider use of cryopreserved donor semen during the early 1970s despite unfounded and misleading concerns over the possible dangers in genetic and functional instability of cryopreserved spermatozoa. It was at about this time that the first commercial human semen cryobanks opened in the United States, aimed at providing "fertility insurance" for the anticipated millions of men who would have vasectomies. The failure to realize the projected market in this area considerably slowed the growth of commercial semen banks until the second half of the 1980s when the absolute need for quarantined donor semen to obviate the risk of AIDS transmission was established.

Cryobanking human semen is now an established procedure worldwide. Probably the most organized country in this regard is France where the Fédération Française des Centres d'Étude et de Conservation du Sperme Humain (Federation CECOS) was created in 1981 (David, 1989; Federation CECOS et al., 1989). From the original center established at Le Kremlin-Bicêtre just outside Paris in 1973, CECOS grew to 14 centers by 1979 and 20 by 1989. In 1989 the name was modified to consider the possible cryopreservation of both sexes of gametes and became the Federation of Centres d'Étude et de Conservation des Oeufs et du Sperme Humain. Cumulative results from CECOS represent some 24,000 live births by 1991.

The longest period of cryopreservation that has resulted in a birth after AIH is now 15 years 9 months (J. H. Olson, personal communication), confirming the opinion of many cryobiologists and the Reproductive Council of the American Association of Tissue Banks (AATB) that semen cryopreservation is a safe process that maintains the reproductive potential of human spermatozoa during effectively indefinite storage in liquid nitrogen at −196°C.

Rigorous standards of operation are essential for all sperm banks. The American Association of Tissue Banks (AATB) has published a set of standards that are also available to nonmembers.

CLINICAL APPLICATIONS

Although human semen cryobanking can be generally divided into the two broad areas of autoconservation (i.e., semen banking for one's own future use) and donor banking, there are many permutations for their clinical application. Artificial insemination by donor used to be known by the acronym AID, but since the advent of human acquired immunodeficiency syndrome (AIDS) other terms have been used, such as (therapeutic) donor insemination with the acronyms TDI or just DI.

Semen Autoconservation

There are various reasons for semen autoconservation.

1. Preservation of reproductive potential before chemical, radiological, or surgical cancer therapy which might, or even will, render an individual sterile, severely subfertile, or impotent
2. "Fertility insurance" for a man before he undergoes surgical sterilization by vasectomy
3. "Convenience cryobanking" to ensure that a man's spermatozoa will be available to treat his partner during his absence (e.g., military service) or as a reserve in case he is unable to provide a fresh ejaculate at the precise moment it is required for an IVF, GIFT, or IUI procedure

Other possible applications, such as the idea of storing and subsequently pooling ejaculates from an oligozoospermic patient, have not proven beneficial, in this case because of the poor cryosurvival of spermatozoa from such men.

Donor Semen Cryopreservation

With the provision of donor semen for therapeutic procedures, cryobanking confers a number of important advantages over the use of fresh semen.

1. Storage of donor semen while awaiting the results of microbiological tests on the ejaculate to ensure that infectious organisms are not transmitted by TDI.
2. The ability to quarantine donor semen to allow for repeat testing of the donor for seroconversion in response to viral infections (e.g., hepatitis or AIDS) that can be transmitted sexually.
3. The ready availability of a wide selection of donor phenotypes and genotypes for use in either TDI or other insemination procedures such as IVF or GIFT. This aspect considers both the improved range of donors available at any point in time and the convenience of constant availability of donor semen, allowing inseminations, especially multiple inseminations, to be performed at perhaps unpredictable times determined by irregular female cycles or the vagaries of ovarian stimulation protocols.

The much debated poor fertility achieved using cryopreserved semen is largely related to comparisons between fresh semen and poor-quality cryobanked semen. This unfounded concern has caused great resistance to the use of cryobanked donor semen, although this debate is now largely academic subsequent to the AIDS epidemic and the demands for adequate and responsible infection control. In fact, several studies have demonstrated that essentially comparable fecundity rates can be achieved using cryobanked semen in the TDI setting.

Strict recruitment and acceptance criteria for semen donors should allow fecundity rates of 10–12% per insemination cycle provided that at least 5×10^6 progressively motile spermatozoa are inseminated into the lower cervical canal on two or three occasions during the periovulatory period (Scott et al., 1990).

TECHNICAL BACKGROUND

Cryoprotectants

Glycerol is by far the most widely used and successful cryoprotectant for human spermatozoa; a final concentration of about 7.5% (v/v) seems to be optimum. Dimethylsulfoxide (DMSO), which should ideally be used at 4°C, not only has direct deleterious effects on human sperm but also requires their exposure to cold shock. Propanediol (PrOH), which is the most successful cryoprotectant for early cleavage human embryos, has seen little application with spermatozoa.

Hen's egg yolk, which is often included in the cryoprotectant medium used for freezing human spermatozoa, is not itself a cryoprotectant but does seem to confer improved sperm plasma membrane fluidity. Indeed, some workers have reported that adequate, even improved, cryosurvival can be obtained with egg yolk in the absence of glycerol (review: Sherman, 1990).

Buffering of the cryoprotectant medium's pH during freezing is essential to avoid damage to the spermatozoa. In Ackerman's GEYC medium buffering is effected by glycine and citrate, but more modern recipes employ a combination of the zwitterionic buffers TES and Tris. TES-Tris is often used in conjunction with egg yolk (TEST-yolk) and also citrate (TESTCY), usually with glycerol as cryoprotectant.

Interindividual Variability

Because there is great interindividual variability in the cryosurvival of spermatozoa from one individual among different cryopreservation methods (Friberg and Gemzell, 1977), no one cryoprotectant or freezing regimen has been proven to be better than any others on a population basis. Studies using pooled semen conceal such interindividual variability and therefore contribute little to establishing an optimized method with broad applicability. For the present we are left with the situation that if one has to cryopreserve semen from a particular man, it may be necessary to try several protocols to establish the one best suited for his spermatozoa.

In terms of donor programs, the problem has been circumvented by simply accepting only those donors that show good cryosurvival by the particular method(s) standard for that cryobank. However, there remain some men who, despite apparently normal sperm quality prefreeze and postthaw, and even proven fertility of their fresh semen, fail to achieve pregnancies when their spermatozoa have been cryopreserved.

Packaging

Although glass ampoules (Fig. 14-1A) were originally used for semen cryopreservation, their use is now strongly discouraged on safety grounds due to fragility. Plastic cryovials with screw caps are used in some laboratories, especially where there is a perceived need from physicians for relatively high-volume insemination aliquots (Fig. 14-1B). However, the large diameter and thick wall of these cryovials cause poor heat transfer and therefore less effective cooling throughout the sample. A small-volume cryovial with a conical base and vanes to improve heat transfer have appeared (Fig. 14-1C) and are reported to give results comparable to those with polypropylene French straws *(paillettes)* invented by the company Instruments de Medicine Veterinaire (IMV) based in L'Aigle, France (Fig. 14-1D).

Straws are probably the most widely used packaging system for human semen (and possibly the only system used for bovine semen) around the world. The French Federation CECOS uses the 0.25 ml size, whereas other organizations have opted for the larger 0.5 ml size (e.g., Canadian Fertility and Andrology Society, 1988, 1992). After filling, straws are sealed using either solid plastic (nylon) plugs, by

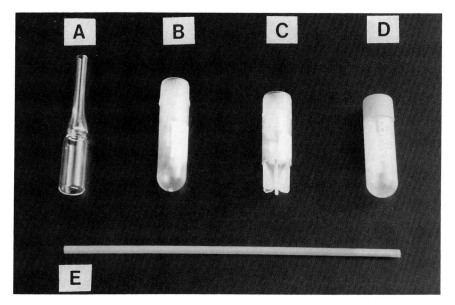

Figure 14-1   Alternatives for packaging frozen semen. (**A**) Glass ampoule. (**B**) Nunc plastic cryovial. (**C**) Nunc small, finned plastic cryovial. (**D**) Corning plastic cryovial. (**E**) French straw, or *paillette*.

heating, or by filling the open end with polyvinyl alcohol powder, which polymerizes on contact with moisture (Fig. 14-2).

Concern has been expressed that straws are more fragile than cryovials, and that for reasons of infection control cryovials must be used. It is my experience that if an appropriate inventory control system is used, i.e., one that does not expose the straws to any bending stress during transfer into, during, or removal from storage, and if straws are not overfilled, broken straws are rare. For example, if straws are stored in narrow tubes (visotubes: 9.2 mm $\varnothing$) attached to canes (Fig. 14-3), as is usual with embryos, many straws are broken when trying to extract them from the

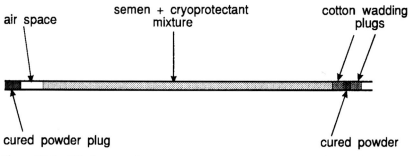

Figure 14-2   Filled semen straw.

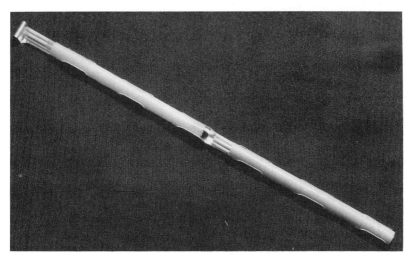

Figure 14-3 Storage of straws in visotubes attached to a cane. Several canes can be stored upright in 11-inch canisters.

visotube because at $-196°C$ straws become rigid with essentially no flexibility. This opinion has been confirmed in discussions with other cryobank directors with experience using straws.

Cryopreservation

The actual cooling curve used for freezing the packaged semen-cryoprotectant mixture depends on the radius of the straw, cryovial, or ampoule. How this cooling curve is achieved is also variable.

Programmable Freezing Systems
Although essential for embryo cryopreservation, in routine use with semen these machines have not been found to produce any better results than the less automated, less expensive alternatives described below. Furthermore, the longer cycle time of these units (i.e., the minimum time between two separate freezing runs) makes them less amenable to use in the andrology laboratory, where several ejaculates may be received for cryopreservation during the course of a few hours. Because spermatozoa have a finite fertile life-span, it is better that they spend it within the female tract after thawing than sitting around the laboratory waiting to be frozen.

Mechanically Assisted Vapor Phase Cooling
Mechanically assisted vapor phase cooling machines cause liquid nitrogen vapor to flow around the samples at a controlled rate so a desired cooling rate can be achieved. Freezing protocols using such systems (Fig. 14-4) must be established empirically.

For example, the Nicool LM-10 unit shown in Figure 14-4 holds one hundred 0.25-ml straws in its freezing chamber, and a variable-speed fan pulls liquid nitro-

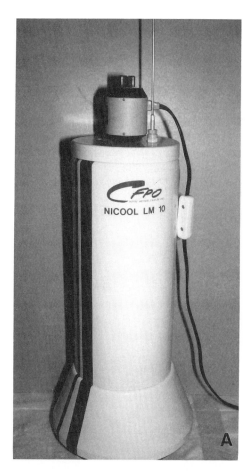

Figure 14-4 (A) Nicool LM-10 mechanically-assisted vapor freezing machine. (B) Its component parts: the base, containing a liquid nitrogen dewar flask *(center)*; the insulated cylinder *(left)*; the variable speed motor on top of the lid underneath which is the inner stainless steel cylinder *(back right)*; and the straw rack, which fits inside the inner cylinder *(front right)*.

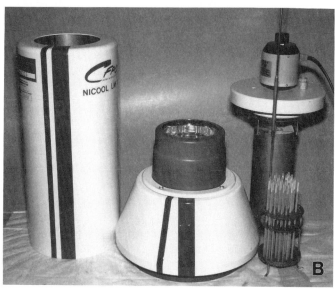

gen vapor past the straws at empirically determined rates to achieve the desired cooling curve. According to the manufacturer's published cooling curves, for human semen with a full load of one hundred 0.25-ml straws, the fan should be set at maximum (i.e., "10") and run for 30 minutes. If fewer than 100 sample straws are to be frozen, the difference must be made up using "ballast" straws, i.e., straws containing only cryoprotectant. The same unit also holds 0.5-ml straws, but here we have found that the optimum cooling curve seems to be achieved with the fan set at maximum but with only 25 straws loaded. Again ballast straws should be used to make up the difference between this number and that of the sample straws to be frozen in a particular freezing run.

Static Vapor Phase Cooling

The static vapor phase cooling method is sometimes referred to as the "garbage can" or "dustbin" method. It requires that a stable temperature gradient be established in the vapor phase above a quantity of liquid nitrogen, obviously in an insulated container, usually a large cylindrical stainless steel dewar vessel (hence the method's nickname). Straws are placed at predetermined heights above the liquid phase for predetermined periods so the desired cooling curve is achieved (Fig. 14-5). Again these protocols must be developed empirically.

For 0.25-ml straws a one-step cooling can be used with the straws placed at 25 cm above the liquid level for 10 minutes before plunging. For 0.5-ml straws, two-step cooling is more common: 15 minutes each at heights of 14 and 6 inches (356 and 152 mm) above the liquid before plunging.

Because there is a temperature gradient established through the vapor phase, straws frozen by this method must be placed horizontally in the vapor so they experience the same cooling effect along their length. It is also important that straws be arranged in a monolayer, not in bundles or multiple layers, so all the straws experience the same cooling effect.

A variation on this method is to place straws in a bundle, usually inside a visotube, in the neck of an open storage dewar vessel for a certain period. This method results in unreliable cryopreservation with marked differences between straws on the outside and inside of the bundle, and even in variations in cryosurvival along the length of each straw. Clearly, this method is not recommended from a cryobiological standpoint.

Inventory Control Systems

The inventory control system to be used depends on the type of storage container being used (review: Richardson, 1976). Cryovials are usually attached to metal canes, which stand free inside the canisters of the storage tank (Fig. 14-6). Straws are usually grouped in plastic tubes (visotubes) arranged in larger plastic goblets so there is an upper and lower level in each canister of the storage tank (Fig. 14-6).

Straws (and cryovials) must be identified individually, so every unit of semen in a cryobank can be positively identified. This step is absolutely essential, and various methods exist for the purpose. The cattle AI industry uses printing devices that

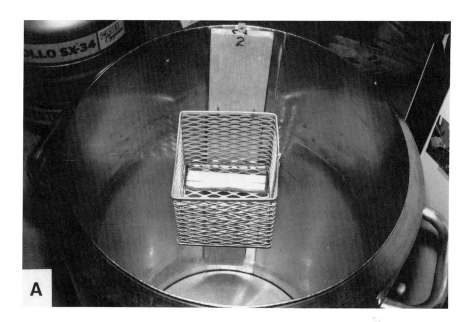

A

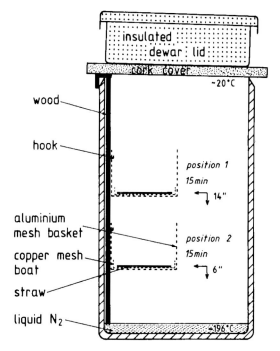

insulated
dewar lid

cork cover

~20°C

wood

hook

position 1
15 min
14"

aluminium
mesh basket

position 2
15 min

copper mesh
boat

6"

straw

liquid N₂

~196°C

B *Vapour Freezing Of 0·5ml Straws*

Figure 14-5 Photograph (**A**) and diagram (**B**) of the "garbage-can" static vapor freezing method. The straws are arranged horizontally in a single layer within a wire mesh "boat" inside the test-tube basket, which is suspended by a pair of nails from the wood batten hung down the inner side of the dewar tank.

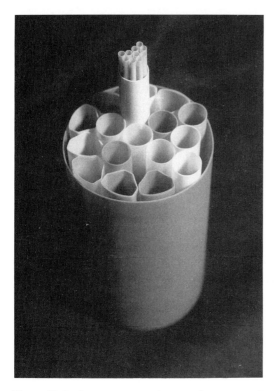

Figure 14-6   Inventory control system for straws using visotubes (usually of different colors and shapes) inside a plastic goblet. Two goblets fit one on top of the other inside an 11-inch canister.

allow a single line of characters along the length of the straw. However, these machines are expensive and cannot be justified for the small batch sizes produced from human ejaculates (*c.f.* the several hundred straws per batch from a bull ejaculate).

A simple method originating from the Federation CECOS uses lines drawn on each straw using a fine-pointed, indelible (spirit-based) marker pen. Lines are drawn at the 1- to 9-cm distances along the straw with the manufacturer's plugged end being taken as zero. Four-digit numbers are normally used, with one line being drawn at the centimeter distance corresponding to the first digit, two lines for the second, three for the third, and four for the fourth (Fig. 14-7). Obviously, numbers containing either one or more zeroes or repeated numbers (e.g., 2013 or 2131) cannot be used. The major disadvantage of this bar-coding system for straw identification is that there is a finite number of (four-digit) permutations available. One possible solution might be to use the number sequence in conjunction with differently colored sealing powders so there are yellow, red, and blue series, for example. Alternatively, the straw color could be used to denote the series.

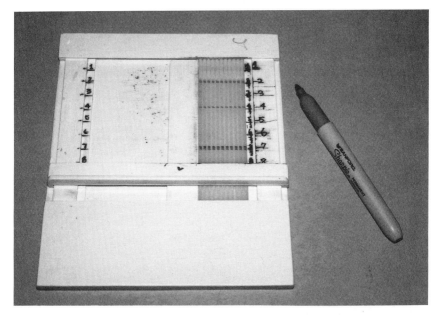

Figure 14-7   Device for marking straws using the bar-code system (see text for details).

An alternative method uses flags attached to each straw. A flag is made from a small self-adhesive label (known to retain its adhesiveness after freezing and thawing), and the required information is written on the flag using a fine ballpoint pen. Although this method allows more information to be attached to each straw, it severely reduces the number of straws that can be stored per visotube in the cryobank. It also makes it more difficult to remove a straw quickly from among its companions in a full visotube.

See also Organization of a Sperm Bank, below. Sample forms are provided in Appendix VII.

CRYOPRESERVATION OF HUMAN SEMEN

Although there has been a resurgence of interest in developing improved methods for cryopreserving human spermatozoa, largely stimulated by acceptance that the risks of HIV transmission makes insemination using fresh donor semen unacceptable, there have not yet been any substantial advances. This section describes a method for cryopreserving human semen that has been widely used, with minimal modification and not inconsiderable success, since the early 1970s.

Glycerol–Egg Yolk–Citrate Method

The method uses a modified Ackerman's cryoprotective medium of the glycerol-egg yolk-citrate (GEYC) formulation and 0.5-ml straws. It is equally applicable for donor or autoconservation uses. Formulations for other cryoprotectants are provided later in this section, although they may require slightly different cooling curves for optimum performance. Examples of the various laboratory forms used for this protocol are provided in Appendix IV.

Reagents

GEYC: Combine 40.0 ml egg yolk (Bacto Egg-Yolk Enrichment, Difco Labs., Cat. No. 3347-72), 30.0 ml glycerol, 2.0 g glycine, 2.6 g glucose, and 2.3 g sodium citrate in 130.0 ml reagent or, better, tissue culture grade water. Heat-inactivate at 56°C for 30 minutes and adjust the pH to 7.2. Divide into aliquots of about 10 ml in sterile plastic Universal containers and store frozen at −20°C or lower until needed. Warm to 37°C before use; do not refreeze for reuse.

Other: All the other materials required for semen cryostorage and cryobank inventory control are obtained from the local agents for the French company BICEF, the human division of IMV, which manufactures them.

Specimen

Semen samples for cryostorage must be produced at the laboratory by masturbation following a recommended (e.g., 3 days) period of ejaculatory abstinence so as to obtain an optimal sample.

Method

1. Prepare the freezing system.
   a. If a static vapor phase system is to be used, prepare the freezing tank (e.g., MVE model TA-60: internal dimensions 70 cm high × 40 cm ∅) (Fig. 14-5) with about 5 liters of liquid nitrogen and allow the temperature gradient to equalize. About 1 hour before use, top up the nitrogen level to the bottom of the freezing rack.
   b. If mechanically assisted vapor phase cooling is to be used (e.g., Nicool LM-10) (Fig. 14-4), transfer liquid nitrogen to the reservoir dewar so it is brim full.
2. Assign the semen sample to be frozen the next batch number in sequence (see Inventory Control Systems, above). For the present purposes we use the barcoding system. Record this number and other required information on the Semen Cryostorage Work Sheet (see Appendix VII).
3. As soon as the ejaculate is liquefied, preferably no later than 30 minutes after ejaculation, a basic semen analysis is performed.
4. From the residual volume of the sample, calculate the number of straws that will be required (the semen will be diluted with an equal volume of GEYC medium, and each straw holds about 0.5 ml.)
5. Mark the straws according to the batch coding. Considering zero as being at the plugged end of the straw, use a fine-pointed, spirit-based marker pen to mark one line at the centimeter distance of the first digit of the batch number, two

lines at the second, three lines at the third, and four lines at the fourth digit (Fig. 14-7).

6. Arrange the straws in the clip holders in groups of multiples of five (i.e., 5, 10, or 15) according to the numbers required (Fig. 14-8A). Alternatively, straws may be filled singly using a single straw suction manifold (see step 8B, below).

7. The semen sample is transferred to a sterile disposable *barquette* (bubbler dish) and diluted with an equal volume of GEYC medium. The GEYC is added slowly with constant swirling of the dish to ensure complete mixing.

8A. Attach the appropriate filling manifold (for 5, 10, or 15 straws) to the plugged end of the straws arranged in the clip. This manifold is attached to a suction line (e.g., a water vacuum pump on the tap). Immerse the open ends of the straw into the semen+GEYC mixture in the dish. Fill the straws by applying suction by placing a finger over the hole in the back of the manifold (Fig. 14-8C). When all the straws are full (i.e. the semen+GEYC mixture has reached the plugs of all the straws), release the suction.

8B. If straws are being filled singly, each straw is inserted into the suction manifold (a 3- or 5-ml syringe with Silastic tubing) (Fig. 14-8D) and suck the semen+GEYC mixture up the straw to the plug by gently pulling back on the syringe plunger. Push the plunger back down only if no straw is attached.

9. Locate the straw(s) over the teeth of the comb (which is over the dish) so that some semen+GEYC mixture is expelled from each straw to leave an air space (Fig. 14-8D). Remove the clips if used.

10. a. Occlude the open ends of the straws by tamping them into the PVC powder (Fig. 14-8E).
   b. Place the straws with the newly sealed end immersed in a shallow dish of water to ensure complete "curing" of the powder (Fig. 14-8F).
   c. After a few minutes remove the straws from the water and wipe off any excess powder from their outside surfaces using paper tissues.

Steps 7–10 are repeated until all the semen+GEYC mixture has been loaded into straws. Additional straws may be needed if insufficient numbers were prepared at step 3.

11.A. Static vapor phase cooling
   a. The straws are placed horizontally as a single layer in a copper wire mesh tray in an aluminum mesh basket within the freezing tank at the upper level (straws at 14 inches above the liquid phase) and left for 15 minutes (Fig. 14-5 and 14-8G).
   b. After this first freezing step the basket is moved to the lower level (straws at 6 inches above the liquid phase) for another 15 minutes.
   c. Finally, the straws (still in the basket) are immersed into the liquid nitrogen at the bottom of the freezing tank. When the bubbling stops they are equilibrated at $-196°C$.

11.B. Mechanically assisted vapor phase cooling
   a. Up to 25 straws are loaded into the LM-10 rack, which is then slid inside

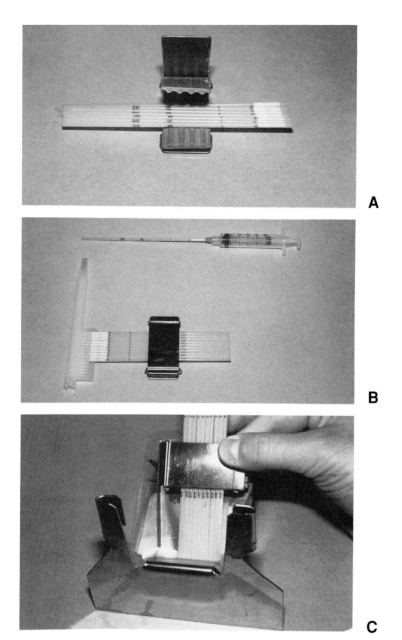

Figure 14-8 Materials used for filling and sealing straws. (**A**) Clip holders for straws. (**B**) Suction devices for filling single straws or groups of straws held in clips. (**C**) Filling a group of straws in a clip holder simultaneously from the bubbler dish, or *barquette.* (**D**) Filling a single straw from the bubbler dish. Note the filled straws placed on the comb device to displace semen + GEYC mixture from the lower part of the straw. (**E**) Tamping a filled straw in the sealing powder. (**F**) Curing a batch of straws by immersion of the powder-sealed ends in water. (**G**) Batch of straws in a wire mesh boat next to a test-tube basket. (**H**) Batch of straws after transfer into a numbered visotube ready for storage in the cryobank.

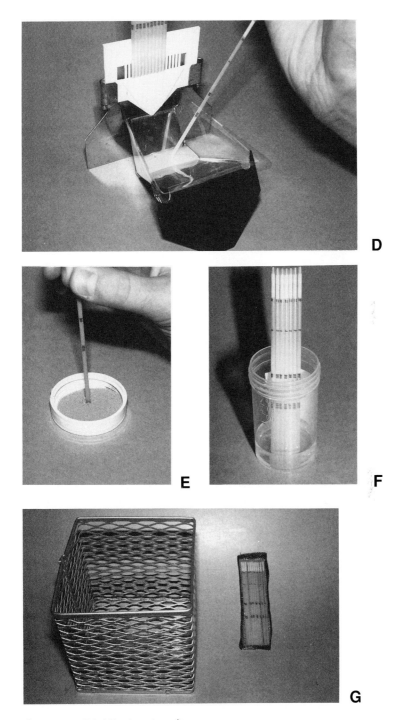

Figure 14-8 (D)–(G) (continued)

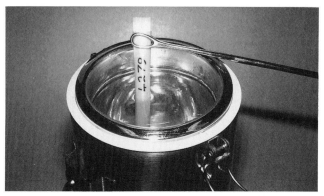

H

Figure 14-8 (H) (continued)

the metal cooling column and held in place by tightening the locking nut around the rack's handle. If 25 straws are not available for a particular freezing run, "ballast" straws filled with cryoprotectant alone must be used to make up the number in order to achieve the correct cooling curve.

b. Once the LM-10 is assembled, the fan is set at "10" for 30 minutes.

c. After 30 minutes plunge the straw rack into the liquid nitrogen dewar (being careful of the dewar's glass lining) and wait until the bubbling stops.

12. Choose an appropriate shape and color visotube (see Organization of a Sperm Bank, below) and write the donor and batch numbers on it using a spirit-based marker pen (Fig. 14-8H).

13. Immerse this visotube in liquid nitrogen in a transfer dewar until the bubbling stops (Fig. 14-8H).

14. Using forceps, rapidly transfer the straws of frozen semen into the visotube (which is full of liquid nitrogen). Protective gloves must be worn.

15. One straw is set aside for assessment (either now or later) of the post-thaw sperm motility.

16. Place the visotube of straws in its appropriate storage location (tank, canister, and goblet locations; see below) in the bank.

17. Make out an Index Card (see Appendix VII) for the batch. This information includes the donor number, straw color, batch number and size (i.e., the number of straws excluding any used for test thawing), date of freezing, storage location (including shape and color of visotube), and the semen analysis laboratory reference number.

18. Enter the batch into the Storage Location Record Form (see Appendix VII); use the donor number not the donor's name or initials. Each page in this book is for a different location (tank, canister, and goblet) and lists the visotubes stored there, along with the batch number and other information relating to their contents. Only occasionally, when a large number of straws is obtained from a sin-

gle donor sample, may there be two visotubes of the same shape and color in the same storage tank location.

19. In the Donor Semen Cryostorage Record Form (see Appendix VII) there is a separate sheet for each donor. Only the donor number is used; the list relating donors' names and numbers is kept separate. Each sample frozen is noted on the appropriate donor's page; information should include the batch number, semen analysis laboratory reference, full storage location, date, and number of straws banked.

20. Thaw out the test straw by transferring it to ambient temperature for 10 minutes and then to 37°C for another 10 minutes. The same thawing procedure is used to thaw straws for insemination or other purposes.

21. Assess the quantitative and qualitative sperm motility and determine the total sperm concentration as described in Chapter 3.

Results

The adequacy of semen cryopreservation is usually assessed using the percentage return of motility, or cryosurvival factor (CSF), which is calculated as:

$$\text{CSF} = \frac{\%\ \text{motile spermatozoa post-thaw}}{\%\ \text{motile spermatozoa pre-freeze}} \times 100$$

If a motility index is used (see Chapter 3), a further assessment can be used that incorporates an appreciation of any declines in sperm progression, not just in the proportion of motile spermatozoa. The return of motility index (RMI) is calculated from the fresh and post-thaw motility index values as:

$$\text{RMI} = \frac{\text{post-thaw motility index}}{\text{pre-freeze motility index}} \times 100$$

Quality Control

The sperm concentration in the test thaw sample must be within ± 10% of half the original semen sperm concentration; otherwise it indicates poor mixing of the semen and cryoprotectant. Batches where this condition is not met may show substantial variability in sperm cryosurvival among straws. For donor semen cryopreservation the additional conditions described in Note 3, below, must also be satisfied.

Notes

1. *Clarified GEYC cryoprotectant.* The presence of egg yolk globules in the GEYC medium precludes the use of CASA instruments to determine the sperm concentration and motility characteristics. To eliminate the problem of mistaking egg yolk globules for immotile, isolated sperm heads, a clarified variant of this traditional recipe is being used in some centers. It simply involves removing the egg yolk globules by filtering the medium through a 0.45 μm Millipore Millex-HV (25 mm ∅) or Swinnex unit (25 or 47 mm ∅) with an HVLP (Durapore) mem-

brane. For high volume use a larger pore size Durapore membrane, or a depth-type glass fiber prefilter is recommended.

2. *Straw colors* are many and varied and contribute to the possible methods for organizing a semen cryobank (see below). As a suggestion, for donor semen cryobanking we use 14 colors of straws, or *paillettes,* which are the easiest to distinguish from each other (Table 14-1). Each color is assigned to a donor in sequence, therefore donors 1, 15, 29, *et seq* have the same straw color. Clear straws may be reserved for autoconservation patients and research purposes.

3. *Criteria of suitability for cryopreservation of donor semen. Before freezing* donor semen must meet ALL the following criteria.

Ejaculate volume	≥ 2.0 ml
Sperm concentration	$> 50 \times 10^6$/ml
Sperm motility (%)	$\geq 50\%$ motile
	$\geq 40\%$ progressively motile
Sperm progression	≥ 3 (scale of 0–4)
Sperm morphology	$\geq 45\%$ normal forms
White blood cells	$< 10^6$/ml

After thawing the sperm motility must fulfill ALL the following criteria; otherwise the sample is discarded.

Cryosurvival (CSF)	$\geq 50\%$
Sperm motility (%)	$\geq 30\%$ motile
	$\geq 25\%$ progressively motile
Sperm progression	≥ 2 (scale of 0–4)

There must be a minimum of 5×10^6 *progressively motile* spermatozoa per straw post-thaw to achieve an adequate fecundity rate with donor semen.

Table 14–1   Colors of straws for semen cryostorage

Color No.	Color	Old IMV No.	BICEF No.
0	Clear	A 101	AUA 013
1	Brown	A 103	CUA 013
2	Red	A 104	DUA 013
3	Green	A 105	EUA 013
4	Blue	A 106	FUA 013
5	Gray	A 107	GUA 013
6	Purple	A 108	HUA 013
7	Yellow	A 109	IUA 013
8	Pink	A 110	JUA 013
9	Dark green	A 111	KUA 013
10	Orange	A 114	NUA 013
11	Light blue	A 115	OUA 013
12	Wine red	A 117	QUA 013
13	Putty	A 118	RUA 013
14	Pistachio green	A 120	TUA 013

Other Cryoprotectant Media Recipes

In addition to the traditional GEYC cryoprotectant medium discussed above, a number of other recipes have been described for use with human spermatozoa. They include formulations using the zwitterionic buffers TES and Tris (TEST) in combination with egg yolk, citrate, or both. Another alternative is the human sperm preservation medium (HSPM), which uses Hepes as the buffering agent. Glycerol is still used as the cryoprotective agent.

TEST-Yolk Buffer

The TEST-yolk buffer (TYB) is commonly used as a refrigeration medium for human spermatozoa (Bolanos et al., 1983; Johnson et al., 1990), although if supplemented with 8% (v/v) glycerol it can be used for cryopreservation.

The TYB medium comprises 4.326 g TES, 1.027 g Tris, and 0.2 g dextrose dissolved in 100 ml reagent water. Penicillin G (1000 IU/ml) and streptomycin (1 mg/ml) may also be added. Yolk from freshly laid chicken eggs is heat-inactivated at 56°C for 60 minutes before adding 25 ml to give 20% (v/v). Centrifuge at 1000 g for 10 minutes, discard the pellet, and adjust the supernatant to pH 7.35–7.45 with Tris and the osmolarity to 290–320 mOsm. Either use immediately or store frozen at −20°C for up to 1 month. TYB can also be purchased commercially (e.g., Cat. No. 9972: Irvine Scientific, Santa Ana, CA, USA).

TEST-Yolk-Citrate Medium

The TEST-yolk-citrate (TESTCY) cryoprotectant medium is a volumetric mixture of 48% TES-Tris (prepared by titrating a 325 mOsm TES solution with a 325 mOsm Tris solution to achieve pH 7.0), 30% 325 mOsm sodium citrate pH 7.0, 20% egg yolk (fresh farm eggs), and 2% 325 mOsm fructose solution (Weidel and Prins, 1987). The formulation must be adjusted to use the Bacto Egg Yolk preparation (see above). Glycerol is added to give a final 6.0% (v/v) concentration after adding to the semen, i.e., 12% in TESTCY buffer if the semen is to be diluted 1:1. The samples are then cooled at −0.5°C/minute to 5°C, packaged in straws, and then placed in a rack at 4 cm above liquid nitrogen (static vapor freeze) for 12 minutes before plunging (Weidel and Prins, 1987).

Human Sperm Preservation Medium

Human sperm preservation medium is a modified, Hepes-buffered Tyrode's medium containing albumin (HSA) and glycerol (Mahadevan and Trounson, 1983). Its composition is 100.0 mM NaCl, 5.365 mM KCl, 2.721 mM $CaCl_2$, 0.492 mM $MgCl_2$, 12.856 mM sodium lactate, 0.321 mM NaH_2PO_4, 30.949 mM $NaHCO_3$, 20.0 mM Hepes free acid, 50.0 mM sucrose, 133.21 mM glycine, 5.506 mM glucose, plus 4.9 g/l HSA and 15.0% (v/v) glycerol. The final solution is filter-sterilized using 0.22-μm Millipore Durapore membranes; antibiotics may be added (e.g., kanamycin sulfate 50 mg/l). The stock is frozen at −20°C in suitable volume aliquots for a maximum of 3 months.

Semen is diluted 1:1 with HSPM, packaged in 0.5-ml straws, and cooled from ambient temperature (about 20°C) to 5°C at −0.5°C/minute. The cooling rate is then increased gradually so that by 0°C it is −10°C/minute, at which it remains until −80°C. Straws are transferred directly from −80°C to liquid nitrogen (Mahadevan and Trounson, 1983).

ORGANIZATION OF A SPERM BANK

Although there are obviously many ways to organize a semen cryobank, as mentioned in Inventory Control Systems, above, there are several basic principles.

1. Every unit of semen (straw or vial) must be individually identifiable so if two insemination doses are removed from the bank and thawed at the same time there is no chance of their being confused.
2. The records identifying the location of a specific batch of semen must be kept in duplicate or in a redundant manner so the information is available in several documents.
3. Records should allow sample identification in both directions. In other words, it must be possible to find a specific batch within the bank; or, starting from a particular storage location in the bank, it must be easy to identify the specimen stored there.
4. The system used to identify storage locations must be easy to use even when the materials are at liquid nitrogen temperatures. For straws, a system based on different shapes and colors of visotubes and different straw and sealing powder colors has proven easy to use. This method is described in detail below. For vials, the canes to which they are attached can be readily identified on their tops and their location within the cryobank identified using tank and canister numbers.
5. For practical purposes it should be possible to find a specific straw or vial quickly.

A simple system for organizing a cryobank using straws.

1. Each *storage dewar* or tank is identified by a roman numeral.
2. Within each tank there are a number of *canisters,* identified using arabic numbers.
3. Depending on tank design, canisters may be short (5 inches ≡ 127 mm) or tall (11 inches ≡ 279 mm). Visotubes are placed directly into the short canisters, but with the tall canisters the use of plastic *goblets* allows each canister to be divided into upper (U) and lower (L) levels.
4. In each goblet are located the *visotubes,* each containing a number of straws from the same ejaculate. Visotubes are available in a number of shapes, sizes, and colors. The number of permutations that are needed can be determined from the maximum number of visotubes that fit into the particular goblet/canister size used in the chosen model of storage dewar. A simple system may employ two shapes—round (R: 13 mm ∅) and polygonal (P)—and one of eight colors: red (R), orange (O), yellow (Y), green (G), blue (B) purple (P), dove gray (D), or white (W). Using this scheme, a full storage location for a batch of straws coded

"R3157" (i.e., "bar-code" number 3157 in the red series of straws (i.e., red straws, or straws sealed with red powder) might be VII-2U-PR, indicating:

Storage tank	VII
Canister	2
Goblet	U (upper)
Visotube shape	P (polygonal)
Visotube color	R (red)

TRANSPORTATION OF CRYOPRESERVED SEMEN

In addition to the long-term storage of semen, cryopreservation allows semen to be transported anywhere in the world. Small numbers of straws or vials can be transported using a "dry shipper," a dewar tank whose inner vessel is filled with a metal honeycomb-like mesh to trap the liquid nitrogen and so reduce its evaporation and minimize possible loss if the tank is tipped over. These dry-shippers, which contain only one small canister, are less easy to fill than a typical storage dewar in that they must be allowed to cool slowly, with repeated addition of liquid nitrogen, over a period of several hours to ensure maximum performance. As an additional precaution, whenever possible straws should be located only in the lower level of the canisters. Obviously larger numbers of straws or vials can be shipped in an ordinary storage-type dewar, although greater care must be taken to prevent it being tipped over. The holding time of the shipping tank being used must be noted and arrangements made for topping up the liquid nitrogen if necessary.

From experience, we have found that the following set of rules eliminates any possible problems with mishandling the shipping tank—or at least transfers liability to the shipping agent. This system also ensures that borderline or substandard batches of straws are not inadvertently sent to consignees.

1. The shipping tank must be capable of being padlocked. Combination padlocks are preferable so as to eliminate possible problems caused by lost keys between the two centers.
2. Weigh the shipping tank empty and then cool and fill it with liquid nitrogen. Monitor its static evaporative loss over a few days to verify tank integrity.
3. The morning before shipment (Monday), transfer the requested straws from the cryobank into the shipping tank after topping it up with liquid nitrogen. Ideally, only the lower half of each canister is used. For each batch of straws include one additional straw for preshipment test-thaw purposes.
4. The afternoon before shipment test-thaw one straw per batch. Copies of these test-thaw results should be sent to the consignee, preferably by FAX. Other information on the donors and batches may be sent by courier or regular mail.
5. The morning of collection (Tuesday) the shipping tank is completely filled with liquid nitrogen to the bottom of the neck plug, padlocked, and weighed. Copies of all shipping documents, including tank and contents weights and expected arrival time are sent to the consignee by FAX.

6. Especially when shipping by air, if the tank weight shows a discrepancy of ≥ 1 kg upon arrival at the freight terminal, it should be returned to the cryobank immediately for investigation.
7. Shipments should be insured for the full replacement value of all straws plus the tank. A supplier cryobank should not be expected to accept any responsibility for any decrease in straw quality after the shipping tank leaves its control.
8. Upon receipt by the consignee, it is strongly recommended that the tank be weighed (before acceptance from the carrier) and post-thaw tests be performed to confirm that the straws have not been damaged during shipment.
9. Any claims for insurance compensation in respect of any damage or loss must be the responsibility of the consignee, who should reasonably be expected to pay the full cost of the shipment in accordance with the previously agreed terms.

References and Recommended Reading

American Association of Tissue Banks (1984). Standards for tissue banking. AATB, Arlington, VA

Bolanos, J. R., Overstreet, J. W., and Katz, D. F. (1983). Human sperm penetration of zona-free hamster eggs after storage of semen for 48 hours at 2°C to 5°C *Fertil. Steril.* **39,** 536.

Canadian Fertility and Andrology Society (1988). *Guidelines for Therapeutic Donor Insemination.* CFAS, Montreal.

Canadian Fertility and Andrology Society (1992). *Revised Guidelines for Therapeutic Donor Insemination.* CFAS, Montreal.

David, G. (1989). Principles et organisation de l'IAD en France: expérience des CECOS. In Englert, Y., Guérin, J. F., and Jouannet, P. (eds): *Stérilité Masculine et Procréations Médicalement Assistées. Progrès en Andrologie 3* Doin, Paris.

Federation CECOS, Le Lannou, D., and Lansac, J. (1989). Artificial procreation with frozen donor semen: experience of the French Federation CECOS. *Hum. Reprod.* **4,** 757.

Friberg, J., and Gemzell, C. (1977). Sperm-freezing and donor insemination. *Int. J. Fertil.* **22,** 148.

Johnson, A., Bassham, B., Lipshultz, L. I., and Lamb, D. J. (1990). Methodology for the optimized sperm penetration assay. In Keel, B. A., and Webster, B. W. (eds): *CRC Handbook of the Laboratory Diagnosis and Treatment of Infertility.* CRC Press, Boca Raton, FL.

Mahadevan, M. M., and Trounson, A. O. (1983). Effect of cryoprotective media and dilution methods on the preservation of human spermatozoa. *Andrologia* **15,** 355.

Polge, C., Smith, U. A., and Parkes, A. S. (1949). Revivial of spermatozoa after vitrification and dehydration at low temperatures. *Nature* **164,** 66.

Richardson, D. W. (1976). Techniques of sperm storage. In Brudenell, J. M., McLaren, A., Short, R. V., and Symonds, E. M. (eds): *Artificial Insemination.* Royal College of Obstetricians and Gynaecologists, London.

Richardson, D. W., Joyce, D., and Symonds, E. M. (eds) (1979). *Frozen Human Semen.* Royal College of Obstetricians and Gynaecologists, London.

Scott, S. G., Mortimer, D., Taylor, P. J., Leader, A., and Pattinson, H. A. (1990). Therapeutic donor insemination using frozen semen. *Can. Med. Assoc. J.* **143,** 273.

Sherman, J. K. (1973). Synopsis of the use of frozen human semen since 1964: state of the art of human semen banking. *Fertil. Steril.* **24,** 397.

Sherman, J. K. (1977). Cryopreservation of human semen. In Hafez, E.S.E. (ed): *Techniques of Human Andrology.* North-Holland, New York.

Sherman, J. K. (1986). Current status of clinical cryobanking of human semen. In Paulson, J. D., Negro-Vilar, A., Lucena, E., and Martini, L. (eds): *Andrology: Male Fertility and Sterility.* Academic Press, Orlando, FL.

Sherman, J. K. (1990). Cryopreservation of human semen. In Keel, B. A., and Webster, B. W. (eds): *CRC Handbook of the Laboratory Diagnosis and Treatment of Infertility.* CRC Press, Boca Raton, FL.

Weidel, L., and Prins, G. S. (1987). Cryosurvival of human spermatozoa frozen in eight different buffering systems. *J. Androl.* **8,** 41.

IV

Laboratory Management

15

Safety in the Andrology Laboratory

People working in andrology laboratories are exposed not only to the usual risks associated with laboratory work but also specific risks related to possible infection from the biological materials being handled. Under the former heading are included such risks as physical injury resulting from the use of electrical equipment, chemical hazards, dropping or lifting heavy objects or boxes, and cuts from broken glassware. Avoiding this type of injury is largely common sense and is not considered further. The use of compressed gases, however, requires specific safety regulations relating to the safe storage and use of cylinders and regulators; the use of cryogenic materials such as liquid nitrogen poses its own additional safety concerns; and biohazard concerns are associated with the risk of infections being transmitted by biological materials including semen, cervical mucus, blood, and urine.

BASIC LABORATORY SAFETY

In addition to common sense aspects, such as not attempting to lift or carry oversized or overweight boxes or pieces of equipment, not stacking cartons too high, using steps instead of climbing onto benches or using chairs with castors as steps, and handling glassware (especially broken glassware) with extreme caution, there are a wide variety of safety concerns when working in a laboratory.

Accident Prevention

Supervisors' responsibilities are to ensure that:

1. All appropriate actions have been taken to correct any safety hazards that might exist is his or her area of responsibility.
2. Proper personal protective clothing and equipment are provided and used.
3. Staff are aware of, and abide by, all federal, provincial, state, and local governmental rules and the institutional safety regulations.
4. Employees receive adequate training in, and information on, safe job procedures.
5. An adequate number of workers are trained in first aid procedures.

Employees' responsibilities are to ensure that:

1. All accidents and injuries are reported to the laboratory supervisor.
2. All federal, provincial, state, and local governmental as well as institutional safety regulations are met.

3. Unsafe procedures and conditions are reported immediately to the laboratory supervisor.
4. They are aware of hazards in their day-to-day work and that appropriate measures are taken to eliminate any risk of accident.
5. Appropriate personal protective clothing and equipment are worn as required, and it is maintained in good condition.

Protective Clothing and Equipment

While performing normal duties a laboratory worker may be exposed to several hazards. If these hazards cannot be controlled at their source(s), personal protective equipment or clothing (or both) must be used (see discussion of responsibilities, above).

Eye Protection

Eye protection must be worn at any time there is a danger of flying particles, irritating substances, liquids, or harmful radiation endangering the eyes. Contact lenses are not a substitute for proper eye protection, and spectacles with plain glass lenses also pose a potential hazard. All workers wearing spectacles who are regularly exposed to this type of hazard should be encouraged to request safety lenses when having prescriptions for new spectacles filled.

Hand Protection

Appropriate gloves must be worn when handling materials or equipment that could be injurious to the skin, such as sharp objects, chemicals, or radioactive, biological, or extremely hot or cold materials.

Respiratory Protection

Although special equipment such as self-contained breathing apparatus or respirators are not required in the andrology laboratory, suitable surgical face masks should be worn whenever there is a possibility of exposure to aerosols of biological material (see Infection Control, below). All flammable or noxious substances such as solvents or fixatives should be handled in a fume hood.

Other Forms of Protective Equipment

Head, foot, and hearing protection should not be required in the andrology laboratory.

Fire Safety

It is the responsibility of the institution to ensure that appropriate fire detection and suppression systems, as required by relevant building and fire safety codes, are installed and serviced, including the provision of portable fire extinguishers. Laboratory supervisors and technical staff, however, also have specific responsibilities.

Supervisors' responsibilities are to ensure that:

1. All staff are informed of fire reporting procedures, the locations of fire-fighting equipment, and evacuation plans.

2. All areas under their responsibility are free of fire hazards and exits are not blocked.
3. Staff are trained in the use of fire extinguishers.

Employees' responsibilities are to ensure that:

1. Fire hazards in the work area are kept to a minimum.
2. Any unsafe conditions or practices are reported immediately to the laboratory supervisor.
3. Evacuation procedures are understood.

Classes of Fire
For the purpose of extinguishing, fires are divided into a number of basic types or classes. In the andrology laboratory, the following three types may be encountered.

Class A: Fires in ordinary combustible materials such as paper, plastics, and rubbish. Live embers are usually associated with this type of fire, which as a result can be deep-seated and require the cooling and quenching effect of water or chemical solutions for effective control.
Class B: Fires in flammable liquids where a blanketing or smothering effect is desirable for extinction.
Class C: Fires in energized electrical equipment, where the use of a nonconductive extinguishing agent is necessary. In many cases, class C fires revert to class A or B fires after the electricity is disconnected.

Types of Fire Extinguisher
To control or extinguish a fire using a portable fire extinguisher, it is essential to know about the types of fire extinguisher (including how to operate and discharge them correctly) and what class(es) of fire on which to use them. All fire extinguishers are labeled with a fire-type rating and operating instructions.

Water extinguishers: For use on class A fires only. Must be protected from freezing.
Dry chemical extinguishers: May be rated for class A, B, or C fires or for only class B and C types: Check label for rating. These extinguishers use nitrogen or carbon dioxide gas pressure as a propellant for the dry chemical powder. The initial discharge should not be aimed directly into the burning material as it could cause it to be spread more widely. When used on a class A fire, this type of extinguisher should be followed by water. There is also the possibility of flash-back or reignition of the flammable material.
Carbon dioxide extinguishers: For use on class B and C fires but may be used to control small class A fires (in which situation they should be followed up with water). Do not let the discharge horn touch the body during or soon after operation as it becomes extremely cold and may cause burns. In confined areas, discharge of this type of extinguisher may displace sufficient air to cause an oxygen-deficient atmosphere. Again there is the possibility of a flashback or reignition of the flammable material.

Halon extinguishers: Effective on class B and C fires but may also be used on class A fires. Halon has low toxicity and can therefore be discharged within enclosed areas. It does not harm fabrics, metals, or other materials, nor does it cause cold burns or leave any residue.

General Fire Safety Rules

The following list of fire safety rules is not exhaustive and should be supplemented by institutional regulations.

1. Never use naked flames when flammable vapors are present. Smoking is forbidden in all laboratories at all times.
2. Never block exit doors, fire/smoke control doors, or access to fire-fighting equipment.
3. Do not store large quantities of flammable solvents in the laboratory. A common regulation is that highly flammable liquids (flash point below 40°C) must not be stored in ordinary glass or metal containers in quantities of more than 4.5 liters. Larger volumes, if essential, must be stored in approved safety containers.
4. Never store equipment or materials in hallways or under stairwells.
5. Use metal or other approved waste containers. Other than for small-scale use (e.g., under-bench locations), plastic waste containers often do not meet fire safety regulations.
6. Always be aware of potential fire or explosion hazards of any chemical or material used in the laboratory.

Hazardous Chemicals

All hazardous materials, whether in transit, storage, or use, must be clearly labeled so as to alert handlers or users of the hazards and safe handling procedures of such materials. Specific relevant information includes the following.

Fire or Explosion Hazard

Relevant information outlines the substance's conditions of flammability (including its flashpoint and means of extinction). Sensitivity to mechanical impact and static discharge in relation to explosion hazards must also be identified, and information on any hazardous combustion products should be available.

Reactivity Data

Reactivity data include descriptions of any conditions under which the substance is chemically unstable or any other substance (or class of substances) with which the substance is incompatible. Information on conditions of reactivity and any hazardous decomposition products is also relevant.

Toxicological Properties

Information on possible routes of entry into the body, including skin contact, skin absorption, eye contact, inhalation, and ingestion, as well as the effects of both acute and chronic exposure to the substance should be available. Other relevant information includes the substance's irritance potential and the likelihood of sensitization to it. Specific information on general toxicity (e.g., poisons), carcinogenicity, teratogenicity, mutagenicity, and reproductive toxicological properties should be clearly identified.

Great care should be taken in the correct handling and disposal of biologically derived materials. They include not only such obvious materials as semen and blood, but blood products (e.g., HSA) and reagents such as enzymes and lectins.

Preventive Measures

The need for personal protective clothing and equipment should be identified, along with procedures to be followed for shipping, storage, handling, and waste disposal. In case of leaks or spills, the protective equipment and clothing must be readily available to users of any hazardous substance. It is the laboratory supervisor's responsibility to ensure that all employees obtain adequate information on all hazardous substances in order to work safely with them. It includes specific training in the safe handling, use, and disposal of such substances.

Radioactive Materials

Any laboratory working with radioactive materials is subject to strict regulations controlling their ordering, shipping, storage, handling, use, and disposal. It is unlikely that a service andrology laboratory needs to use radioactive materials. Laboratory procedures involving radioimmunoassay (RIA) techniques may be employed for the measurement of circulating (blood serum or plasma) or urinary hormone levels. Such techniques are not generally considered an integral function specific to the andrology laboratory, and regulations and guidelines for clinical laboratories are widely available. Consequently, this aspect is not considered further in this text except to note that with the advent of modern fluorescence or enzyme-linked immunoassay (EIA) technology the need for RIAs in laboratories providing routine diagnostic services in the field of reproductive medicine will soon be nonexistent.

Compressed Gases

Safe handling of compressed gases includes not only the cylinders themselves but also the regulators used to control the flow and pressure of the gas at delivery. Gas cylinders must be transported only on special dollies with safety straps or chains around them. In the storage location or during use in the laboratory, cylinders must be stood upright and attached by safety straps to mounting brackets fixed to the bench or wall. Cylinders must be protected from mechanical shock and extremes of heat or cold.

Regulators must be attached and removed using the correct wrench, spanner, or key. Ensure that the main (inlet) valve is tightly closed before attaching a regulator to a gas cylinder. Take great care not to damage the screw threads when attaching or removing a regulator. Regulators should be serviced regularly to ensure accurate, reliable, safe performance. When gas is not flowing, close the inlet valve from the cylinder to the regulator and open the outlet valve. Maintaining pressure inside the regulator when not in use greatly shortens its life.

Always use appropriate tubing or piping for the gas being used and its purpose. For flammable gases use butyl rubber tubing; for high-pressure gases use a tubing with a suitable pressure rating as well as any necessary security fittings (e.g., terry clips where the tubing is attached to the regulator outlet).

For sensitive applications such as carbon dioxide or its mixtures for in vitro fertilization or embryo culture (e.g., 5% CO_2 in air or 5% CO_2/5% O_2/90% N_2), never use copper piping; as Cu^{2+} ions are highly embryotoxic. Use piping made of an inert material such as stainless steel or high grade PVC.

CRYOGENICS

Because of its extremely cold temperature ($-196°C$), the handling and use of liquid nitrogen (LN_2) requires extreme care and attention. Always wear appropriate protective clothing and equipment, including long sleeves, suitable gloves, and splash-proof goggles or, preferably, a whole-face visor or faceshield. Whenever possible, LN_2 should be transferred from its supply dewar vessel by transfer hose or other delivery device; open pouring should be discouraged.

Touching the inside of dewar vessels containing LN_2 or any object that has been in recent contact with LN_2 using bare fingers can cause severe cold burns. If frostbite does occur, warm the affected skin in warm water at a temperature of about 40°C. Encourage the victim to exercise the affected part while it is being warmed and allow the circulation to return naturally.

Dewar vessels must be protected from mechanical insult. Glass dewar vessels must be treated with extreme caution, and it is worth considering the use of styrofoam boxes for short-term uses involving small volumes of LN_2. Plastic-encased dewar vessels are perfectly suitable, except that spilling LN_2 over the plastic casing, especially at the vessel's open neck, often causes it to split. Even steel storage dewar tanks can be punctured, and the loss of vacuum between the outer and inner walls results in rapid evaporative loss of the LN_2 and hence loss of the cryopreserved material.

Never seal or enclose a dewar vessel containing LN_2, as evaporation of the LN_2 causes a substantial buildup of internal pressure that will certainly explode glass dewar vessels (e.g., thermos flasks or jugs). All lids or caps for LN_2 dewars must be loose-fitting or include an emergency pressure release valve.

Straws or vials that have been immersed in LN_2 must be very carefully handled as there is a genuine risk of explosion. If a vial is not completely sealed, LN_2 enters it during its period of immersion; this liquid rapidly turns to gas when returned to ambient temperature and the sudden huge increase in its volume causes the vials to explode. This possibility is a serious concern if glass cryovials or ampoules are used—and, along with the risk of breakage while opening, good reason not to use glass ampoules at all. With straws, evaporation of the liquid that permeates the cotton plug at the top of the straw often causes violent expulsion of this plug the first time the straw is transferred, even for a few seconds, from the liquid phase to ambient temperature (e.g., while searching for a particular straw or batch of straws). Consequently, protective goggles or a visor must also be worn when thawing straws or cryovials.

INFECTION CONTROL

Modern infection control regulations require that all human tissue samples be considered potentially pathogenic; this clearly includes all specimens handled in an andrology laboratory. Therefore all andrology laboratories, semen banks, IVF laboratories, and the like must have adequate safety programs to protect their staff against accidental contamination. It also dictates that laboratory workers recognize the potential dangers of their profession (review: Schrader, 1989).

The notoriety of HIV has resulted in many individuals being preoccupied with the possibility of AIDS transmission by handling semen or blood. Although it is a significant concern, it must not be allowed to overshadow the wide range of other pathogens commonly found in specimens handled by andrology laboratories. In fact, AIDS is substantially less infective through this route than hepatitis, which is the most frequently occurring infection of laboratory workers (Pike, 1976). Hepatitis B virus has been detected in semen, urine, and saliva as well as blood; and infection can occur from contamination of even a small area of infected skin if an open lesion such as a scratch or graze is present. Because an effective hepatitis B vaccine is now available (Recombivax HB: Merck, Sharp & Dohme), all health care professionals should be vaccinated.

In addition, the organisms causing many traditional sexually transmissible diseases are found in semen (see Chapter 6). Cases of accidental gonorrhea or *Chlamydia, Mycoplasma,* or *Streptococcus* infection in laboratory personnel have been documented.

Cytomegalovirus and papillomavirus have also been isolated in semen. However, although no documented laboratory-associated infections have been reported, the possibility of transmission of these pathogens by exposure to mucous membranes (e.g., ingestion or inhalation of aerosolized material) or accidental innoculation (e.g., fingerstick or contamination of an open wound) does exist.

Specific Recommendations

The following recommendations are adapted from those published by Schrader (1989) and the World Health Organization (1992).

1. Vaccination of all laboratory personnel handling human tissues and body fluids should be encouraged in accordance with the recommendations for medical personnel in general.
2. Laboratory personnel must handle every specimen of human tissue or body fluid as if it were contaminated with an infectious organism.
3. Extraordinary precautions must be taken to avoid accidental wounds from (contaminated) sharp instruments in the laboratory, including any sharp edges or

corners of microscope slides and coverslips. Hypodermic needles should be eliminated from general laboratory use to minimize the risks of fingerstick injury.

4. Avoid contact between biological materials and open skin lesions. Disposable rubber or plastic gloves must be worn at all times when handling fresh or frozen semen, seminal plasma, blood plasma or serum, cervical mucus, and urine, as well as any containers or handling devices (e.g., pipettes) that have come into contact with these materials. Gloves must be removed and discarded as contaminated waste when leaving the laboratory, handling the telephone, and so on. Never reuse gloves.

5. A laboratory coat or gown must be worn, fastened, in the laboratory. This protective clothing must be removed on leaving the laboratory. Under no circumstances should such clothing be worn in social rooms or cafeterias.

6. Hands must be washed after removing gowns and gloves. Hands must be washed thoroughly and immediately if they become contaminated with biological material. All hand washing must be with a disinfectant soap and hot water.

7. If the outside of any sample container is contaminated, it must be washed with a disinfectant solution, such as a 1:10 dilution of 5.25% sodium hypochlorite (household bleach) with tap water.

8. Disposable laboratory supplies should be used whenever and wherever possible. After use they should be collected in special *Biological Hazard* containers and properly disposed of as for other infectious material, e.g., by incineration or autoclaving.

9. All laboratory equipment that could potentially be contaminated by biological material must be disinfected or sterilized (e.g., by alcohol spray) after a spill or after work activity is completed, including equipment handled while wearing protective gloves, e.g., microscopes and pipetting devices.

10. Mechanical pipetting devices must be used for the manipulation of all liquids in the laboratory. Although practically all laboratories totally prohibit pipetting by mouth, some authorities still accept the use of mouth pipetting for fine control of extremely small volume transfers (e.g., when handling eggs). Under these situations a 0.22-μm filter must be placed in the suction line and the mouthpiece sterilized with alcohol before each use. In general there must be no risk of aerosol formation or the aspiration of a volume large enough to contaminate the filter directly.

11. All procedures and manipulations of biological fluids must be performed so as to minimize the creation of droplets and aerosols. Surgical masks should be worn when procedures are conducted that have a high potential for creating airborne droplets or aerosols. Such procedures include centrifugation or vigorous mixing (especially vortex mixing) of open containers. Centrifuges should be covered or placed in biohazard cabinets during the centrifugation of biological fluids.

12. Laboratory work surfaces must be decontaminated with a disinfectant (see item 7, above) immediately after any spill occurs and on completing work with biological fluids each day.

13. Eating, drinking, smoking, applying cosmetics, and so on are prohibited in all laboratories.

IMPLEMENTATION OF LABORATORY SAFETY

Institutional policies regarding general safety, fire drills, and so on must be observed, including any relevant legal statutes. Specific safety requirements for laboratory personnel handling cryogenic materials and biological samples including body fluids must also be clearly explained and documented in the laboratory manual. Any necessary training must be provided, and it should be made clear to all employees that all safety requirements must be strictly observed. Employers should monitor employee compliance to ensure adherence to all safety procedures and offer additional education, counseling, and retraining as necessary (see Basic Laboratory Safety, above).

Employers must provide any and all safety equipment (e.g., laboratory coats or gowns, gloves, masks, protective clothing for handling cryogenics) and other materials (e.g., disinfectants, disinfectant soap) as required. The institution must also arrange for the proper disposal of the various types of laboratory waste, including sharp instruments, broken glass, used solvents and other chemicals, and contaminated waste.

CONCLUSIONS

It is a fact of life that no safety program can guarantee complete protection from all physical, chemical, or pathogenic hazards encountered by laboratory personnel in the course of their work. However, it is not only common sense and good practice to make every practical effort to minimize all such risks, it is often a legal requirement of the employer and employee. Federal governments and agencies have passed laws or issued specific recommendations that regulate laboratories and laboratory practice. In many areas both professional societies and labor organizations have taken leading roles in the recommendation and implementation of safety precautions. The recommendations in this chapter are simple to implement and should be routine in an andrology laboratory. All laboratory personnel should ensure that they are aware of all regulations that might pertain to their particular location and circumstances.

References and Recommended Reading

Pike, R. M. (1976). Laboratory-associated infections: summary and analysis 3921 cases. *Health Lab. Sci.* **13**, 105.

Schrader, S. M. (1989). Safety guidelines for the andrology laboratory. *Fertil. Steril.* **51**, 387.

World Health Organization (1992). *WHO Laboratory Manual for the Examination of Human Semen and Sperm-Cervical Mucus Interaction, 3rd ed.* Cambridge University Press, Cambridge.

16

Technician Training and Quality Control Aspects

It is a fundamental principle of laboratory tests that they are never entirely free from error. However, understanding the source(s) and extent of such errors is a prerequisite for correct appreciation and interpretation of test results in the diagnostic process. To evaluate these errors, quality control (QC) has been introduced into clinical laboratory tests and has become routine practice (Cembrowski and Carey, 1989).

To date, the preconditions for QC in the andrology laboratory have not been met for various reasons, primarily related to the general belief that "it can't be done." Certainly there are difficulties in dealing with live gametes as analytes and in their use for standard preparations, but these difficulties are not insurmountable if one is prepared to make a commitment to the concept of QC. Furthermore, the perceived lack of definitive and reference methods for the determination of semen characteristics has now been addressed by the various editions of the WHO's *Laboratory Manual* (Belsey et al., 1980; World Health Organization, 1987, 1992), although there do remain some concerns in the practical implementation of some procedures (see below).

Although absolute reference methods are slowly being introduced, e.g., flow cytometry for the estimation of sperm concentration, the worldwide acceptance and use of the WHO *Laboratory Manual* has already led to a greatly increased standardization of semen analysis techniques (World Health Organization, 1987, 1992). This standardization provides a basis for the application of QC procedures in semen analysis. Indeed, several laboratories have started to introduce internal QC as suggested by some investigators (Mortimer et al., 1986; Dunphy et al., 1989; Knuth et al., 1989); and the first modern ring trial for external QC has been performed (Neuwinger et al., 1990). The various mathematical models for quality control (e.g., Bland and Altman, 1986; Cembrowski and Carey, 1989) require further evaluation before general recommendations can be made, but many laboratories will start using internal QC schemes in the near future.

TECHNICIAN TRAINING

Obviously quality control must begin with adequate training of the staff performing semen analyses and other andrology laboratory procedures. The various editions of the WHO *Laboratory Manual* have provided more or less standardized methods, but in practice they have not been implemented identically in different laboratories. Indeed, in certain areas there have been eloquent misinterpretations or obscurities. For example, it was certainly unclear that the Second Edition was encouraging the use of multiparametric sperm morphology assessments, and the lack of any definition as to the meaning of "linear" motility made the Second Edition's motility classification scheme of "rapid and linear motility" (class **a**) versus "slow, linear or nonlinear motility" (class **b**) impossible to establish objectively. It was for just this reason that Dunphy et al. (1990) found that class **b** motility was the most significant predictor of in vivo fertility because they included all spermatozoa showing significant lateral head displacement in class **b** as "nonlinear"—it being well known that spermatozoa showing larger ALH values penetrate cervical mucus more successfully (see Chapters 7 and 11). These problems have been resolved in the Third Edition.

Certainly the increased activity of the WHO and various national fertility and andrology societies in organizing andrology workshops will address the problem of uniform implementation of semen analysis and other methods. It is anticipated that during the 1990s we shall see a dramatic increase in the worldwide availability of standardized diagnostic procedures in andrology.

Goal-Orientated Training Scheme for Semen Analysis

As an adjunct to any QC program there must exist a structured training scheme whereby new laboratory staff can achieve not only competence in their duties but also comparability with others already performing the same procedures. The method described below has been used by me to train andrology technicians to perform semen analyses to uniformly high standards of accuracy and reproducibility.

Preliminaries
New technical staff are initially exposed to the performance of semen analyses by trained technicians and given free access to the laboratory's procedures manual and other resource texts (e.g., current WHO *Laboratory Manual,* appropriate book chapters, and monographs). Once they have gained a general idea of what is being done, each component of a semen analysis is fully explained in detail and the new technician allowed adequate time to gain preliminary hands-on experience to become comfortable with each component procedure.

Goal-Oriented Learning
Upon gaining initial confidence, the new technician then performs assessments of the various components of semen analysis on clinical material in duplicate to those being carried out by the trained staff. These duplicate assessments are performed in groups of 30, and the discrepancies between the novice and expert results are analyzed appropriately for continuous or discrete variables.

Discrete variables, such as modal progression ratings or subjective rankings of debris or round cells, should never differ by more than one rank, and should be identical in > 90% of cases. In other words, no more than two ratings can be different in a group of 30 assessments and then by no more than ± 1 rank each.

Continuous variables, such as sperm concentration and the percentages of sperm motility, vitality, and morphological normality, are amenable to analysis using techniques such as paired *t*-tests or the method described by Bland and Altman (1986). The latter method considers the average discrepancy between two sets of values (calculated as the mean of a series of individual difference values) compared to the average of the individual paired measurements. However, this analysis assumes that both methods of measurement (or individuals making the measurements in this case) are equally likely to be correct. When training novice technicians, the following variation is more useful, although for subsequent quality control analyses, the original method using technician-average values should be employed (see Quality Control of Semen Analysis, below).

Sperm Motility, Vitality, and Normal Morphology Assessments

1. For each of the 30 pairs of counts (percent motility, percent progressive, percent live, percent normal), the difference between the novice and expert values is determined by subtraction:

$$\text{Difference} = X_{\text{NOVICE}} - X_{\text{EXPERT}}$$

The sign of the difference indicates whether the novice is counting high (a positive difference) or low (a negative difference) compared to the expert (Table 16-1).

2. Calculate the mean and standard deviation (SD) of the 30 difference values.

Sperm Concentration Values

For sperm concentration evaluation, each difference value is expressed as a percentage of the expert's value, as the range of sperm concentration values is wide. Again the sign of the difference value is retained and the mean and SD of the 30 difference values are calculated (Table 16-2).

Interpretation of Results

The aim is to achieve consistency between the novice and the trained expert(s). Consequently, the novice's goal is to achieve a zero mean difference and a 95% range of differences that is within a predetermined level of acceptability, e.g., ± 5%. The 95% range of discrepancy is calculated by multiplying the SD by the value of the *t* statistic for that number of observations and the appropriate level of significance. For example, for a 5% significance level with $n = 30$, $t = 2.042$. The SD is not multiplied by 2.0 until $n = 60$.

Typically, on the first set of counts, the novice shows a large average difference and a wide range of discrepancy. With subsequent sets of counts these values decrease, and usually the average difference reduces to zero before the range of discrepancy decreases to 5% (Figs. 16-1 to 16-4). The novice is not allowed to contribute to clinical results until this condition has been reached. With each successive group of 30 assessments novices can see a reduction in the degree and extent of discrepancy between their assessments and those of the expert(s).

Table 16–1 Sample training data and calculations for assessment of the percent motile spermatozoa

Sample	Novice	Expert	Difference
1	68	65	3
2	62	59	3
3	20	21	−1
4	63	61	2
5	32	33	−1
6	45	48	−3
7	55	58	−3
8	45	43	2
9	56	59	−3
10	42	42	0
11	39	36	3
12	34	37	−3
13	59	55	4
14	48	48	0
15	46	48	−2
16	64	61	3
17	35	38	−3
18	58	59	−1
19	42	39	3
20	48	50	−2
21	54	52	2
22	46	46	0
23	51	56	−5
24	58	60	−2
25	61	64	−3
26	67	66	1
27	48	49	−1
28	70	68	2
29	49	46	3
30	51	48	3

Mean difference	0.03
SD of difference	2.57
95% Range of differences upper limit	5.27
95% Range of differences lower limit	−5.21

Table 16–2 Sample training data and calculations for assess ments of sperm concentration. Novice and Expert values are ×10⁶/ml.

Sample	Novice	Expert	Diff.	%Diff.
1	24.8	24.5	0.3	1.2
2	87.3	89.5	−2.2	−2.5
3	121.3	123.0	−1.7	−1.4
4	83.0	80.3	2.7	3.3
5	53.5	53.5	0.0	0.0
6	64.8	63.8	1.0	1.6
7	38.3	37.0	1.3	3.4
8	27.8	28.5	−0.7	−2.5
9	190.5	183.8	6.7	3.6
10	63.0	61.8	1.2	1.9
11	123.5	127.8	−4.3	−3.4
12	212.5	209.0	3.5	1.7
13	97.0	98.0	1.0	1.0
14	89.5	92.8	−3.3	−3.6
15	189.5	182.5	7.0	3.8
16	12.5	12.6	−0.1	−0.8
17	141.3	137.8	3.5	2.5
18	123.0	122.8	0.2	0.2
19	164.0	169.5	−5.5	−3.3
20	157.5	162.5	−5.0	−3.1
21	23.2	22.8	0.4	1.7
22	77.5	76.3	1.2	1.6
23	110.0	110.5	−0.5	−0.5
24	40.8	40.0	0.8	2.0
25	117.5	113.5	4.0	3.5
26	70.0	72.3	−2.3	−3.2
27	61.3	63.0	−1.7	−2.7
28	59.3	59.0	0.3	0.5
29	32.5	31.8	0.7	2.2
30	30.5	31.5	−1.0	−3.2

Mean difference	0.18
SD of differences	2.50
95% Range of differences upper limit	5.29
95% Range of differences lower limits	−4.93

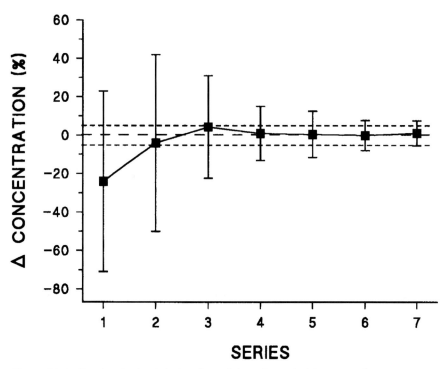

Figure 16-1 Results obtained during the training of a technician to perform sperm concentration determinations using the volumetric dilution and hemocytometry method (see text for details). The *long-dashed line* denotes zero average difference, and the two *short-dashed lines* denote ± 5% average differences. See text for explanation.

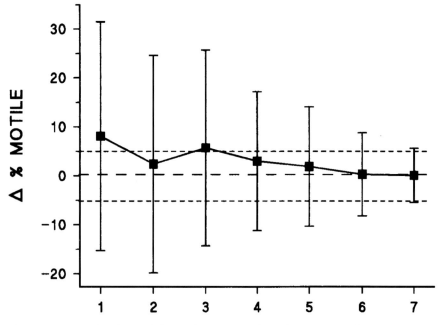

Figure 16-2 Results obtained during the training of a technician to perform visual sperm motility counts (see text for details). The *long-dashed line* denotes zero average difference, and the two *short-dashed lines* denote ± 5% average differences. See text for explanation.

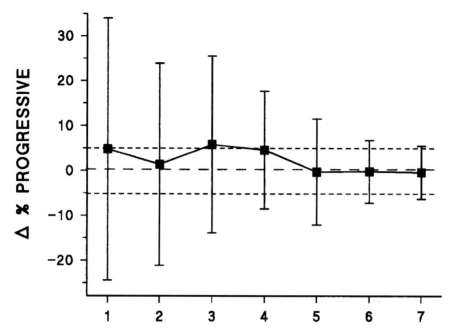

Figure 16-3 Results obtained during the training of a technician to perform visual sperm progressive motility counts (see text for details). The *long-dashed line* denotes zero average difference, and the two *short-dashed lines* denote ± 5% average differences. See text for explanation.

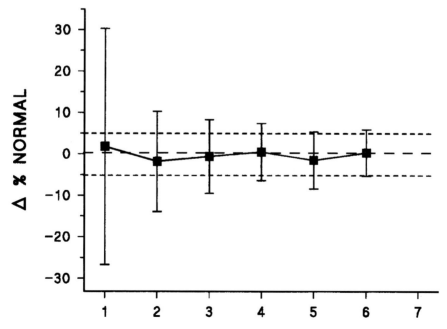

Figure 16-4 Results obtained during the training of a technician to perform visual assessments of normal sperm morphology (see text for details). The *long-dashed line* denotes zero average difference, and the two *short-dashed lines* denote ± 5% average differences. See text for explanation.

QUALITY CONTROL AND QUALITY ASSURANCE

Basic Concepts

The terms quality control and quality assurance are used to refer to the control of the testing process to ensure that test results meet their quality requirements. Their definitions overlap to some degree. *Quality Control (QC)* includes establishing specifications for each aspect of the testing process, assessing the procedures used in the testing process to determine conformance to these specifications, and taking any necessary corrective actions to bring procedures into conformance. *Quality assurance (QA)* is more expansive and not only encompasses quality control of the testing process but involves monitoring and control of the ultimate outcomes of the testing process, including aspects such as financial costs attributable to the laboratory, clinical relevance (diagnostic sensitivity and specificity), and user satisfaction.

Coefficient of Variation
The **coefficient of variation (CV)** for a series of measurements (ideally at least 10) is calculated according to the equation:

$$CV\ (\%) = \frac{\text{standard deviation}}{\text{mean}} \times 100$$

Intraindividual and interindividual CVs exist for any testing procedure and may be used to calculate an optimal *analytical coefficient of variation* (CV$_A$) as:

$$CV_A = 0.5 \times \sqrt{[(CV_{INTRA})^2 + (CV_{INTER})^2]}$$

Extension of the Goal-Oriented Training Method
The method of Bland and Altman (1986; see also above) can also be used to assess the maintenance of standardization between trained technicians. In this situation, because all trained individuals are equally likely to be correct, the average of the two or more observers is used to calculate the individual technician's discrepancies (Table 16-3).

Quality Control of Semen Analysis

The precision of the techniques used in andrology laboratories should be determined by estimates of intra- and intertechnician variability of estimates at regular intervals. These measurements should consider not so much the degree of agreement between observations or between observers but, rather, the potential for discrepancy between intra- or interobserver measurements. QC measurements can be made at a number of levels.

Intraindividual = within an individual technician.
Interindividual = *intralaboratory* = between technicians within a laboratory
Interlaboratory = between laboratories

Table 16–3 Sample quality control data and calculations for assessments of sperm vitality (percent live spermatozoa) by four trained technicians (A–D)

Sample	Actual Counts				Average	Differences from Average			
	A	B	C	D		A	B	C	D
1	65	69	64	67	66.25	1.25	−2.75	2.25	−0.75
2	82	83	76	81	80.50	1.50	2.50	−4.50	0.50
3	90	89	84	91	88.50	1.50	0.50	−4.50	2.50
4	74	73	66	67	70.00	4.00	3.00	−4.00	−3.00
5	79	75	83	81	79.50	−0.50	−4.50	3.50	1.50
6	89	92	92	92	91.25	−2.25	0.75	0.75	0.75
7	89	83	82	84	84.50	4.50	−1.50	−2.50	−0.50
8	67	70	69	71	69.25	−2.25	0.75	−0.25	1.75
9	72	76	72	72	73.00	−1.00	3.00	−1.00	−1.00
10	91	87	86	89	88.25	2.75	−1.25	−2.25	0.75
11	92	91	88	87	89.50	2.50	1.50	−1.50	−2.50
12	85	87	90	86	87.00	−2.00	0.00	3.00	−1.00
13	80	85	89	87	85.25	−5.25	−0.25	3.75	1.75
14	80	82	84	84	82.50	−2.50	−0.50	1.50	1.50
15	91	79	83	81	83.50	7.50	−4.50	−0.50	−2.50
16	74	78	77	82	77.75	−3.75	0.25	−0.75	4.25
17	82	75	85	86	82.00	0.00	−7.00	3.00	4.00
18	89	88	86	84	86.75	2.25	1.25	−0.75	−2.75
19	80	80	87	81	82.00	−2.00	−2.00	5.00	−1.00
20	76	71	73	75	73.75	2.25	−2.75	−0.75	1.25
21	48	50	46	48	48.00	0.00	2.00	−2.00	0.00
22	83	82	84	90	84.75	−1.75	−2.75	−0.75	5.25
23	82	88	87	91	87.00	−5.00	1.00	0.00	4.00
24	76	80	71	77	76.00	0.00	4.00	−5.00	1.00
25	76	74	73	72	73.75	2.25	0.25	−0.75	−1.75
26	63	58	62	65	62.00	1.00	−4.00	0.00	3.00
27	68	79	76	77	75.00	−7.00	4.00	1.00	2.00
28	76	72	74	71	73.25	2.75	−1.25	0.75	−2.25
29	70	63	64	71	67.00	3.00	−4.00	−3.00	4.00
30	78	83	89	80	82.50	−4.50	0.50	6.50	−2.50
Mean difference from average						0.03	−0.46	−0.13	0.61
SD of difference from average						3.27	2.72	2.83	2.38

Source: Unpublished data from the University of Calgary Diagnostic Semen Laboratory.

For the present, andrology laboratories rarely determine either intra- or interindividual CVs at the technician level, and no attempt has been made to establish these concepts at the interlaboratory level. Consequently, scientists, physicians, and epidemiologists alike have little confidence in the reliability of semen analysis data. Established QC practices are also vital for establishing expected performance limits prior to implementing any program of providing standard reference preparations to andrology laboratories.

The aspects of semen analysis most in need of QC standards are the quantitative and qualitative aspects of sperm production: sperm concentration, motility, vitality, and morphology assessments. In addition, some consideration should also be given to making available positive and negative control sera and seminal plasma samples for the detection and titration of antisperm antibodies on a broader basis than previously available. This point is especially important in light of the rapidly increasing number of laboratories performing direct and indirect Immunobead tests.

Practical Considerations

For the purposes of internal QC, aliquots of semen samples diluted for hemocytometry can be stored and analyzed at regular intervals for sperm concentration. For long-term applications, aliquots of (pooled) semen samples could be frozen (i.e., stored at $-20°$ to $-30°C$, in contrast to cryopreserved) and diluted after thawing.

For sperm morphology and vitality, sets of stained, mounted slides can be prepared and reanalyzed at intervals either by the same or different observers. Such preparations could be used repeatedly over considerable periods.

To determine the precision of sperm motility estimates, different technicians may make independent observations on the same fresh sample, or aliquots of (pooled) semen samples may be cryopreserved and analyzed at intervals. Obviously, the cryopreservation approach should use a clarified cryoprotectant (see Chapter 14), although there is the limitation that few samples with exceptional progressive motility are available, as cryopreservation usually causes a reduction in qualitative sperm progression as well as in the proportion of motile cells.

In the absence of semen cryobanking facilities, video recordings of semen samples could be used as surrogates, although observers' perceptions of video images on a television monitor is likely different from that when looking through a microscope. If this method is chosen for future standardization, it may be necessary that andrology laboratories have at least a limited videomicroscopy capability (e.g., a small CCD camera with C-mount and a small, surveillance-type monochrome monitor; a video camera recorder, or VCR, is not essential) and perform all visual motility counts off the monitor screen rather than directly through the microscope.

Serum and seminal plasma samples for antisperm antibody assays would best be provided frozen (at $-20°$ to $-30°C$, or in liquid nitrogen if convenient), although lyophilized standards could also be considered for the indirect Immunobead test.

Potential Problems

There are a number of potential sources of problems to be faced when considering distribution of QC materials along the lines described above.

1. Safe shipment by mail or courier service to each destination laboratory of glass microscope slides for morphology and vitality assessments and plastic vials of diluted semen for hemocytometry
2. Need for transporting frozen material on dry ice, including the availability of freezer space at each destination laboratory
3. Need for transporting cryopreserved material in liquid nitrogen, including the availability of liquid nitrogen cryostorage facilities at each destination laboratory
4. Need for videotaped material to be available in different television standards (e.g., PAL, SECAM, NTSC) and videocassette formats (e.g., VHS, S-VHS,

Beta-I, Beta-IS, Beta-II, Video-8, or Hi-8) to accommodate the equipment available to each destination laboratory

In addition, there is the need to establish the "correct" result for each reference preparation according to the predetermined methodology that is to be used and by an absolute reference method if available (e.g., flow cytometry for determining sperm concentration). Although the preparation and "calibration" of each reference preparation should be performed by one expert andrology laboratory, access to highly specialized equipment need not be on site if collaboration with another, suitably equipped laboratory is established beforehand.

CONCLUSIONS

From the discussions in the previous section it is apparent that intraindividual, intralaboratory, and even interlaboratory standardization and QC of semen analysis are attainable. What is needed is commitment by the andrology laboratories and some organization for providing interlaboratory QC materials. Interlaboratory and intratechnician QC can be achieved locally relatively easily.

References and Recommended Reading

Belsey, M. A., Eliasson, R., Gallegos, A. J., Moghissi, K. S., Paulsen, C. A., and Prasad, M.R.N. (1980). *Laboratory Manual for the Examination of Human Semen and Semen-Cervical Mucus Interaction.* Press Concern, Singapore.

Bland, J. M., and Altman, D. G. (1986). Statistical methods for assessing agreement between two methods of clinical measurement. *Lancet* 1, 307.

Cembrowski, G. S., and Carey, R. N. (1989). *Laboratory Quality Management: QC ⇌ QA.* American Society of Clinical Pathologists, Chicago.

Dunphy, B. C., Kay, R., Barratt, C.L.R., and Cooke, I. D. (1989). Quality control during the conventional semen analysis, an essential exercise. *J. Androl.* 10, 378.

Dunphy, B. C., Li, T.-C., Macleod, I. C., Barratt, C.L.R., Lenton, E. A., and Cooke, I. D. (1990). The interaction of parameters of male and female fertility in couples with previously unexplained infertility. *Fertil. Steril.* 54, 824.

Knuth, U. A., Neuwinger, J., and Nieschlag, E. (1989). Bias to routine semen analysis by uncontrolled changes in laboratory environment—detection by long-term sampling of monthly means for quality control. *Int. J. Androl.* 12, 375.

Mortimer, D., Shu, M. A., and Tan, R. (1986). Standardization and quality control of sperm concentration and sperm motility counts in semen analysis. *Hum. Reprod.* 1, 299.

Neuwinger, J., Behre, H. M., and Nieschlag, E. (1990). External quality control in the andrology laboratory: an experimental multicenter trial. *Fertil. Steril.* 54, 308.

World Health Organization (1987). *WHO Laboratory Manual for the Examination of Human Semen and Semen-Cervical Mucus Interaction, 2nd ed.* Cambridge University Press, Cambridge.

World Health Organization (1992). *WHO Laboratory Manual for the Examination of Human Semen and Sperm-Cervical Mucus Interaction, 3rd ed.* Cambridge University Press, Cambridge.

Appendix I: Semen Analysis Procedural Schedule and Sample Laboratory Form

Procedural Schedule

Time After Ejaculation	Action
0–5 Minutes	1. Register sample in the laboratory.
	2. Place sample in incubator at 37°C.
20–25 Minutes	3. Examine sample for completion of liquefaction, appearance, and odor.
30 Minutes	4. Measure semen pH.
	5. Measure ejaculate volume and assess viscosity.
	6. Prepare specimens for microbiological evaluation if requested.
	7. Make eosin-nigrosin smears.
	8. Make and examine a wet preparation; assess:
	a. Sperm motility and progression
	b. Sperm aggregation/agglutination
	c. Presence of other cells and debris
	9. Make video recordings for subsequent sperm movement and analysis, if required.
	10. Make the dilutions for the hemocytometric determination of sperm concentration.
	11. Prepare smears to be stained for sperm morphology.
	12. Take any aliquots for antibody titrations and biochemistry assays (including the spot test for fructose, if performed.
	13. Prepare a washed sperm population for the direct Immunobead test.
	14. If indicated from the wet preparation use one of the specific methods for detecting leukocytes.
As soon as possible	15. Complete the preparation of aliquots for antibody titrations and biochemistry assays, if performed.
	16. Perform the spot test for fructose, if requested.
3 Hours[a]	17. Make more eosin-nigrosin smears.
	18. Reassess sperm motility and progressivity in a fresh wet preparation.
Subsequently	19. Hemocytometer counts.
	20. Vitality scoring.
	21. Morphology scoring.
	22. Any antibody titrations (sperm agglutination or cytotoxicity).
	23. Any biochemistry batch assays requested.

[a]Usually omitted when analyzing samples provided for assisted reproduction purposes.

349

Normal Values of Semen Variables (WHO, 1992)

Standard Tests

Volume	2.0 ml or more
pH	7.2–8.0
Sperm concentration	20×10^6 spermatozoa/ml or more
Total sperm count	40×10^6 spermatozoa/ejaculate or more

Standard Tests

Motility	50% or more with forward progression (i.e., categories a and b) or 25% or more with rapid progression (i.e., category a) within 60 minutes of ejaculation
Morphology	30% or more with normal form[a]
Vitality	75% or more live (i.e., excluding dye)
White blood cells	$< 1 \times 10^6$/ml
Immunobead test	< 20% spermatozoa with adherent particles
MAR test	< 10% spermatozoa with adherent particles

Optional tests

α-Glucosidase (neutral)	20 mU or more/ejaculate
Zinc (total)	2.4 µmol or more/ejaculate
Citric acid (total)	52 µmol or more/ejaculate
Acid phosphatase (total)	200 U or more/ejaculate
Fructose (total)	13 µmol or more/ejaculate

[a]Although no clinical studies have been completed, experience in a number of centers suggests that percent normal forms should be adjusted downward when more strict criteria are applied. An empirical reference value is suggested to be 30% or more with normal forms.

ANDROLOGY LABORATORY

Semen Analysis

Lab. Ref. No. (YRxxxx)

NAME:	DoB:	DATE:
REFERRED BY:	SAMPLE:	TIME:

SAMPLE INFO:		SPERM MORPHOLOGY	PREP:
Abstinence (days)		Normal forms (%)	
Place of production (coded; 1 = lab)		Head defects (%)	
Method of production (coded; 1 = mast)		Neck / midpiece defects (%)	
Completeness (0 = no; 1 = yes)		Tail defects (%)	
Appearance (coded)		Cytoplasmic droplets (%)	
Odour (coded)		Teratozoospermia Index	
Liquefaction (coded; 1 = by 30 min)		Leukocytes (per 100 sperm)	
Viscosity (coded; 1 = normal)		Germinal line cells (per 100 sperm)	
pH		SPERM VITALITY (% live)	
WET PREP: Debris (coded)		At _____ mins post-ejac'n	
"Round cells" (coded; <2 = normal)		At _____ mins post-ejac'n	

	%	Site
Epithelial cells (coded; <2 = normal)	DIRECT IMMUNOBEAD TEST	
Erythrocytes (coded; 0 = normal)	Combined (GAM) bead screen	
Bacteria / Protozoa (coded)	Isotype-specific: IgG	
Clumping: % of spermatozoa	IgA	
type (coded)	IgM	

		COMMENTS:-
Volume (ml)		
Sperm concentration (M/ml)	INDIRECT IMMUNOBEAD TEST	
Total sperm count (M/ejac)	SPERMAGGLUTINATION (titre)	
Leukocytes (M/ml)	SPERMIMMOBILIZATION (titre)	

Microbiological analysis (coded; 0 = no)	
MOTILITY : minutes post-ejac'n	
(a) Rapid progressive (%)	
(b) Slow progressive (%)	
(c) Non-progressive (%)	
(d) Immotile (%)	
Progression rating (0-4)	
Motility Index (0-300)	
MOTILITY : minutes post-ejac'n	
(a) Rapid progressive (%)	
(b) Slow progressive (%)	
(c) Non-progressive (%)	
(d) Immotile (%)	
Progression rating (0-4)	
Motility Index (0-300)	

Sign & Date:

DM:02/92

Figure App I-1 Sample laboratory form.

351

Appendix II: Microscope Field Calibration

Preparations of known depth are essential for performing objective counts of cells under the microscope. Although this is easily achieved using volumetric chambers (e.g., hemocytometers, Makler chambers, Microcells), it is not so easy when working with viscous materials such as cervical mucus. This problem led to the concept of low and high power fields (10× and 40× objectives, respectively), except that the field of view is not necessarily constant for objectives of the same magnification among microscope manufacturers. Add to this difference the influence of different eyepieces, other microscope components incorporating intermediate magnification, or "tube factors," and the likelihood of different laboratories working with the same field area becomes increasingly remote.

The commonest unit, the high power field (HPF), used a 40× objective. However, the oculars (usually 10×) used in the classic studies typically had apertures of 14 mm, giving substantially smaller field areas than modern wide-field oculars with apertures of about 20 mm. The diameter of the microscopic field of view can be calculated by dividing the diameter of the aperture of the ocular by the magnifying power of the objective. Hence the traditional HPF would have had a diameter of 0.35 mm (and a radius of 175 μm), giving an area of 0.0962 mm^2 (96,211 μm^2) calculated using the formula: **area** $= \pi r^2$. However, a typical modern microscope (eg, Olympus BH2) at a nominal 400× magnification would have a field area of 0.1963 mm^2, which is 2.041 times that of the older model. Consequently, the numbers of cells per HPF should be interpreted after correction by a factor of 2, so that twice as many would now be expected per HPF to produce a given result.

This appendix explains the two steps required to obtain reliable counts under the microscope that can be converted to concentrations. First, it is necessary to calibrate the area of the field of view (so objects can be determined per unit area); and, second, one must know how to make fixed-depth preparations suitable for working with cervical mucus.

CALIBRATING THE FIELD AREA

Calibration of the field area requires access to a stage micrometer slide. These devices typically have a 1 mm line subdivided into one-tenth and one one-hundredth parts so the smallest divisions are 10 μm. For each combination of optics (i.e., objective, oculars, and intermediate magnification), focus on the micrometer scale and measure the diameter of the field of view as accurately as possible. Using these diameter values, calculate the area of each field of view using the formula

Table AppII–1 Field areas for the Olympus BH2 microscope using WHK10× oculars and a BH2-CA magnification changer

Objective	Field Area ($\times 10^6 \ \mu m^2$)		
	× 1.0	× 1.25	× 1.5
10 ×	3.033 (0.330)	1.953 (0.512)	1.354 (0.739)
20 ×	0.741 (1.350)	0.484 (2.066)	0.334 (2.995)
40 ×	0.189 (5.302)	0.122 (8.203)	0.085 (11.76)
100 ×	0.030 (33.78)	0.020 (51.02)	0.013 (75.19)

Multiply the number of objects per field by the correction factor in parentheses to obtain the number per square millimeter.

given above. A table of such measurements for the Olympus BH2 microscope is provided (Table AppII-1).

If the preparation depth is known (e.g., when using a 20-μm Microcell), the volume of the preparation within the field of view can be calculated by:

$$\text{Volume (mm}^3 \equiv \mu l) = \text{field area (mm}^2) \times \text{preparation depth (mm)}$$

Table AppII-2 shows the field volumes for 20- and 50-μm Microcells used in conjunction with an Olympus BH2 microscope. From these field volumes a series of correction factors can be calculated to convert the number of objects per field of view to per unit volume. Table AppII-3 presents the correction factors derived from the values in Table AppII-2 to convert to $10^3/\mu l$ ($\equiv 10^6/ml$).

Counting cells, especially motile spermatozoa, in the entire field of view is not easy when there are more than a moderate number per field. Consequently, it is recommended to use an eyepiece reticle or graticule to define a smaller area to be counted. For applications with Microcells, a special reticle is available that subdivides the center part of the field into a 10 × 10 array analogous to the grid of a Makler chamber. A detailed description of how to calibrate this reticle and perform reliable sperm concentration counts using Microcells was available from their distributor (Fertility Technologies Inc., Natick, MA, USA).

Table AppII–2 Field volumes for the Olympus BH2 microscope using Microcells.

Objective	Field Volume (μl) with 20-μm Microcell			Field Volume (μl) with 50-μm Microcell		
	× 1.0	× 1.25	× 1.5	× 1.0	× 1.25	× 1.5
10 ×	0.0607 (16.5)	0.0391 (25.6)	0.0271 (37.2)	0.1517 (6.59)	0.0977 (10.2)	0.0677 (14.8)
20 ×	0.0148 (67.5)	0.0097 (103)	0.0067 (150)	0.0371 (26.9)	0.0242 (41.3)	0.0167 (59.9)
40 ×	0.0038 (265)	0.0024 (410)	0.0017 (588)	0.0095 (106)	0.0061 (164)	0.0043 (235)

Values are given for WHK10× oculars and 1.0 ×, 1.25 ×, and 1.5 × intermediate magnifications. Multiply the number of objects per field by the correction factor in parentheses to obtain the number per cubic millimeter (i.e., per microliter, equivalent to $10^3/ml$).

Table AppII–3   Grid volumes for the Olympus BH2 microscope fitted with the eyepiece reticle for use with Microcells

	Grid Volume (μl $\times$ 10^{-3}) with 20-μm Microcell			Grid Volume (μl $\times$ 10^{-3}) with 50-μm Microcell		
Objective	$\times$ 1.0	$\times$ 1.25	$\times$ 1.5	$\times$ 1.0	$\times$ 1.25	$\times$ 1.5
10 $\times$	19.721 (50.7)	12.736 (78.5)	8.924 (112)	49.302 (20.3)	31.840 (31.4)	22.311 (44.8)
20 $\times$	4.901 (204)	3.168 (316)	2.204 (453)	12.251 (81.6)	7.920 (126)	5.511 (181)
40 $\times$	1.210 (826)	0.784 (1276)	0.545 (1835)	3.026 (330)	1.960 (510)	1.361 (735)

Multiply numbers of objects per grid by the correction factor in parentheses to obtain number per cubic millimeter (i.e., per microliter). Note that only about one-third of the field of view is counted using the eyepiece reticle.

FIXED DEPTH PREPARATIONS OF CERVICAL MUCUS

Fixed depth preparations of cervical mucus use ordinary slides and coverslips. The coverslip is supported a fixed distance above the slide by silicone grease impregnated with glass beads of a known diameter.

Washing the Beads

Glass beads are purchased from Sigma (G4649: Ø 100 μm) and are washed according to the method described below (Drobnis et al., 1988; World Health Organization, 1992).

1. Cover the beads with acetone in a glass beaker. Swirl vigorously and decant the acetone. Repeat twice more.
2. Rinse the beads four to six times using reagent water.
3. Soak the beads in 1 M HCl for 20 minutes with stirring.
4. Decant the acid and rinse the beads four to six times using reagent water.
5. Cover the beads with a 2 M aqueous NaCl solution (116.88 g/l) and stir for 10 minutes.
6. Decant the saline and rinse twice using fresh 2 M NaCl.
7. Rinse the beads 10 times using reagent water, stirring 2–5 minutes for each change of water.
8. Spread the beads out in a Pyrex baking dish or other flat container and dry in a 200°C oven.
9. The beads may be autoclaved, if desired, and stored sterile.

Preparing the Support Material

1. Mix the washed beads with high vacuum silicone grease (e.g., Dow Corning Corporation; Edwards High Vacuum) in approximate 1:5 proportions.
2. Remove the plunger from a 5- or 10-ml plastic syringe and, using a weighing spatula, fill the syringe barrel with the glass beads-silicone grease mixture.

3. Replace the plunger and expel as much air as possible from the syringe.
4. Fit the syringe with a 10-gauge *blunt* needle.

Making Fixed Depth Preparations

1. Prepare a cleaned microscope slide with four "posts" of the glass beads/silicone grease mixture arranged in a square pattern in the center of the slide with sides of about 20 mm.
2. Place a drop (*ca.* 3 mm $\emptyset$) of endocervical mucus in the center of this square and cover it with a 22 × 22 mm coverslip.
3. Press down gently on the coverslip so the "posts" are flattened, and the coverslip is fixed with a single layer of beads between it and the slide.

N.B.   a. If a sealed preparation is required, it can be achieved by pipetting mineral oil under the edges of the coverslip between the support posts.

      b. Obviously, other depths of preparations can be produced using beads of different diameter. It is essential to establish the diameter of the *largest beads* in a batch as they are the ones that control the preparation depth, not the average diameter.

Calculating Cell Concentrations

Cell concentrations are calculated as described above, using a 0.1 mm depth value. Consequently, the field volumes are 2.0 times those shown in Table AppII-2 for 50-μm Microcells. For a 100 μm deep preparation, the field volume for a modern microscope using a 40× objective and widefield oculars is 0.0196 mm^3, so a traditional count of 10 cells/HPF is equivalent to 500 cells/mm^3.

References

Drobnis, E. Z., Yudin, A. L., Cherr, G. N., and Katz, D. F. (1988). Hamster sperm penetration of the zona pellucida: kinematic analysis and mechanical implications. *Dev. Biol.* **130,** 311.

World Health Organization (1992). *WHO Laboratory Manual for the Examination of Human Semen and Sperm-Cervical Mucus Interaction,* 3rd ed. Cambridge University Press, Cambridge.

Appendix III: Epifluorescence

Fluorescence is the luminescence of a substance that has been excited by radiation. Stokes' law dictates that the wavelength of the emitted fluorescent light is longer than that of the exciting radiation owing to its loss of energy. Consequently, a fluorescent substance can be excited by near-UV invisible radiation and seen in the visible spectrum, and many substances can be excited by blue or green radiation, resulting in green, yellow, or red fluorescence. A dye that fluoresces is called a fluorochrome. For example, the widely used fluorochrome fluorescein isothiocyanate (FITC) is excited with blue radiation and produces a green fluorescent emission.

At the simplest level, fluorescence microscopy requires the following.

1. A **light source** that supplies adequate intensity of the required excitation wavelength.
2. An **exciter filter** that transmits only the required wavelength and suppresses all the other parts of the light source's emission spectrum.
3. A specimen, either inherently fluorescent or labeled with a **fluorochrome.**
4. A **barrier filter,** which absorbs the excess exciting light not absorbed by the specimen so it does not interfere with observation of the specimen's fluorescence. This filter may be more specific so it can isolate a particular spectral range.

Because only a small part of the field of view emits fluorescence, and fading (sometimes called photobleaching) occurs steadily after a relatively short period of irradiation of the fluorochrome, it is important to optimize the fluorescent light available for observation. This process can be helped if the light source and illumination path are kept short, are exactly aligned, and contain as few glass faces as possible (and certainly no ground-glass surfaces). High numerical aperture objectives should be used, and low power oculars minimize the reduction in fluorescence intensity (as fluorescence intensity decreases exponentially with an increase in total magnification). From a practical standpoint, always work with the microscope in a dark room or screened corner of the laboratory to promote adaptation of the eyes.

Transmitted light fluorescence is not considered here, as it has been largely replaced by incident light fluorescence, or epifluorescence, which is far more effective. With epifluorescence the objective acts as the condenser, thereby obviating the need for its centering. Also, the exciting light passes on down through the specimen and is lost; hence it does not interfere with the fluorescent image. Nothing comes free, however, and epifluorescence requires an additional optical component, a chromatic beam splitting mirror or dichroic mirror. Although it can replace the barrier filter, additional suppression filters are often used.

Dichroic mirrors reflect certain spectral ranges, which therefore reach the specimen unattenuated in intensity while allowing complete transmission of others. The dividing line between reflection and transmission is set at the optimum wavelength for the particular fluorochrome, specifically midway between the maxima of the excitation and emission spectra. In modern epifluorescence systems the exciter filter, dichroic mirror, and barrier filter are combined into a single optical unit, or "cube," which often allows incorporation of a supplementary exciter filter and additional barrier filter to make the set more specific. These cubes are usually arranged in a slider or rotator so fluorescence sets can be quickly and easily interchanged (e.g., Olympus BH2-RFCA attachment, or the Leitz Ploemopak module).

CHARACTERISTICS OF COMMON FLUOROCHROMES

Table AppIII-1 shows the characteristics of the most common fluorochromes used in andrology laboratories, as well as the suggested filter sets, or "cubes," for Olympus, Leitz, and Zeiss epifluorescence microscopes.

ANTIFADING MOUNTANTS FOR FLUORESCENCE MICROSCOPY

To reduce the loss of fluorescence intensity during observation, especially during photomicrography, due to bleaching of the fluorochrome by the incident irradiation, special fluorochrome "recycling" agents can be incorporated into the mountant. Two alternatives are suggested.

Phenylenediamine Mountant

Phenylenediamine mountant (Johnson and Nogueira Araujo, 1981) is prepared by adding 200 mg *p*-phenylenediamine (PDA) to 20 ml of a 150 mM saline solution

Table AppIII–1 Optical requirements for epifluorescence microscopy of common fluorochromes used in andrology laboratories

	Wavelength (nm)			Suggested Filter Sets		
Fluorochrome	**Excitation**	**Emission**	**Barrier**[a]	**Olympus**	**Leitz**	**Zeiss**
Acridine orange	487 (blue)	510	510–515	B	I2	09, 10, 11
Chlortetracycline (CTC)	395 (UV + violet)	520	455	V	D	05, 09
Ethidium bromide	482 (green)	616	580	G	N2	14, 15
Fluorescein diacetate (FDA)	489 (blue)	514	510–515	B	I2	09
Fluorescein isothiocyanate (FITC)	494 (blue)	520	510–515	IB (or B)	I2	09, 10, 11 16, 17, 19
Hoechst 33258	343 (UV)	480	400	U	A2	01, 02
Hoechst 33342	343 (UV)	483	400	U	A2	02
Propidium iodide	493 (green)	639	570–580	G	N2	14, 15
Quinacrine mustard	440 (blue)	510	455	B	E2	05, 06
Rhodamine (TRITC)	541 (green)	572	570–580	G	N2.1	14, 15

[a]Barrier indicates the wavelength at which the dichroic mirror operates.

(173 mg NaCl in 20 ml reagent water) and stirring in the dark until dissolved. To a 1.0 ml aliquot of this solution add 2.7 mg of KH_2PO_4 and mix in the dark until dissolved. To the remaining 19.0 ml of PDA/NaCl solution add 54 mg of Na_2HPO_4 and again mix in the dark until dissolved. Recombine the two solutions to make the $10\times$ strength stock mountant solution, which should be stored frozen at $-20°C$ in small (e.g., 1.0 ml) aliquots until needed. For use, add 1.0 ml of the $10\times$ PDA stock to 9.0 ml of glycerol and adjust to pH 8.0 with a carbonate buffer comprising Na_2CO_3 53 g/l and $NaHCO_3$ 42 g/l in reagent water. Correct pH adjustment usually requires about 200 μl carbonate buffer per 10 ml of mountant. The mountant may be used until its color changes to dark brown-black. If the $10\times$ stock has turned black, it must be discarded.

Propyl Gallate Mountant

Propyl gallate is a simpler mountant than the PDA recipe (Giloh and Sedat, 1982), comprising 5% (w/v, about 250 mM) n-propylgallate (Sigma P3130) in glycerol adjusted to pH 8.0 using the same carbonate buffer as for the PDA mountant described above.

References

Giloh, H., and Sedat, J. W. (1982). Fluorescence microscopy: reduced photobleaching of rhodamine and fluorescein protein conjugates by n-propyl gallate. *Science* **217,** 1252.

Johnson, G. D., and Nogueira Araujo, G. M. de C (1981). A simple method of reducing the fading of immunofluorescence during microscopy. *J. Immunol. Methods* **43,** 349.

Appendix IV: Sample Antisperm Antibody Laboratory Report Form

A sample form for reporting antisperm antibody test results according to the procedures described in Chapter 5 is provided. This form is intended for use with blood serum (male or female) or solubilized cervical mucus. Results of tests on seminal plasma or direct Immunobead tests on spermatozoa are reported on the Semen Analysis Form (see Appendix I).

ANDROLOGY LABORATORY

ANTISPERM ANTIBODIES REPORT

PATIENT INFO	SURNAME, Forename(s)		CLINIC No.
MALE PARTNER			
FEMALE PARTNER			

PARTNER & SAMPLE	DATES (ddmmyy)		ANTIBODY ASSAYS		
	SAMPLE	TEST	TYPE	TITRE	SITE
MALE SERUM			INDIRECT IBT		
			AGGLUT'N		
			CYTOTOXIC		
FEMALE SERUM			INDIRECT IBT		
			AGGLUT'N		
			CYTOTOXIC		
CERVICAL MUCUS			INDIRECT IBT		
			AGGLUT'N		
			CYTOTOXIC		

COMMENTS:

SIGNED: DATE:

BINDING SITES: H-H = head-to-head MP-MP = midpiece-to-midpiece	T-T = tail-to-tail H-T = head-to-tail tt-tt = tail tip-to-tail tip	MIXED = unidentifiable	DM:02/92

Figure App IV-1 ASAB test report form.

Appendix V: Sample Semen Donor Screening Forms

Two suggested forms are provided for semen donor screening according to the guidelines described in Chapter 6 (Figs. AppV-1 and AppV-2).

INITIAL SCREENING

Sample/Date	Test	Result
BLOOD	Group	A / B / AB / O Rh+ve / Rh−ve
___ / ___ / ___	CBC	Normal/abnormal: _____
	SMA 6	Normal/abnormal: _____
	SMA 12	Normal/abnormal: _____
	HBsAg	Negative/positive
	VDRL	Negative/positive
	HIV-I Ab	Negative/positive
	HIV-II Ab	Negative/positive
	HTLV-I Ab	Negative/positive
	Hep-C Ab	Negative/positive
	CMV Ab	Negative/positive
URETHRA	*Chlamydia*	Negative/positive
___ / ___ / ___	Gonococcus	Negative/positive
	Ureaplasma	Negative/positive
	Mycoplasma	Negative/positive
URINE	Routine	Negative/positive: _____
___ / ___ / ___		
SEMEN	C & S	Negative/positive: _____
___ / ___ / ___	*Mycoplasma*	Negative/subculture/slight/moderate/heavy
	Ureaplasma	Negative/subculture/slight/moderate/heavy
	Gonococcus	Negative/positive
OTHERS	_____
	_____

TREATMENT	_____
	_____

Completed by: _____   Date:___ / ___ /19___

Figure App V–1   Initial screening report form.

REPEAT SCREENING

Sample/Date	Test	Result
BLOOD	HbsAg	Negative/positive
__ / __ / __	VDRL	Negative/positive
	HIV-I Ab	Negative/positive
	HIV-II Ab	Negative/positive
	HTLV-I Ab	Negative/positive
	Hep-C Ab	Negative/positive
	CMV Ab	Negative/positive
URETHRA	*Chlamydia*	Negative/positive
__ / __ / __	Gonococcus	Negative/positive
	Ureaplasma	Negative/positive
	Mycoplasma	Negative/positive
URINE	Routine	Negative/positive: _____
__ / __ / __		
SEMEN	C & S	Negative/positive: _____
__ / __ / __	*Mycoplasma*	Negative/subculture/slight/moderate/heavy
	Ureaplasma	Negative/subculture/slight/moderate/heavy
	Gonococcus	Negative/positive
OTHERS		_____
		_____
TREATMENT		_____
		_____
COMMENTS		_____
		_____

Completed by: _____   *Date:* __ / __ /19__

Figure App V–2   Repeat screening.

Appendix VI: Sample Sperm–Mucus Interaction Testing Laboratory and Report Forms

A series of forms comprises laboratory forms for each of the following procedures as described in Chapter 9 (Figs. AppVI-1 to AppVI-5): Kremer test; slide tests (Kurzrok-Miller test, sperm–cervical mucus contact test); crossed hostility testing; postcoital test. In addition, there is a suggested combined Mucus Tests Report Form.

ANDROLOGY   LABORATORY

KREMER   TEST   FORM

PATIENT INFO	SURNAME, Forename(s)	CLINIC	LAB REF No. FOR SMIT
MALE PARTNER			
FEMALE PARTNER			

EVENT	DATE	CALCULATIONS
L.M.P.		Abstinence = ____ days
Mucus taken for test		Test day = ____ of a ___ day cycle
N.M.P.		Usual cycle = _____ days

INSLER SCORE

Cervical os	
Mucus quantity	
Spinnbarkeit	
Ferning	
Leukocytes	
T o t a l s c o r e	/ 15
Mucus pH	

MICROSCOPY

Make/model = _____

Objective = ____ x   Intermediate = ____ x

Oculars = ____ x   Graticule = _____

Field area = _____ μm^2

Correction factor = x _____ to mm^2

Sperm contamination per field =
_____ *motile +* _____ *immotile*

PENETRATION ASSESSMENT

Distance (mm)	10	40	70	Vanguard sperm
Field #1				migration distance
Field #2				= _____ mm
Field #3				
Total in 3 fields				**RESULT**
Average / field				**Penetration**
Corrected / field				**score** =
Sperm / mm^2				_____ / **20**

COMMENTS:	SEMEN ANALYSIS
	LAB REF No.
Signed: Date:	DM:02/92

Figure App VI-1

ANDROLOGY LABORATORY

K-M & SCMC TESTS FORM

PATIENT INFO	SURNAME, Forename(s)	CLINIC No.	LAB REF No. FOR SMIT
MALE PARTNER			
FEMALE PARTNER			

EVENT	DATE	CALCULATIONS
L.M.P.		Abstinence = _____ days
Mucus taken for test		Test day = _____ of a _____ day cycle
N.M.P.		Usual cycle = _____ days

INSLER SCORE

Cervical os	
Mucus quantity	
Spinnbarkeit	
Ferning	
Leukocytes	
Total score	/ 15
Mucus pH	

MICROSCOPY

Make/model = _____

Objective = _____ x   Intermediate = _____ x

Oculars = _____ x   Graticule = _____

Field area = _____ $\mu m\hat{}2$

Correction factor = x _____ to mm^2

Sperm contamination per field =
_____ motile + _____ immotile

	OBSERVATIONS	Readings at =>	mins	mins	RESULT
K–M TEST	No penetration into mucus				Negative
	Penetrate but show "shaking"				Abnormal
	Penetrate but no migration				Poor
	Penetrate with good migration				Normal

	OBSERVATIONS	Readings at =>	mins	mins	
SCMC TEST					0 to 25% Negative
	Immotile spermatozoa (%)				26 to 50 % Positive (+)
	"Shaking" spermatozoa (%)				51 to 75 % Positive (+ +)
	Test rated as				76 to 100 % Highly Positive

COMMENTS:	SEMEN ANALYSIS
	LAB REF No.

Signed:	Date:	DM:02/92

Figure App VI-2

ANDROLOGY LABORATORY

CROSSED HOSTILITY TEST FORM

PATIENT INFO	SURNAME, Forename(s)		CLINIC No.	LAB REF No. FOR SMIT
MALE PARTNER				
FEMALE PARTNER				

EVENT	DATE	CALCULATIONS
L.M.P.		Abstinence = ____ days
Mucus taken for test		Test day = ____ of a ____ day cycle
N.M.P.		Usual cycle = _____ days

INSLER SCORE	Patient	Donor	MICROSCOPY
Cervical os			Make/model = _____
Mucus quantity			Objective = ____ x Intermediate = ____ x
Spinnbarkeit			Oculars = ____ x Graticule = _____
Ferning			Field area = _____ μm^2
Leukocytes			Correction factor = x _____ to mm^2
T o t a l s c o r e	/15	/15	*Sperm contamination* per field =
Mucus pH			PATIENT: ____ motile + ____ immotile DONOR: ____ motile + ____ immotile

PENETRATION TEST ASSESSMENTS

MUCUS	SEMEN	KREMER TEST	SCMC TEST	K-M TEST
Patient	Patient	___/20		
Patient	Donor	___/20		
Donor	Patient	___/20		
Donor	Donor	___/20		

COMMENTS:	SEMEN ANALYSIS
	LAB REF No.
	DONOR REF.
Signed: Date:	DM:02/92

Figure App VI-3

367

PATIENT MUCUS / PATIENT SEMEN			
DISTANCE (mm)	10	40	70
Field #1			
Field #2			
Field #3			
Total in 3 field			
Average / field			
Corrected / field			
Sperm / mm^2			
OBSERVATIONS Read at =>		min	min
No penetration into mucus			
Penetrate but show "shaking"			
Penetrate with good migration			
OBSERVATIONS Read at =>		min	min
Immotile spermatozoa (%)			
"Shaking" spermatozoa (%)			
Test rated as			

(KREMER TEST, K-M TEST, SCMC TEST)

PATIENT MUCUS / DONOR SEMEN			
DISTANCE (mm)	10	40	70
Field #1			
Field #2			
Field #3			
Total in 3 field			
Average / field			
Corrected / field			
Sperm / mm^2			
OBSERVATIONS Read at =>		min	min
No penetration into mucus			
Penetrate but show "shaking"			
Penetrate with good migration			
OBSERVATIONS Read at =>		min	min
Immotile spermatozoa (%)			
"Shaking" spermatozoa (%)			
Test rated as			

(KREMER TEST, K-M TEST, SCMC TEST)

DONOR MUCUS / PATIENT SEMEN			
DISTANCE (mm)	10	40	70
Field #1			
Field #2			
Field #3			
Total in 3 field			
Average / field			
Corrected / field			
Sperm / mm^2			
OBSERVATIONS Read at =>		min	min
No penetration into mucus			
Penetrate but show "shaking"			
Penetrate with good migration			
OBSERVATIONS Read at =>		min	min
Immotile spermatozoa (%)			
"Shaking" spermatozoa (%)			
Test rated as			

(KREMER TEST, K-M TEST, SCMC TEST)

DONOR MUCUS / DONOR SEMEN			
DISTANCE (mm)	10	40	70
Field #1			
Field #2			
Field #3			
Total in 3 field			
Average / field			
Corrected / field			
Sperm / mm^2			
OBSERVATIONS Read at =>		min	min
No penetration into mucus			
Penetrate but show "shaking"			
Penetrate with good migration			
OBSERVATIONS Read at =>		min	min
Immotile spermatozoa (%)			
"Shaking" spermatozoa (%)			
Test rated as			

(KREMER TEST, K-M TEST, SCMC TEST)

Figure App VI-3   (back)

ANDROLOGY   LABORATORY

POST-COITAL   TEST   FORM

PATIENT INFO	SURNAME, Forename(s)	CLINIC	LAB REF No. FOR SMIT
MALE PARTNER			
FEMALE PARTNER			

EVENT	DATE	CALCULATIONS
L.M.P.		Abstinence = _____ days
Previous ejac'n or coitus		PCT delay = _____ hours
Coitus for test		
P.C.T. performed		Test day = ____ of a ___ day cycle
N.M.P.		Usual cycle = _____ days

INSLER SCORE

Cervical os	
Mucus quantity	
Spinnbarkeit	
Ferning	
Leukocytes	
T o t a l s c o r e	/ 15
Mucus pH	

MICROSCOPY

Make/model = _____

Objective = _____x   Intermediate = _____x

Oculars = _____x   Graticule = _____

Field area = _____ $\mu m\char94 2$

Correction factor = x _____ to mm$\char94$2

ASSESSMENT OF POST-COITAL MUCUS

COUNTS	1	2	3	4	5	6	7	8	9	10	SUM	MEAN	#/mm^2
Progressive													
Non-prog													
"Shaking"													
Immotile													
TOTAL													

COMMENTS:

RESULT =   negative / poor / average / good / e xcellent

Signed: Date: DM:02/92

Figure App VI-4

ANDROLOGY LABORATORY

SPERM - MUCUS TESTING REPORT

PATIENT INFO	SURNAME, Forename(s)	CLINIC	LAB REF No. FOR SMIT
MALE PARTNER			
FEMALE PARTNER			

EVENT	DATE	CALCULATIONS
L.M.P.		Abstinence = _____ days
Previous ejac'n or coitus		PCT delay = _____ hours
Coitus for test		Test day = ____ of a ____ day cycle
P.C.T. performed		
N.M.P.		Usual cycle = _____ days

INSLER SCORE	Patient	Donor	SEMEN ANALYSIS INFO					
Cervical os			Patient					
Mucus quantity			Donor					
Spinnbarkeit			POSTCOITAL TEST RESULT					
Ferning			INSUFFICIENT MUCUS FOR TEST					
Leukocytes								
Total score	/15	/15	NEGATIVE / POOR					
Mucus pH			AVERAGE / GOOD / EXCELLENT					

PENETRATION TEST ASSESSMENTS

MUCUS	SEMEN	KREMER TEST	SCMC TEST	K-M TEST
Patient	Patient	___/20		
Patient	Donor	___/20		
Donor	Patient	___/20		
Donor	Donor	___/20		

COMMENTS:

Signed:	Date:	DM:02/92

Figure App VI-5

Appendix VII: Semen Cryopreservation Forms

The semen cryopreservation forms (Figs. AppVII-1 to AppVII-4) are for use in conjunction with the method for human semen cryopreservation described in Chapter 14. The series comprise a semen cryostorage work sheet, a batch index card, a storage location record, and a donor semen cryostorage record.

SEMEN CRYOSTORAGE WORK SHEET					
BATCH	LAB.REF.	DATE	DONOR	STRAW COLOUR	STORAGE LOCATION

Figure App VII-1

DONOR	STATUS	LAB. REF.	BATCH

DATE	STORAGE LOCATION	STRAWS	RELEASED FOR	LEFT

Figure App VII-2 Batch index card.

| STORAGE LOCATIONS | | | | TANK | CANISTER | GOBLET |

VISO-TUBE	BATCH	STRAW COLOUR	No. OF STRAWS	SAMPLE INFORMATION
P R				
P O				
P Y				
P G				
P B				
P P				
P W				
P D				
R R				
R O				
R Y				
R G				
R B				
R P				
R W				
R D				

Figure App VII-3

BATCH	LAB.REF	STORAGE LOCATION	DATE	No. OF STRAWS

DONOR CRYOSTORAGE RECORD

Figure App VII-4

Appendix VIII: Equipment Required for a Basic Andrology Laboratory

This appendix lists the minimum equipment required to establish a basic diagnostic andrology laboratory. Where specific manufacturers or models are described it merely expresses my preference, it does *not* indicate that other sources are unsuitable. The list is divided into per work station, per laboratory, and access only sections to indicate the recommended level of availability required for efficient working of the laboratory.

PER WORK STATION

Microscope	Olympus BH2-S compound microscope with phase contrast optics (detailed specifications given below). A BH2-T unit is acceptable provided that no photo or videomicrography capability is required with phase-contrast optics.
Slide warmer:	Large slide warmer/drier, preferably with hinged cover, to keep slides, coverslips, Microcells, Makler chambers, pipette tips, and so on warm before use.
Pipetters:	1. Gilson Pipetman (P10, P100, and P1000 models), each with tip ejector, and rack.
	2. Positive displacement pipetter, 50 µl but digitally adjustable.
	3. "Pi-Pump" hand controllers for serological pipettes.
Counters:	1. Single-channel tally counter for hemocytometer counts.
	2. Multichannel counter for differential counts. The new multifunction manual counter from Hamilton-Thorn Research, specially designed for andrology laboratories, is preferable to the older Clay-Adams mechanical units.
Counting chambers:	*Either* Makler chamber with spare cover glass *or* an extra microscope eyepiece fitted with a special reticle for use with disposable Microcells.
Vortex mixer:	Essential to ensure thorough mixing of diluted specimens for hemocytometry.

PER LABORATORY

Centrifuge:	Benchtop model with swing-out rotor and biological containment buckets (i.e., protection from aerosol contam-

376

ination). Carriers/adapters are required for the following Falcon tubes: Nos. 2095, 2070, 2001, 2003; and 1.5-ml Eppendorf tubes. Digital speed and time settings are recommended for ease of use. Depending on the workload, a second centrifuge may be necessary; it is also important as a backup.

Heated stage(s): At least one (preferably each) microscope should be fitted with a heated stage to regulate at 37°C in order to make motility analyses more reliable (and essential if making videorecordings for CASA analysis). There are various "stand-alone" units on the market but it is preferable to have one built into the Olympus BH2 microscope stage (e.g. JC Diffusion International, La Ferté-Fresnel, France; or Minitüb, Tiefenbach, Germany).

Hemocytometers: Improved Neubauer design, an initial complement of 10 is recommended (with spare cover glasses).

Incubators: Gravity convection type. Ideally, one of small to medium size for specimen reception and one (perhaps larger) for running tests. For incubating sperm preparations, sperm function tests, and so on under a 5% CO_2 atmosphere anaerobic jars (with *two* vents in the lid: gas in and gas out) are usually adequate for andrology purposes and certainly less expensive than a CO_2 incubator.

Hot plate: Capable of at least 55°C for running the fructose spot test.

Waterbath: For heat-inactivating sera and seminal plasma samples.

Oven: For drying and heat-sterilizing (up to 200°C), about 200-liter capacity.

Inverted microscope: For reading sperm-agglutination tray tests, e.g., Olympus CK model, preferably with phase-contrast optics.

Pipetters: For sperm-agglutination titration assay:
1. Repeat 25-μl dispenser.
2. Eight-way 25-μl pipetter for making serial dilutions in a microtiter tray.
3. Hamilton No. 702N 5-μl microsyringe dispenser with fixed needle and spring Chaney adapter.
4. Hamilton PB-600-$\frac{1}{50}$ microsyringe dispenser and No. 705-SN 50-μl syringe with a fixed, blunt needle.

N.B. Spare Hamilton syringes are advisable.

Video system: For motility counts and quality control. Monochrome surveillance type camera and monitor are sufficient. For eventual CASA analysis the system should also include an HQ-VHS VCR (HiFi not necessary) and a time-date or other character generator for encoding numbers/text (i.e., sample identification information) into the video signal.

Stage micrometer: For calibration of microscope field sizes.

ACCESS ONLY

pH meter: Ion selective capabilities are not needed.
Balance: Capable of weighing to 0.1 mg.
Heated stirrer: Combined hot plate and magnetic stirrer for making solutions.
Fume hood: To exhaust fixative and other solvent fumes to exterior (safety requirement). Easy access only is required.
Water system: At least a Milli-RO system is required to prepare reagent grade water. Access to a more elaborate system, equivalent to those used by clinical IVF laboratories is required for tissue culture grade water if culture media are to be prepared at the laboratory.

Suggested Olympus BH2-S Configuration for Andrology Applications

BHS-F   Microscope stand with power cord and cover
BHS-LSH   Halogen lamp 100 W housing (+ spare lamps)
BH2-SVR/L   Right- or left-hand mechanical stage
BH2-HL   Slide holder
BH2-PC   Phase-contrast turret condenser
BH2-6RE   Sextuple (six-place) revolving nosepiece
BH2-CA   Magnification changer
BH2-TR30   Trinocular tube
Eyepieces   WHK10×, one pair, plus perhaps an extra pair for use with reticles (e.g., one for photomicrography showing the camera field sizes, one for the 10 × 10 ruled box reticle).
                   NFK 3.3×LD Photo eyepiece 3.3×
                   NFK 5×LD Photo eyepiece 5×
                   NFK 6.7×LD Photo eyepiece 6.7×
Objectives: Either: 10×, 20×, and 40× D-Achromat PL phase contrast
                   Or: 10×, 20×, and 40× S-Plan PL phase contrast
                   Also: S-Plan 100× *non*-phase (for morphology scoring)
                           10× D-Achromat NH phase contrast for CASA use
BH2-FH   Filter holder with: green (45G533: IF550) filter, daylight filter, diffuser filter
MTV-W   C-mount video camera adapter
MOM-L   Adapter-L for OM-series camera, if required

Notes: (1) No phase centering telescope is required, as the Bertrand lens in the magnification changer fulfills this function; and (2) an epifluorescence system for at least one microscope is required for fluorescence methods for sperm vitality, acrosome status, antisperm antibody, and leukocyte tests (see Appendix III).

Index

Key: "f" after a page number indicates a figure; "t" after a page number indicates a table